Ocular Manifestations of Neurologic Disease

Ocular Manifestations of Neurologic Disease

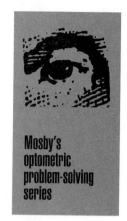

Mosby's
optometric
problem-solving
series

Edited by

Bernard H. Blaustein
OD, FAAO

Associate Professor of Optometry
Pennsylvania College of Optometry
Philadelphia, Pennsylvania

Series Editor
Richard London
MA, OD, FAAO

Diplomate in Binocular Vision and Perception
Pediatric and Rehabilitative Optometry
Oakland, California

*with 120 illustrations
and 19 color plates*

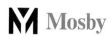 Mosby

St. Louis Baltimore Boston Carlsbad Chicago Naples New York Philadelphia Portland
London Madrid Mexico City Singapore Sydney Tokyo Toronto Wiesbaden

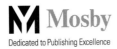

Dedicated to Publishing Excellence

A Times Mirror
Company

Executive Editor: Martha Sasser
Associate Developmental Editor: Amy Dubin
Project Manager: John Rogers
Production Editor: Helen Hudlin
Design Coordinator: Renée Duenow
Series Design: Jeanne Wolfgeher
Manufacturing Supervisor: Theresa Fuchs
Editing and Production: Carlisle Publishers Services
Cover Photography: From Ciba-Geigy, Ciba Collection of Medical Illustrations, Summit, New Jersey

Copyright © 1996 by Mosby–Year Book, Inc.

Printed in the United States of America
Composition by Carlisle Communications, Ltd.
Printing/binding by R. R. Donnelley & Sons Company

Mosby–Year Book, Inc.
11830 Westline Industrial Drive
St. Louis, Missouri 63146

Library of Congress Cataloging-in-Publication Data
Blaustein, Bernard H.
    Ocular manifestations of neurologic disease / edited by Bernard H.
Blaustein.
        p.   cm. — (Mosby's optometric problem-solving series)
    Includes bibliographical references and index.
    ISBN 0-8151-0507-X
    1. Ocular manifestations of general diseases.
  2. Neuroophthalmology.   I. Title   II. Series.
    [DNLM: 1. Eye Manifestations. 2. Nervous System Diseases-
    -diagnosis.   WW 460 B6450 1996]
    RE65.B56   1996
    616.07′5—dc20
    DNLM/DLC   95-50441
    for Library of Congress   CIP

98 99 00 / 9 8 7 6 5 4 3

Contributors

James M. Aylward, OD, FAAO
Chief, Optometry Section
Worcester Outpatient Clinic—Division of
The Brockton/West Roxbury Veterans
Administration Medical Center
Worcester, Massachusetts

Bernard H. Blaustein, OD, FAAO
Associate Professor of Optometry
Pennsylvania College of Optometry
Philadelphia, Pennsylvania

Andrew S. Gurwood, OD, FAAO
Assistant Professor
Department of Clinical Sciences
Pennsylvania College of Optometry
Philadelphia, Pennsylvania

Barbara J. Jennings, MA, OD, FAAO
Research Consultant
Vitreo Retinal Foundation
Memphis, Tennessee

Anthony B. Litwak, OD, FAAO
Residency Program Director
Veterans Administration Medical Center
Baltimore/Fort Howard, Maryland

Bruce G. Muchnick, OD, FAAO
Assistant Professor of Optometry
The Eye Institute
Pennsylvania College of Optometry
Philadelphia, Pennsylvania

Jeffrey S. Nyman, OD, FAAO
Associate Professor
Department of Clinical Science and
Biomedical Sciences
The Eye Institute
Pennsylvania College of Optometry
Philadelphia, Pennsylvania

Gerald Selvin, OD, FAAO
Professor of Optometry
New England College of Optometry
Boston, Massachusetts

Joseph Sowka, OD, FAAO
Associate Clinical Professor
School of Optometry
Southeastern University of the Health
Sciences
Miami Beach, Florida

Preface

Optometry is intimately related to neurology. In fact, the diagnosis of many neurologic entities can be made on the basis of eye signs or symptoms. A significant percentage of the nerve fibers in the central nervous system pass within the optic chiasm and are directly concerned with visual function. Moreover, the nerve fibers to the extraocular muscles comprise a significant part of the brain stem, and, like the visual fibers, travel through the brain in a lengthy, circuitous route. The course of these fibers brings them in close proximity to many important neurologic structures, and pathologies within these structures may influence the visual or ocular motility system. Finally, many of the cranial nerves are concerned with visual or oculomotor function.

Thus, cerebral vascular disease often will manifest as transient visual loss. An intracranial mass may produce disc edema or headache. Brain stem disease may cause ocular motility or eyelid dysfunction. In fact, many patients with neurologic disease are apt to present to the optometrist thinking that their problems represent ocular or visual dysfunction, and the routing optometric evaluation includes many tests to determine the integrity of the patient's neurologic status.

Ocular Manifestations of Neurologic Disease is written for the optometric clinician who desires a concise overview of the area. The topics are broad-based and cover those areas that are of major concern to the primary care optometrist. This book does not pretend to be encyclopedic nor is it meant to be a substitute for more comprehensive texts on the subject of neuro-ocular disease.

If optometrists gain more insight into the ocular manifestations of neurologic disease and are stimulated to increase their knowledge of this fascinating and challenging subject, the long hours spent editing will have been worth the effort.

I wish to express my deepest appreciation to my wife, Paula, for her continuous encouragement and support. I also should like to thank Martha Sasser, Amy Dubin, and Kellie White at Mosby, who have had to put up with my editorial anxieties.

Bernard H. Blaustein, OD, FAAO

Contents

stand the presenting complaints for these patients, as well as the appropriate treatment and referrals to make when necessary.

1

Cranial Nerve Disease

James M. Aylward

Key Terms

anosmia	Tolosa-Hunt	gasserian ganglion
optic atrophy	syndrome	Bell's palsy
optic nerve	Duane's retraction	tinnitus
meningiomas	syndrome	cerebellopontine
Benedikt's	Millard-Gubler	angle tumor
syndrome	syndrome	gag reflex
third nerve palsy		

The 12 cranial nerves are responsible for the sensory, motor, and autonomic innervation to the structures of the head, as well as to the visceral organs of the thorax and abdomen. Six of the twelve pairs are intimately related to ocular function, and a significant portion of the routine optometric examination pertains to the evaluation of these nerves and the structures they innervate.

Understanding the anatomic characteristics of the cranial nerves, including the relationships that exist between the various nerves and their neighboring structures, becomes critically important when assessing patients who present with cranial nerve palsies. The ability to appropriately evaluate the cranial nerves provides the clinician with the diagnostic tools needed to localize pathologic conditions that lead to cranial nerve impairment.

From an optometric standpoint, several of the cranial nerves can be considered "secondary"; however, understanding the structure and function of these nerves can occasionally provide valuable clinical information, and most of these nerves can be quickly assessed in a clinical setting. They are included here for the sake of completeness.

Olfactory Nerve

The olfactory nerve (I) conveys the sensation of smell from the nasal mucosa to the temporal lobe; disruption of the olfactory nerve leads to anosmia. Anosmia can be unilateral or bilateral, although unilateral cases are rarely noticed by the patient. The sense of smell frequently is affected by local disorders of the nasal mucosa, and conditions such as chronic rhinitis cause anosmia much more frequently than does intracranial pathology.[1] Because of the nonspecific nature of the results, the sense of smell is not typically tested in clinical settings.

In its course, the olfactory nerve lies on the underside of the frontal lobe, just superior to the prechiasmal optic nerve (Figure 1-1). Space-occupying lesions of the frontal lobe or meningiomas of the olfactory groove commonly cause disruption of the first cranial nerve. The resulting anosmia may be accompanied by optic nerve signs such as pallor and central scotoma, and in cases of frontal lobe tumors, the patient may display changes in personality and mental status.[1,2]

CLINICAL PEARL

Space-occupying lesions of the frontal lobe or meningiomas of the olfactory groove commonly cause disruption of the first cranial nerve. The resulting anosmia may be accompanied by optic nerve signs.

Optic Nerve

The optic nerve (II) is the principal pathway for the afferent visual system, and its origin is within the sensory retina. The nerve may be damaged at any point from the optic nerve head to the lateral geniculate body, and symptoms of optic nerve dysfunction can range from minor blurring or dimming of vision to an absolute loss of sight.

Optic nerve function can be evaluated accurately by investigating three general areas: visual perception, including visual acuity, color vision, and brightness comparison; visual field analysis; and pupillary responses. The results of these tests provide valuable information regarding the location of pathology that affects the optic nerve.

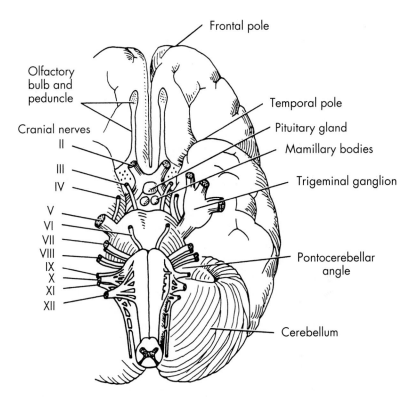

Frontal pole

Olfactory bulb and peduncle

Cranial nerves
II
III
IV
V
VI
VII
VIII
IX
X
XI
XII

Temporal pole

Pituitary gland

Mamillary bodies

Trigeminal ganglion

Pontocerebellar angle

Cerebellum

FIGURE 1-1 Position of the cranial nerves as they exit the brain stem. (Modified from deGroot J, Chusid JG: Cranial nerves and pathways. In deGroot J, Chusid JG, eds: *Correlative neuroanatomy,* ed 20, 1988, East Norwalk, Conn, Appleton-Lange. Reprinted by permission of Appleton-Lange, 1988.)

Anatomic Considerations

The innermost layer of the sensory retina is composed of approximately 1 million ganglion cell bodies, and it is the axons of these cells that make up the retinal nerve fiber layer and ultimately form the optic nerve.[3]

Three to four millimeters nasal to the fovea, the axons of the retinal nerve fiber layer merge and exit through the scleral canal to form the optic nerve head. The nerve head is typically 1.5 to 2.0 mm in diameter.[4] Variations in the size of the scleral opening and the angle at which the nerve exits the globe produce optic nerve head characteristics such as cupping and pigmented or scleral crescents.

The axons pierce through fenestration within the scleral connective tissue (lamina cribrosa) and form the intraorbital portion of the optic nerve. At 30 mm, the intraorbital optic nerve constitutes the longest section of the nerve. Its excess length is necessary for free movement of the globe, and it also serves to permit 6 to 8 mm of unrestrained proptosis.[5]

Behind the lamina cribrosa, the optic nerve becomes myelinated, and therefore its diameter increases to approximately 4 mm. At this point the nerve also becomes sheathed by pial, arachnoid, and dural tissue extending from the intracranial meninges. As it exits the sclera, the intraorbital nerve is surrounded by multiple branches from both the ciliary nerve and the ciliary artery.[4]

At the apex of the orbit, the optic nerve passes through the annulus of Zinn surrounded by the connective tissue of the four recti muscles and in the company of the oculomotor nerve (III), the abducens nerve (VI), and the nasociliary branch of the trigeminal nerve (V_1). The nerve enters the optic foramen just lateral to the superior orbital fissure and travels through the optic canal within the sphenoid bone. The periosteum of the canal and the dura of the optic nerve sheath are fused, and therefore the nerve is tethered within the canal. The intracanalicular optic nerve is in close approximation with the sphenoidal sinus, being separated by only 0.5 mm of bone.[5]

Leaving the canal, the optic nerve rises toward the chiasm at approximately a 45° angle. Here the frontal lobe is directly above the optic nerve with the anterior cerebral and anterior communicating arteries lying between the nerve and the cerebral tissue. The optic nerve is adjacent to the internal carotid artery as the artery leaves the cavernous sinus (Figure 1-2). At this point the optic nerve is also in relatively close proximity to cranial nerves III, IV, and VI as they exit the cavernous sinus to enter the superior orbital fissure.

The two optic nerves converge to form the optic chiasm, which sits approximately 10 mm above the sella turcica and the pituitary gland. There is considerable variation in the anterior-posterior positioning of the chiasm, and this factor partially accounts for the variable nature of visual field defects seen in chiasmal pathology.[6]

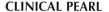

CLINICAL PEARL

The two optic nerves converge to form the optic chiasm, which sits approximately 10 mm above the sella turcica and the pituitary gland. There is considerable variation in the anterior-posterior positioning of the chiasm, and this factor partially accounts for the variable nature of visual field defects seen in chiasmal pathology.

Posteriorly, the optic chiasm is contiguous with the anterior tip of the third ventricle (Figure 1-2). Laterally, the internal carotid arteries flank the uncrossed temporal fibers from each optic nerve, and within

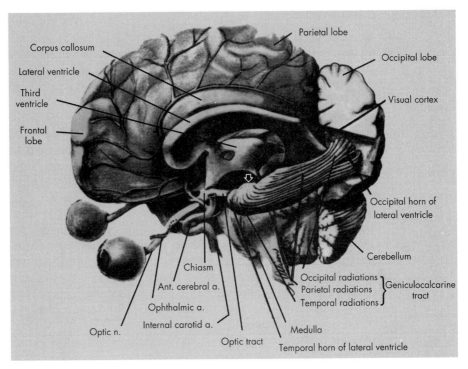

Corpus callosum

Lateral ventricle

Third ventricle

Frontal lobe

Parietal lobe

Occipital lobe

Visual cortex

Occipital horn of lateral ventricle

Cerebellum

Chiasm

Ant. cerebral a.

Ophthalmic a.

Optic n.

Internal carotid a.

Optic tract

Occipital radiations
Parietal radiations ⎱Geniculocalcarine
Temporal radiations ⎰ tract

Medulla

Temporal horn of lateral ventricle

FIGURE 1-2 Anterior and posterior visual pathway. (From Glaser JS: Anatomy of the visual sensory system. In Glaser JS, ed: *Neuroophthalmology*, ed 2, Philadelphia, 1990, JB Lippincott, 62. Reprinted by permission of JB Lippincott, 1990.)

the central portion of the chiasm the nasal fibers cross to meet the temporal fibers of the contralateral optic nerve. During this crossing, the inferior nasal fibers deviate anteriorly to briefly enter the opposite nerve (von Willebrand's loop). This unique pattern is responsible for junctional scotomas seen in anterior chiasmal disease.

Once decussation has occurred, the axons exit the chiasm to form the optic tracts. The two diverging tracts are separated by the pituitary stalk and the wall of the third ventricle. The optic tracts incline slightly, passing lateral to the cerebral peduncles, and enter the lateral geniculate body on either side of the thalamus (Figure 1-2). Before reaching the lateral geniculate body, axons responsible for the afferent pupillary reflex leave the optic tract and proceed to the Edinger-Westphal nucleus. The lateral geniculate body is the terminal point for the optic nerve and the anterior visual pathway. Here visual information from the nerve fiber layer will be rearranged in a precise topographic manner before continuing on to the posterior visual system.

Pathologic Considerations

Because the optic nerve is a culmination of the retinal ganglion cell axons, lesions that affect the retinal nerve fiber layer will produce visual field defects that occasionally appear neurologic in nature. Arcuate or wedge-shaped scotomas can be caused by chorioretinal lesions that interrupt the overlying nerve fiber layer; central or cecocentral scotomas may be seen in lesions affecting the papillo-macular bundle; and arcuate, altitudinal, or quadrantlike defects can develop after retinal arterial occlusions.[7-9] Fortunately, the pathology responsible for these field defects is usually evident during fundus evaluation, and vision is reduced only to the extent that the macula is involved. Other neurologic signs, such as an afferent pupillary defect, are absent unless the pathology is extensive (see Chapter 8).

Congenital anomalies frequently occur at the optic nerve head and can affect the function of the retinal nerve fibers as they pass through the scleral canal. These anomalies include coloboma, optic pits, tilted discs, and optic nerve head drusen. As with lesions of the retinal nerve fiber layer, the various congenital optic nerve defects are readily visible on funduscopic examination, and patients normally lack pupillary findings or other neurologic symptoms.

Posterior to the lamina cribrosa, the optic nerve is susceptible to an assortment of pathologic processes, including ischemia, inflammation, and compression. Impairment of the optic nerve at any point anterior to the chiasm will produce unilateral signs and symptoms, with scotomas and vision loss being the most common (see Chapter 6).

Patients with Graves' disease may develop optic nerve symptoms secondary to compression of the nerve at the apex of the orbit by the congested extraocular muscles. These patients usually exhibit notice-able proptosis and have restrictive muscle signs such as an inability to rotate the eye during forced duction testing. Optic nerve symptoms include a monocular or binocular decrease in vision, reduced color vision, and central or arcuate field defects.[10] The nerve head may be completely normal or may present with varying degrees of edema.

Because of the optic nerve's position just lateral to the sphenoid sinus, any pathology involving the sinus also may secondarily involve the nerve. A mucocele within the sphenoid sinus may cause inflammation of the optic nerve or, after bony destruction of the optic canal and superior orbital fissure, may cause direct compression of the nerve. In either case, the patient usually will suffer a slowly progressive monocular vision loss and central scotoma, and will eventually develop optic atrophy. Diplopia may occur from involvement of the neighboring cranial nerves (III, IV, and VI).[11,12]

Regardless of the cause, compression of the optic nerve can produce a central scotoma or large arcuate defect that extends to the periphery. Optic atrophy is the hallmark of compression and, in chronic cases, the initial atrophy is often followed by the appearance of optociliary shunt vessels.

> **CLINICAL PEARL**
>
> *Optic atrophy is the hallmark of compression and, in chronic cases, the initial atrophy is often followed by the appearance of optociliary shunt vessels.*

Optic nerve glioma is a fairly uncommon tumor. It is most frequently seen in children, and an association with neurofibromatosis has been identified.[13] Gliomas may occur at any point along the optic nerve, and they occasionally extend from one nerve into the chiasm. Orbital gliomas usually become symptomatic during a phase of rapid growth that causes proptosis, optic atrophy, and occasionally strabismus.[14] Afflicted patients will manifest a monocular decrease in vision, afferent pupillary defect, and possibly a central scotoma. Chiasmal gliomas tend to be more static and may present with bilateral vision loss and bilateral field defects, although not usually bitemporal hemianopsia.[15]

Optic nerve meningiomas arise from the arachnoid layer and therefore can affect the optic nerve at any point in its course. Meningiomas may occur in all age groups, but are seen most frequently in middle-aged women.[16] These tumors exhibit very slow growth, and the resulting compression is often unrecognized until significant damage has occurred to the optic nerve. Patients report a slowly progressive dimming of vision, exhibit an afferent pupillary defect and decreased color vision, and eventually develop optic atrophy, with optociliary shunt vessels possible.[17] Primary optic nerve meningiomas usually involve the intraorbital nerve and may cause a concurrent slowly progressive proptosis. Secondary meningiomas, which typically arise from the sphenoid bone, tend to be clinically silent; however, when bilateral optic nerve signs are present, extension of the tumor to the chiasm should be suspected.[18]

The optic nerve's close association with the internal carotid artery as it exits the cavernous sinus, and with the anterior cerebral and anterior communicating arteries in the circle of Willis, renders the nerve susceptible to the ischemic, compressive, and inflammatory changes that can occur in these vessels. Aneurysms of the internal carotid artery can become quite large, and those that occur outside the cavernous sinus frequently produce visual symptoms without other neurologic abnormalities.[19,20] The resulting compression leads to the typical signs of unilateral progressive vision loss with nasal or central field defects and optic atrophy.

As the optic nerves merge to form the chiasm, the unique pattern of the visual fibers in this area provides the clinician with valuable localizing information. The hallmark of perichiasmal disease is bitemporal hemianopsia, and, although complete bitemporal defects are rarely seen except in trauma, a variety of bitemporal patterns, with varying degrees of asymmetry, are typical of chiasmal disease (see Chapter 8).

Lesions responsible for chiasmal syndromes are often asymptomatic early on. Patients may complain of vague visual symptoms, including decreased central acuity, dimness to their vision, and changes in their depth perception. Systemic symptoms include headaches and lethargy. Clinical findings other than the visual field defects are often unremarkable; however, patients with highly asymmetric fields may exhibit an afferent pupillary defect on the more involved side. Optic atrophy is seen in approximately 50% of cases, and, when present, takes on a band pattern, leaving the superior and inferior areas of the nerve unaffected.[21]

The chiasm can be affected by aneurysms, meningiomas, and craniopharyngiomas, but by far the most frequent lesion involving the chiasm is the pituitary adenoma.[22] Pituitary tumors classically invade the chiasm from below and lead to bitemporal hemianopsias, which begin superiorly. The distance of the chiasm from the pituitary gland, however, suggests that field defects will occur only after considerable enlargement of the tumor has taken place. These patients are more likely to notice symptoms of fatigue, cold intolerance, weight gain, impotency in men, and amenorrhea in women before they present with visual symptoms.

Posterior to the chiasm, the optic tracts carry the combined information from the right and left hemifields a short distance to the lateral geniculate body. Lesions in this area produce bilateral signs such as incongruous homonomous hemianopsia. Visual acuity is frequently spared; however, when acuity is affected it may be unilateral or bilateral, with the worse vision in the eye contralateral to the tract lesion. Similarly, an afferent pupillary defect may be seen on the contralateral side.[23,24]

Approximately two thirds of the way to the lateral geniculate body, the afferent pupillary fibers leave the optic tract, and lesions after this point do not produce any pupillary abnormalities.

The optic nerves terminate by synapsing in the lateral geniculate body. From this point, optic nerve findings such as decreased acuity, afferent pupillary defects, and optic atrophy are not seen. Topical diagnosis relies on bilateral visual field findings, systemic neurologic signs and symptoms, and the results of radiologic studies.

Oculomotor Nerve

The oculomotor nerve (III) is responsible for stimulus to most of the extraocular muscles. It also provides parasympathetic stimulation to the ciliary muscle, effecting changes in accommodation and to the iris sphincter to control miosis. Complete paralysis of the oculomotor nerve is clinically obvious. Patients exhibit marked ptosis, a dilated, nonreactive pupil, and the classic "down and out" eye turn. Incomplete paralysis is not uncommon, however, and may present with more subtle pupil, lid, or extraocular muscle signs. Consequently, all aspects of third nerve function should be carefully tested in patients with abnormal signs attributable to any portion of the third nerve. Furthermore, evidence of involvement of neighboring cranial nerves or the presence of central nervous system signs provides critical information regarding the location of any suspected pathology.

Clinical investigation of the oculomotor nerve includes red lens test, Bielschowsky head tilt test in cases of vertical diplopia, and evaluation of the pupils, with special attention paid to any anisocoria that is greater in bright illumination.

Anatomic Considerations

The third nerve nucleus is the largest of the cranial nerve nuclei and is situated within the brain stem in the floor of the aqueduct of Sylvius (Figure 1-3). Warwick[25] investigated the topographic organization of the nucleus and identified both paired and midline structures. The nucleus is the origin for fibers innervating the superior, inferior, and medial recti, the inferior oblique, and levator palpebrae, as well as the parasympathetic system. The nucleus is unique in that its innervation to the superior rectus muscle is largely crossed and the levator nucleus is midline rather than paired.[25] These details contribute to some of the clinical signs seen in nuclear lesions of the third nerve.

Leaving the brain stem between the cerebral peduncles, the third nerve passes beneath the posterior cerebral and posterior communicating arteries adjacent to the optic tracts. The nerve proceeds within the subarachnoid space and passes to the top of the petrous bone, where it penetrates the dura to enter the cavernous sinus (Figures 1-1 and 1-4).

Within the cavernous sinus the third nerve is the most superior structure, lying just above the fourth cranial nerve in the lateral wall of the sinus (Figure 1-5).

The nerve leaves the cavernous sinus, passes through the superior orbital fissure, and enters the orbital apex along with cranial nerves IV, VI, and V_1. Once in the orbital apex, the third nerve is joined by the optic nerve as it passes through the annulus of Zinn. Before this point the third nerve has divided into superior and inferior branches. The superior branch divides further to innervate the superior rectus and levator. The inferior branch divides and innervates the medial rectus, inferior rectus, and inferior oblique. A separate branch of the inferior division supplies the parasympathetic innervation to the ciliary ganglion.[26]

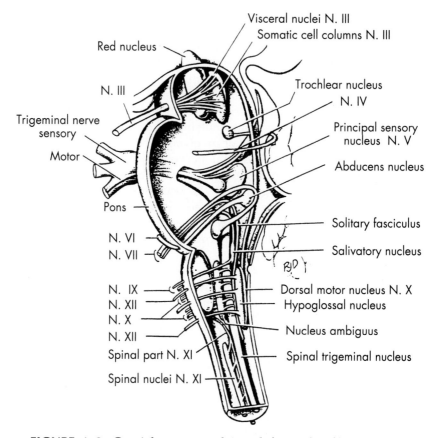

FIGURE 1-3 Cranial nerve nuclei and fascicular fibers within the brain stem. (From Carpenter MB, Sutin J: The medulla. In *Human neuroanatomy,* ed 8, Baltimore, 1983, Williams & Wilkins, 338. Reprinted by permission of Williams & Wilkins, 1983.)

Pathologic Considerations

Nuclear lesions affecting the third nerve are rare and are usually caused by occlusion of branches from the basilar artery or by brain stem compression. Because of the levator's midline position, patients usually suffer bilateral, symmetric ptosis. Unilateral weakness of the respective extraocular muscles is seen; however, because of the crossed innervation to the superior rectus, upgaze will be restricted on the contralateral side as well.[27]

Lesions that alter the third nerve fibers within the brain stem (fascicular lesions) are normally diagnosed on the basis of the presence of other neurologic signs. Benedikt's syndrome is characterized by an ipsilateral third nerve palsy with a contralateral hemitremor or other involuntary movement disorder. Weber's syndrome is recognized by the combination of an ipsilateral third nerve palsy with

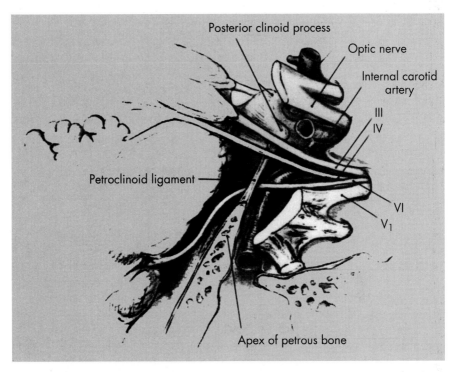

Posterior clinoid process

Optic nerve

Internal carotid artery

III

IV

Petroclinoid ligament

VI

V₁

Apex of petrous bone

FIGURE 1-4 Course of cranial nerves III, IV, V, and VI as they proceed toward and through the cavernous sinus. Notice the position of VI at the tip of the petrous bone. (From Miller NR: The embryology and anatomy of the ocular motor system. In *Clinical neuro-ophthalmology,* vol 2, Baltimore, 1985, Williams & Wilkins, 582. Reprinted by permission of Williams & Wilkins, 1985.)

contralateral hemiplegia (Table 1-1). The lesions that cause these various syndromes are frequently vasoocclusive in origin.[28]

CLINICAL PEARL

Lesions that alter the third nerve fibers within the brain stem (fascicular lesions) are normally diagnosed on the basis of the presence of other neurologic signs.

From the cerebral peduncles to the cavernous sinus, the oculomotor nerve travels within the subarachnoid space. Possible pathologic processes include aneurysms, ischemic disease, tumors, and trauma.[29,30]

Aneurysms of the posterior communicating artery are responsible for many cases of acute third nerve palsy, and these almost always include some degree of pupillary dysfunction.[30] Patients typically

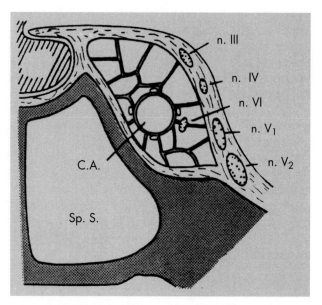

FIGURE 1-5 Position of cranial nerves III, IV, VI and V_1, V_2 in the cavernous sinus. Notice the position of VI near the carotid artery. (Modified from Umansky F, Nathan H: The lateral wall of the cavernous sinus, *J Neurosurg* 56:228-234, 1982. Reprinted by permission of the American Association of Neurological Surgeons, 1982.)

present with pain in and around the eyes and severe headache of fairly rapid onset. Although compression of the nerve may produce symptoms relatively slowly, rupture of the aneurysm usually causes symptoms within hours, and these patients frequently lose consciousness.

CLINICAL PEARL

Aneurysms of the posterior communicating artery are responsible for many cases of acute third nerve palsy, and these almost always include some degree of pupillary dysfunction.

Diabetes is a common cause of third nerve palsy.[29] These patients also may present with symptoms of pain. Often the pain occurs 2 to 3 days before the onset of the extraocular muscle symptoms and ceases abruptly once the palsy develops. This is not always the case, and the pain may be difficult to distinguish from the pain associated with aneurysms. In contrast to aneurysms, however, third nerve palsies secondary to diabetes almost always spare the pupil.[31] This is true of other types of ischemic insult to the nerve as well, and this characteristic is thought to be related to the preferential sparing of blood flow to the peripherally located pupillary fibers.

TABLE 1-1
Brain Stem Syndromes

Syndrome	Site	Signs	Etiology
Benedikt's	Midbrain-fascicular fibers of CN III	CN III palsy and either contralateral tremor or cerebellar ataxia	Tumor; hemorrhage
Weber's	Midbrain-fascicular fibers of CN III	CN III palsy and contralateral hemiplegia	Occlusion; aneurysm; tumor
Möbius'	Midbrain-nucleus of CN VI	Bilateral horizontal gaze palsies and bilateral CN VII palsies	Congenital absence of abducens nuclei
Duane's	Midbrain-nucleus of CN VI	Unilateral or bilateral CN VI palsies and co-contraction of CN III	Congenital abnormality of CN VI nerve or nucleus
Foville's	Base of ponsfascicular fibers	CN VI, CN VII, and CN VIII palsies and possible Horner's syndrome	Ischemia; inflammation; infiltration; compression of brain stem
Raymond's	Base of ponscorticospinal tract	CN VI palsy and contralateral hemiplegia	
Millard-Gubler	Base of ponscorticospinal tract	CN VI palsy, CN VII palsy, and contralateral hemiplegia	

Diabetic third nerve palsies usually resolve spontaneously within 2 to 3 months, and cases that fail to show improvement require a complete neurologic evaluation, including computed tomography scan or magnetic resonance imaging to rule out more serious pathology.

The third nerve is vulnerable to stretching and compression, especially at its position over the petrous apex before entering the cavernous sinus. A fixed, dilated pupil may be seen early in cases of compression, but more subtle pupillary signs are also frequent. Therefore any anisocoria that is greater in bright illumination should be suspect. Extraocular muscle palsies secondary to compression may be complete or partial. Ptosis and restricted supraduction are common early signs, and progression is typical.[28]

Pathology within, or extending to, the cavernous sinus does not typically involve the third nerve in isolation. Unilateral polyneuropathies involving the oculomotor, trochlear (IV), and abducens (VI) nerves, the first two divisions of the trigeminal nerve (V_1, V_2), and the autonomic innervation to the pupil are more characteristic of cavernous sinus syndromes (Table 1-2).[32] Nevertheless, isolated third nerve palsies may be seen early in cavernous sinus disease, and monitoring for progressive involvement of neighboring cranial nerves is critical.

TABLE 1-2
Cranial Nerve Syndromes

Syndrome	Site	Signs	Etiology
Cavernous sinus	Cavernous sinus	Varying combinations of CN III, CN IV, CN V (divisions 1 and 2), and CN VI palsies and possible Horner's syndrome	Aneurysm; fistula; tumors: nasopharyngioma, others
Tolosa-Hunt	Same as above	Same as above	Nonspecific granulomatous inflammation (pseudotumor)
Orbital apex/ superior orbital fissure	Orbital apex or superior orbital fissure	Proptosis and varying combinations of CN III, CN IV, CN V (division 1), and CN VI palsies and occasional CN II involvement	Meningioma; osteoma; dermoid cyst; glioma; aneurysm; nonspecific granulomatous inflammation (orbital pseudotumor)
Petrous apex	Tip of petrous bone	Varying combinations of CN V (all divisions) and CN VI palsies, occasional CN VII palsy and possible dry eye	Tumors of the middle cranial fossa; nasopharyngioma
Gradenigo's	Same as above	Same as above	Otitis media with mastoiditis/petrousitis
Cerebellopontine	Junction of pons and cerebellum	Varying combinations of CN V, CN VII, CN VIII palsies and sometimes CN IX and CN X palsies	Tumors: acoustic neuroma, meningioma, others
Ramsay Hunt	CN VII geniculate ganglion	CN VII palsy and periauricular vesicles	Herpes zoster
Vernet's	Jugular foramen	Varying combinations of CN IX, CN X, and CN XI palsies	Nasopharyngioma; meningioma; aneurysm

Painful ophthalmoplegia or numbness in the distribution of the first (V_1) and second (V_2) divisions of the trigeminal nerve suggests an oculomotor-trigeminal combination. Simultaneous paralysis of III and VI is evident by the globe's position and its inability to abduct. Involvement of the sympathetic fibers carried by the nasociliary branch of V_1 is more difficult to detect because a concurrent parasympathetic lesion resulting in pupillary dilation may mask the presence of a sympathetic defect. In these cases, close examination may show a pupil that is smaller in dim light and poorly reactive to bright light.

Lesions commonly causing cavernous sinus syndrome include aneurysms, pituitary tumors, craniopharyngiomas, nasopharyngiomas, and metastatic disease.[28]

Aneurysms of the cavernous sinus generally show slowly progressive extraocular muscle involvement, variable pain, and variable pupillary findings[32] (see Chapter 2). Expanding pituitary tumors may invade the cavernous sinus from above or laterally, impinging on the third nerve. Optic nerve and chiasmal signs, however, are almost always evident by this stage.[22] Nasopharyngiomas are relatively uncommon tumors, yet they are frequently responsible for cavernous sinus disease. This carcinoma causes bony destruction and direct infiltration from below the sinus, producing trigeminal symptoms early in its course[33] (see Chapter 2).

Lesions of the third nerve in the area of the superior orbital fissure or orbital apex present with symptoms very similar to cavernous sinus syndrome, and precise localization may be difficult (Table 1-2). Orbital and superior orbital fissure lesions typically produce proptosis, although 2 to 3 mm of proptosis may be seen in patients with complete third nerve palsy of any cause because of the loss of normal muscle tone. Third nerve palsies accompanied by visual symptoms and signs of optic neuropathy are more likely to occur in this region.[34] Pain or numbness may be restricted to the superior region innervated by the ophthalmic branch of the trigeminal nerve (V_1), because the maxillary branch (V_2) does not proceed through the superior orbital fissure.

Idiopathic granulomatous inflammation involving the orbit (orbital pseudotumor) or the anterior cavernous sinus (Tolosa-Hunt syndrome) is characterized by pain and ophthalmoplegia (Table 1-2). These inflammatory reactions mimic intracranial pathology and are usually diagnosed only after radiologic studies have excluded the presence of mass lesions or aneurysms.

Restricted superior gaze seen in Graves' disease may be confused with a partial third nerve palsy; however, the presence of bilateral signs, as well as other associated thyroid signs, usually makes the distinction clear.

Aberrant regeneration is a unique feature of third nerve palsies. This misdirection of fibers is usually seen 6 months to 1 year after disruption of the nerve. Aberrant regeneration is most frequently related to trauma or aneurysms; it is seen less frequently in patients with tumors, and is never seen in diabetic third nerve palsies.[35] Abnormal lid signs include upper lid retraction on downgaze (pseudo von Graefe's sign) and lid retraction on adduction (lid gaze dyskinesia). The pupil also may be affected, showing miosis on adduction unrelated to convergence.

Trochlear Nerve

The trochlear nerve (IV) innervates the superior oblique muscle, which is responsible for intorsion and depression of the globe.

Patients suffering from fourth nerve palsies typically complain of vertical diplopia, and in the absence of frank diplopia, may report difficulty with near tasks. Most patients develop a compensating head tilt to the side opposite the affected eye. This head tilt is not always diagnostic, however, because some patients will develop head tilts to the ipsilateral side to maximize image separation and facilitate suppression. Furthermore, patients with monocular vision loss would not be expected to adopt any head tilt.

CLINICAL PEARL

The trochlear nerve innervates the superior oblique muscle, which is responsible for intorsion and depression of the globe.

The Maddox rod is extremely useful in evaluating fourth nerve function; in addition, the Bielschowsky head tilt test (Parks three step) can help discriminate weakness of the superior oblique from other causes of vertical diplopia (see Chapter 4).

The clinical signs of fourth nerve paralysis include vertical diplopia in primary gaze, increased separation with downgaze, increased separation of the images on adduction, and increased separation with head tilt toward the affected side. Loss of intorsion is best seen behind the slit lamp and is most apparent while observing vertical movements with the eye abducted.[36]

Anatomic Considerations

The paired nuclei of the fourth cranial nerve lay just caudal to the third nerve nuclei, in the floor of the cerebral aqueduct (Figure 1-3). The fascicular portions of the nerves bend around each side of the aqueduct and then decussate within the roof of the aqueduct before exiting from the dorsal aspect of the brain stem. In this manner each nucleus projects to the contralateral superior oblique (Figure 1-1).

The fourth nerve is the only cranial nerve to exit from the dorsal surface of the brain stem, and, as a result, it has the longest intracranial course. The nerve, however, is protected from the effects of compression throughout much of its length by the overlying tentorium.[26]

After exiting the brain stem, the trochlear nerve proceeds laterally around the midbrain, passes between the superior cerebral and posterior cerebral arteries, and pierces the dura mater to enter the cavernous sinus slightly inferiorly to the oculomotor nerve (Figure 1-4). Like the third nerve, the fourth nerve is located within the lateral wall of the sinus (Figure 1-5).

Leaving the cavernous sinus, the trochlear nerve crosses over the third nerve to enter the superior orbital fissure. Within the orbit, the nerve turns superiorly, outside the annulus of Zinn, to innervate the superior oblique muscle.

Pathologic Considerations

Trochlear nerve palsies are the most common cause of acquired vertical diplopia, and they may be seen in all age groups.[37]

Patients with congenital trochlear palsies usually develop abnormally high fusional reserves and a compensating head tilt to overcome the resulting vertical disparity. These palsies often go undiagnosed until a breakdown in the patient's fusional reserves leads to diplopia. Decompensation may follow trauma or illness, and also may occur with no antecedent event.[38] Evidence of a head tilt in old photographs, or vertical fusional reserves of 10 to 20 prism diopters, suggests the presence of a long-standing fourth nerve palsy.

Isolated trochlear nerve palsies, both unilateral and bilateral, are frequently related to trauma. Closed head trauma, with a resulting contrecoup effect, may injure both fourth nerves as they exit the midbrain, causing bilateral defects. Orbital trauma may injure the fourth nerve, but just as frequently injures the tendon or the muscle itself.[29,30] Regardless of the site of damage, unilateral signs of superior oblique weakness will result.

CLINICAL PEARL

Isolated trochlear nerve palsies, both unilateral and bilateral, are frequently related to trauma.

Diabetes can cause ischemic insult to the fourth nerve and lead to an isolated superior oblique palsy.[29,39] These patients usually show good recovery within 3 months.

Fourth nerve palsies can occur in the company of other neuropathies, especially in the case of cavernous sinus pathology.[32] The closest association is between the third and fourth cranial nerves. The resulting combination of oculomotor and trochlear paralysis may be difficult to detect grossly; however, it can be identified behind the slit lamp by observing a lack of intorsion on abduction.[36]

Abducens Nerve

The abducens nerve (VI) provides uncrossed innervation to the lateral rectus, and therefore it controls abduction of the globe. In addition, the nucleus of the abducens nerve plays a role in coordinating the two eyes during horizontal gaze movements. Interruption of the abducens nerve results in an esotropia that is greater at distance, secondary to the unopposed action of the medial rectus. Patients with abducens palsies frequently will complain of diplopia while driving and may develop a compensating head turn toward the side of the affected eye.

As with cranial nerves III and IV, the function of the abducens nerve is best tested using a red lens or Maddox's rod, and the image separation will be greatest in the field of action of the paretic muscle (see Chapter 4).

Anatomic Considerations

The paired nuclei of the abducens nerves are situated in the floor of the fourth ventricle, caudal to the nuclei of the oculomotor (III) and trochlear (IV) nerves (Figure 1-3). Fibers from the nucleus of the facial nerve (VII) curve over the abducens nucleus, and the fascicular fibers of these nerves pass adjacent to one another to exit ventrally near the junction of the pons and the medulla (Figures 1-1 and 1-3). The abducens nucleus also sends fibers to the contralateral third nerve nucleus by way of the medial longitudinal fasciculus. These fibers contribute to the innervation of the contralateral medial rectus and facilitate horizontal conjugate gaze movements.[40]

As the nerve exits the brain stem, it turns upward along the base of the pons and ascends the face of the clivus within the subarachnoid space. It perforates the dura near the tip of the petrous bone and bends acutely over the apex of this bone to enter the cavernous sinus (Figure 1-4). Unlike cranial nerves III and IV, which are located within the lateral wall, the abducens nerve lies in the body of the cavernous sinus, adjacent to the internal carotid artery (Figure 1-5). Sympathetic fibers from the carotid plexus briefly fuse with the abducens nerve before joining the first division of the trigeminal nerve (V_1), which runs parallel to the abducens nerve within the cavernous sinus. The abducens nerve enters the orbit through the superior orbital fissure and continues through the annulus of Zinn to innervate the lateral rectus muscle.[26]

Pathologic Considerations

Nuclear lesions of the abducens nerve never produce isolated abducens palsies; instead they result in paralysis of the ipsilateral lateral rectus and the contralateral medial rectus during horizontal gaze movements, and therefore produce horizontal gaze palsies. (Convergence action of the medial rectus is spared.) These horizontal conjugate gaze palsies are almost always seen in association with other neurologic signs or systemic abnormalities, frequently including paralysis of the ipsilateral facial nerve (VII).[40]

Möbius' syndrome is caused by a congenital malformation of the abducens nuclei (Table 1-1). These patients manifest bilateral horizontal gaze palsies in which the eyes exhibit a complete lack of horizontal movements. The facial muscles are also involved bilaterally, which results in the inability to close the mouth and abnormal closure of the lids. Other congenital defects may include deafness, webbed fingers or toes, mental retardation, and skeletal abnormalities.[41]

Duane's retraction syndrome is also a congenital disorder involving the abducens nucleus (Table 1-1). This syndrome is characterized by a lack of abduction with limited adduction on the affected side, and retraction of the globe with narrowing of the palpebral fissure on attempted adduction. The syndrome is usually unilateral, vision is typically normal, and patients are often asymptomatic. Duane's retraction syndrome is thought to be caused by abnormal innervation of the lateral rectus by the third nerve, in the absence of the abducens nucleus or nerve.[42]

Horizontal gaze palsies also can be seen in patients with Wernicke-Korsakoff syndrome secondary to metabolic injury to the abducens nucleus.[43]

Lesions affecting the fascicular portion of the abducens nerve usually damage neighboring structures as well, and abducens palsies are included in a variety of brain stem syndromes. Foville's syndrome consists of ipsilateral abducens and facial palsies (VI and VII), loss of hearing on the affected side (VIII), and an ipsilateral Horner's syndrome (central). Raymond's syndrome is characterized by an ipsilateral abducens palsy with contralateral hemiplegia secondary to involvement of the corticospinal tract in the area of the abducens nucleus. The addition of an ipsilateral facial palsy constitutes Millard-Gubler syndrome (VI, VII, and contralateral hemiplegia).[44] These syndromes may develop secondary to ischemia, compression, infiltration, or inflammation of the brain stem (Table 1-1).

In its course through the subarachnoid space, the abducens nerve is susceptible to a wide variety of intracranial pathology. The nerve is in close contact with the anterior inferior cerebral artery and the basilar artery, and is vulnerable to atherosclerotic changes and aneurysms of these vessels.[29,39] As the nerve ascends the clivus, it can be affected from below by basal tumors or intracranial extension of nasopharyngeal carcinoma. It may be affected from above by compression resulting from space-occupying lesions, and it may be stretched or injured in cases of head trauma.[29,39]

The abducens nerve is particularly sensitive to changes in intracranial pressure, either because of its long and exposed course, or because of its precarious position over the tip of the petrous bone (Figure 1-4). Increased intracranial pressure of any origin can cause unilateral or bilateral abducens paralysis.[45] A sixth nerve palsy in the presence of disc edema and associated with symptoms of headache is highly suggestive of increased intracranial pressure.

CLINICAL PEARL

Increased intracranial pressure of any origin can cause unilateral or bilateral abducens paralysis.

As the sixth nerve curves over the apex of the petrous bone, it is directly adjacent to the gasserian ganglion of the trigeminal nerve (V). Inflammation, tumors, or aneurysms affecting this area can produce an abducens palsy, facial pain, and decreased corneal sensation (petrous apex syndrome). Infective processes, especially otitis media in children and mucormycosis in diabetics, may lead to a severe mastoiditis and subsequent inflammation of the petrous bone, producing Gradenigo's syndrome. This syndrome includes the abducens and trigeminal signs of the petrous apex syndrome, but also may include an ipsilateral facial palsy secondary to inflammation of the facial nerve within the petrous pyramid of the temporal bone (Table 1-2).[44]

Within the cavernous sinus, abducens palsies are most commonly associated with other neurologic signs and symptoms. These include multiple extraocular muscle palsies from involvement of the oculomotor and trochlear nerves, periorbital and facial pain or numbness from involvement of the first two divisions of the trigeminal nerve, and occasionally, an ipsilateral Horner's syndrome from involvement of the sympathetic fibers.[32] As mentioned previously, the cavernous sinus can be affected by meningiomas, craniopharyngiomas, nasopharyngiomas, pituitary adenomas, and metastatic carcinomas[28] (see Chapter 2).

Sixth nerve palsies secondary to lesions involving the superior orbital fissure or orbit occur with multiple cranial nerve signs as well, and the distinction between an orbital lesion and cavernous sinus lesion is not always apparent.

Despite the propensity for abducens palsies to occur in the company of multiple cranial nerve signs, isolated sixth nerve palsies are not at all uncommon. Diabetes is a frequent cause of acute unilateral abducens paralysis, as are other conditions that cause small vessel disease and ischemia (hypertension, atherosclerosis).[46] These palsies usually follow a benign course, resolving over a 2- to 3-month period.

CLINICAL PEARL

Diabetes is a frequent cause of acute unilateral abducens paralysis, as are other conditions that cause small vessel disease and ischemia (hypertension, atherosclerosis). These palsies usually follow a benign course, resolving over a 2- to 3-month period.

Other causes of isolated sixth nerve palsies include viral infections in children, cavernous sinus aneurysms, giant cell arteritis, sarcoidosis, multiple sclerosis, nasopharyngeal carcinoma, and syphilis.[29,39,46]

In evaluating patients with acute or chronic abducens paralysis, it is critically important to search for involvement of other cranial nerves and to recognize their localizing significance. The appearance of additional signs on follow-up suggests a progressive lesion, and palsies that are initially considered benign, but do not improve over a 3-month period, require a thorough neurologic workup to rule out the presence of intracranial pathology.[47,48]

Trigeminal Nerve

The trigeminal nerve (V) is the largest of the cranial nerves. It is primarily a sensory nerve composed of three major branches and their multiple subdivisions. In addition, it contains a small motor root that supplies innervation to the muscles of mastication. The nerve conveys afferent sensory stimulation from the skin of the face, the conjunctiva and cornea, the mucosal membranes of the nasal and oral cavities, the anterior two thirds of the tongue, and the teeth. It is also responsible for the sensory innervation of the intracranial meninges and major cerebral vessels. As with other sensory nerves, the pattern of distribution is divided along the vertical midline and impulses pass to the ipsilateral ganglion.

Disruption of the trigeminal nerve typically results in unilateral pain. The pain may correspond to one or more of the trigeminal branches and can become quite intense. Loss of sensation, although slightly less common, is often well localized to a specific subdivision of the nerve.

Symptoms of pain are difficult to objectively evaluate; however, anesthesia can be tested by examining the patient's response to light touch (cotton-tipped applicator) or pinprick. Testing should be done close to the midline on each side of the face in all three divisions of the trigeminal nerve. The results may be more reliable if the patient closes his or her eyes. Corneal and conjunctival sensation can be tested by stimulating corresponding areas in each eye with a wisp of cotton while observing the blink response (Figure 1-6). Because the motor component of the blink response is bilateral (VII), results can be obtained even in the event of a concurrent facial or ocular motor nerve palsy.

Motor function of the trigeminal nerve can be tested by asking the patient to clench the jaw tightly while the examiner palpates the masseter muscles for loss of muscle mass or noticeable weakness on either side (Figure 1-6). Lateral movements of the jaw also are controlled by the motor component of the trigeminal nerve, and

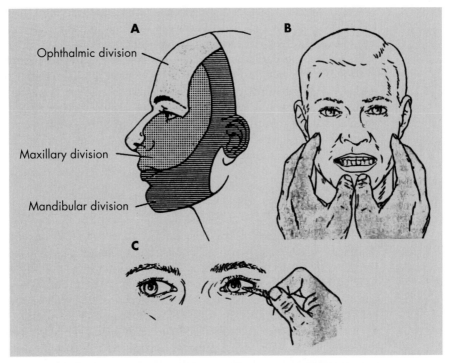

FIGURE 1-6 A, Distribution of the three branches of the trigeminal nerve V. **B,** Testing motor division of V. **C,** Testing corneal sensitivity. (Modified from Rodnitzky RL: The basic neurologic examination. In Rodnitzky RL, ed: *Van Allen's pictorial manual of neurologic tests*, ed 3, Chicago 1988, 27. Reprinted by permission of Mosby, 1988.)

muscle strength can be tested by cupping each side of the patient's jaw in the examiner's palms and comparing the force of movements to the left and right. Weakness to the right indicates involvement of the left side.

Anatomic Considerations

The principal sensory nucleus and the motor nucleus of the fifth cranial nerve both lie within the pons (Figure 1-3). The sensory nucleus extends caudally to the spinal cord and, through a complex network of synapses with second- and third-order neurons, communicates information to the contralateral cerebral cortex.[49]

The motor and sensory roots of the trigeminal nerve exit the lateral pons as distinct branches (Figure 1-3). Together they travel a short distance in the subarachnoid space, crossing over the facial (VII) and auditory (VIII) nerves as they enter the internal acoustic meatus. The trigeminal nerve then pierces through the dura over the top of the petrous bone just lateral to the abducens nerve (VI). After crossing the tip of the petrous bone, the sensory portion of the nerve fans out to form the gasserian ganglion (Figures 1-7 and 1-8). The gasserian ganglion lies between two layers of dura mater in a shallow depression of the petrous bone known as Meckel's cave. The motor root is positioned on the underside of the ganglion.[26]

From the gasserian ganglion, the trigeminal nerve divides into three prominent branches, the ophthalmic (V_1), the maxillary (V_2), and the mandibular (V_3).

The ophthalmic division enters the cavernous sinus adjacent to the internal carotid artery and proceeds within the lateral wall of the sinus, inferior to the trochlear nerve (IV) (Figure 1-5). While in the cavernous sinus, the ophthalmic nerve receives sympathetic fibers from the carotid plexus after their brief course with the abducens nerve (VI).[50] Just before exiting the cavernous sinus, the ophthalmic nerve divides further into three main branches: the lacrimal, the frontal, and the nasociliary. All three branches enter the orbit through the superior orbital fissure.

The lacrimal nerve continues above the lateral rectus to enter the lacrimal gland. The frontal nerve passes above the superior rectus and bifurcates to form the supratrochlear nerve, which innervates the medial portions of the upper lid and forehead. The frontal nerve then continues forward through the supraorbital notch to become the supraorbital nerve. In its course, the supraorbital nerve supplies the

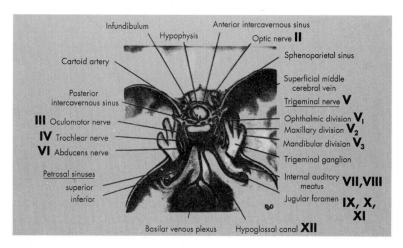

FIGURE 1-7 The exit points of the cranial nerves within the middle and posterior cranial fossa and their relationship to the cavernous sinus. (From Carpenter MB, Sutin J: The blood supply of the central nervous system. In *Human neuroanatomy*, ed 8, Baltimore, 1983, Williams & Wilkins, 346. Reprinted by permission of Williams & Wilkins, 1983.)

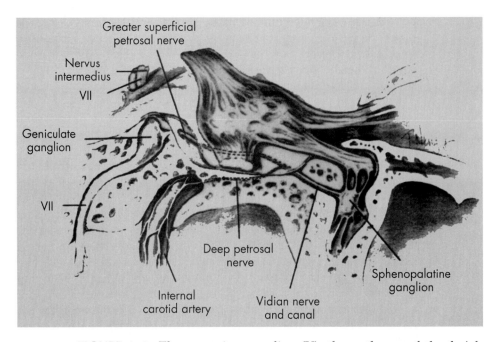

FIGURE 1-8 The gasserian ganglion (V), the pathway of the facial nerve (VII), and the sympathetic route to the sphenopalatine ganglion. (From Miller NR: Anatomy, physiology and testing of normal lacrimal secretion. In *Clinical neuro-ophthalmology,* vol 2, Baltimore, 1985, Williams & Wilkins, 464. Reprinted by permission of Williams & Wilkins, 1985.)

forehead, the upper lid, the frontal sinus, and the skin on the side of the nose. The nasociliary branch travels through the annulus of Zinn, passes beneath the superior rectus, and continues on a long and branching course. Within the orbit, the nasociliary nerve gives rise to the short posterior ciliary nerves, which run to the ciliary ganglion, and to the long posterior ciliary nerves, which pass to each side of the optic nerve, enter the sclera, and continue forward to innervate the iris sphincter, ciliary body, and cornea. The long ciliary nerves also carry sympathetic fibers to the iris dilator muscle.

The maxillary division (V_2) of the trigeminal nerve enters the cavernous sinus and is situated at the inferior border of the sinus (Figure 1-5). It exits the cranial cavity through the foramen rotundum and enters the orbit through the inferior orbital fissure. The nerve travels forward as the infraorbital nerve and exits the orbit through the infraorbital foramen, where it sends terminal branches to the inferior lid, the lateral aspect of the nose, and to the medial upper lip. In its course, the maxillary nerve also supplies the upper teeth, the roof of the mouth, and portions of the soft palate.[26]

The mandibular division (V_3), along with the motor root, exit the cranial cavity through foramen ovale. Sensory innervation is supplied to the skin and mucous membranes of the cheek, portions of the external and internal ear, the lower teeth and lip, and the anterior two thirds of the tongue. Motor innervation is supplied to the pterygoid, masseter, and temporalis muscles.[26]

Pathologic Considerations

The cause of facial pain or anesthesia often can be determined by recognizing the various neurologic signs and additional cranial nerve defects that frequently accompany pathology involving the trigeminal nerve.

Lesions within the brain stem usually cause ipsilateral signs; however, the pattern of distribution of these signs may not correspond to the typical divisions of the three main branches of the trigeminal nerve. Furthermore, brain stem lesions frequently cause a diminished perception to pain and temperature, while sparing the sensation of pressure and light touch.[51] The presence of a concurrent horizontal gaze palsy (nuclear VI) or movement disorder (corticospinal tract) is highly localizing to the brain stem. Pontine tumors or occlusion of the vertebral-basilar circulation are frequent causes of trigeminal lesions at this level.

Lesions of the trigeminal sensory root and gasserian ganglion are difficult to separate from one another, because both will affect all three divisions of the nerve. The sensory root may become involved in cases of cerebellopontine tumors, such as acoustic neuromas and meningiomas. In these cases, paralysis of the facial (VII) and vestibulocochlear (VIII) nerves usually precedes trigeminal involvement, leading to a syndrome of decreased hearing (VIII), ipsilateral facial palsy (VII), and pain or decreased sensation in all three divisions of the fifth nerve (cerebellopontine syndrome) (Table 1-2).[52]

Decreased corneal sensation is frequently caused by herpetic infection of the cornea or follows intraocular surgery. Reduced sensation also can develop secondary to impairment of the trigeminal sensory root or gasserian ganglion. Pathologic insult to the ganglion often results in loss of corneal sensitivity, and the resulting neurotrophic keratopathy can be one of the earliest objective signs of a cerebellopontine tumor.

Facial pain or anesthesia accompanied by paralysis of the lateral rectus (VI) suggests interference with either the sensory root or the ganglion in the area of the petrous apex.[53] Common causes include tumors, aneurysms, inflammation, and mastoiditis in Gradenigo's syndrome. Tumors of the base of the skull, including nasopharyngioma, may impinge on all three branches simultaneously through the ganglion, or may affect the maxillary (V_2) and mandibular (V_3) branches separately as they depart through their respective foramina.[33]

Concurrent signs of facial pain and an extraocular muscle palsy, including any combination of cranial nerves III, IV, VI, or the presence of a painful Horner's syndrome, suggest pathology within the cavernous sinus.[31] The pain would be expected to involve only the first two divisions of the trigeminal (V_1, V_2), because the mandibular division (V_3) exits through the foramen ovale without entering the cavernous sinus. Carotid artery disorders may affect V_1 and V_2 preferentially because of their close proximity to the artery as they enter the posterior cavernous sinus. Pain restricted to the ophthalmic division (V_1), along with extraocular muscle palsies, suggests a more anterior cavernous sinus lesion or a lesion within the superior orbital fissure.[32] The addition of optic nerve signs may suggest involvement of the orbit; however, extensive cavernous sinus disease also can lead to optic nerve damage.

Pathology affecting the three major divisions of the trigeminal nerve outside of the ganglion and cavernous sinus usually can be localized by the pattern of involvement. Facial trauma and skull fractures are the most common causes of damage to the individual branches.[44] Injuries to the supraorbital or supratrochlear branch of the frontal nerve (V_1) are common in trauma to the superior orbital rim and result in anesthesia of the forehead and upper lid. Injury to the inferior orbital rim or an orbital "blow-out" fracture frequently cause damage to the infraorbital nerve (V_2), resulting in anesthesia to the lower lid. In the absence of trauma, however, decreased sensation in the distribution of the maxillary division (V_2) may suggest carcinoma of the maxillary sinus.[54]

Facial pain not associated with any of the neurologic signs mentioned above may be attributed to trigeminal neuralgia, also known as tic douloureux. This condition is usually seen in patients 50 to 60 years of age and is more common in women. Symptoms include sharp stabbing pains, usually involving only the maxillary (V_2) and mandibular (V_3) divisions of the trigeminal nerve, and the symptoms are frequently brought on by chewing, exposure to cold, or stimulation of other "trigger points." Trigeminal neuralgia can become severe enough to require medical or surgical intervention.[44]

Facial Nerve

The facial nerve (VII) provides innervation to the muscles of facial expression, including the orbicularis oculi and the frontalis. In addition, it supplies parasympathetic (secretomotor) fibers to the lacrimal gland. In its course the seventh nerve also innervates the stapedius muscle of the inner ear and the salivary glands, and it contains a small sensory branch that conveys taste sensation from the anterior two thirds of tongue (Figure 1-9). Paralysis of the facial nerve can present

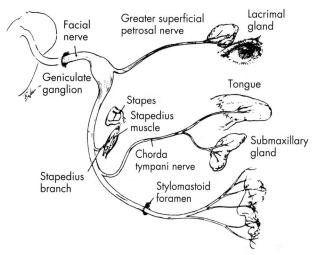

FIGURE 1-9 The branches and end organs of the facial nerve (VII). (From Alford BR: Neurophysiology of facial nerve testing, *Arch Otolaryngol Head Neck Surg* 93:214, 1973. Reprinted by permission of the American Medical Association, 1973.)

in a variety of forms, depending on the site of injury. The most common and most noticeable features, however, are a unilateral loss of the normal facial creases and folds, widening of the palpebral fissure and laxity of the lower lid with an inability to close the eye properly, and downturning of one corner of the mouth (Figure 1-10). Patients also may experience decreased lacrimation and salivation, and a painful response to sound in the affected ear (hyperacusis).[44]

CLINICAL PEARL

The facial nerve provides innervation to the muscles of facial expression, including the orbicularis oculi and the frontalis.

Testing the seventh cranial nerve involves observing a set of voluntary contractions of the facial muscles (Figure 1-11, *A* to *D*). Patients should be asked to raise their eyebrows, tightly close their eyes, and smile widely or bare their teeth. Any unilateral asymmetry will be noticeable, and orbicularis strength may be tested by attempting to open the patient's eyelids during forced closure (Figure 1-11, *D*). Unilateral weakness may involve all the muscles on one side of the face, or may be partial, with the lower face being affected more commonly than the upper. Schirmer's tear testing is helpful in

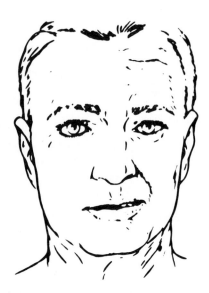

FIGURE 1-10 Right facial nerve palsy: loss of furrows on the forehead, widening of the palpebral fissure, loss of the nasolabial fold, and downturning of the corner of the mouth. (Modified from Rodnitzky RL: Abnormal signs and symptoms: basis and interpretation. In Rodnitzky RL, ed: *Van Allen's pictorial manual of neurologic tests*, ed 3, Chicago, 1988, Mosby, 101. Reprinted by permission of Mosby, 1988.)

assessing the secretomotor function of the nerve. Evaluating taste sensation is less reliable and is not generally useful in a clinical setting.

Anatomic Considerations

The nucleus of the facial nerve lies within the pons, lateral to nucleus of the abducens nerve (VI). The fascicular fibers of the facial nerve hook medially around the abducens nucleus and then return laterally to exit at the caudal border of the pons. After exiting the brain stem, both the motor and sensory (intermediate nerve) branches of the facial nerve, along with the vestibulocochlear nerve (VIII), enter the internal auditory meatus within the petrous portion of the temporal bone (Figures 1-7 and 1-8). Within the temporal bone, the facial and intermediate nerves separate from the eighth cranial nerve, and together the two branches of the facial nerve enter the facial canal. Within this long bony channel, the facial nerve traverses its way through the temporal bone and gives rise to three small branches.[49]

The first branch originates shortly after the nerve enters the facial canal and passes through the geniculate ganglion (Figure 1-8). Here a branch of the intermediate nerve containing parasympathetic as well as sensory fibers separates and travels anteriorly as the greater

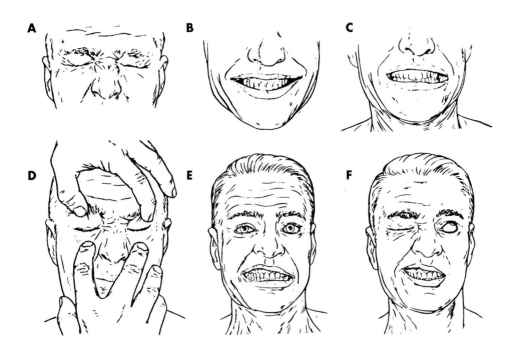

FIGURE 1-11 **A** to **D**, Testing cranial nerve VII. **E** and **F**, Appearance of central (**E**) vs. peripheral (**F**) facial palsy. Notice sparing of the superior muscles. (Modified from Rodnitzky RL: The basic neurologic examination. In Rodnitzky RL, ed: *Van Allen's pictorial manual of neurologic tests,* ed 3, Chicago, 1988, Mosby, 29. Reprinted by permission of Mosby, 1988.)

superficial petrosal nerve. The greater superficial petrosal nerve passes under the gasserian ganglion (V) and continues through the foramen lacerum (entry point of the carotid artery), where it is joined by the deep petrosal nerves, which carry sympathetic fibers from the carotid plexus. United, these two petrosal nerves form the vidian nerve. The vidian nerve proceeds to the sphenopalatine ganglion. From this ganglion, the sensory, sympathetic, and parasympathetic fibers travel toward the orbit with the maxillary nerve (V_2); they then separate from the maxillary nerve and combine with sensory fibers from the ophthalmic nerve (V_1). This combination ultimately produces the lacrimal nerve, which innervates its respective gland.

The main trunk of the facial nerve leaves the geniculate ganglion and continues in the facial canal, passing adjacent to the structure of the inner ear. Here the second branch of the facial nerve, the stapedius nerve, originates and innervates the stapedius muscle.

Continuing through the mastoid region of the temporal bone, the terminal branch of the intermediate nerve separates from the facial nerve to become the chorda tympani nerve. The chorda tympani eventually innervates the salivary glands and also transmits taste sensation from the anterior two thirds of the tongue.[44]

The facial nerve continues through the canal until exiting the cranial cavity through the stylomastoid foramen. External to the skull, the facial nerve enters the parotid gland and bifurcates at the angle of the jaw to innervate the various muscles of the face.

Pathologic Considerations

One interesting feature of the seventh cranial nerve is the organization of its supranuclear innervation. The contralateral cerebral cortex supplies innervation to all portions of the facial nucleus. That portion of the nucleus that corresponds to the orbicularis and the frontalis muscles, however, receives ipsilateral innervation as well. Because of this bilateral cerebral innervation to the upper facial muscles, any central lesion such as a stroke will produce contralateral paralysis of the lower face, with sparing or only slight weakness of the upper face.[44] In contrast, a peripheral lesion, i.e., nuclear or infranuclear, usually will produce complete facial paralysis on one side (Figure 1-11, E to F). Central (supranuclear) seventh nerve palsies are most commonly seen after cerebral vascular accidents.

Lesions affecting the nuclear or fascicular portions of the seventh cranial nerve are recognized by the presence of a unilateral or bilateral facial palsy along with a variety of brain stem signs. These may include an ipsilateral gaze palsy (nuclear VI), abducens palsy (VI), decreased corneal sensitivity (V root or ganglion), or movement disorder (spinal tract involvement). Facial palsies are a component of several cranial nerve syndromes, including Möbius', Foville's, Millard-Gubler, and cerebellopontine angle syndrome (Tables 1-1 and 1-2).[41,44,52]

CLINICAL PEARL

Lesions affecting the nuclear or fascicular portions of the seventh cranial nerve are recognized by the presence of a unilateral or bilateral facial palsy along with a variety of brain stem signs.

Leaving the brain stem at the cerebellopontine angle, the seventh nerve is in close association with the eighth cranial nerve, and lesions at this level, particularly acoustic neuromas, affect hearing, balance, and all functions of the facial nerve.[55] Patients may complain of facial paralysis, decreased tearing, and decreased salivation and taste sensation, as well as auditory and vestibular disturbances.

Lesions of the geniculate ganglion produce symptoms identical to those listed above, with the exception of disturbed balance. Balance is a function of the eighth cranial nerve, which separates from the facial nerve before the facial canal. Patients may continue to report auditory symptoms such as hyperacusis secondary to paralysis of the stapedius muscle. The geniculate ganglion can be infected by the herpes zoster virus, and these patients typically develop herpetic vesicles around the ear at the time of the facial palsy (Ramsay Hunt syndrome) (Table 1-2).[56]

Pathology in this area may affect the greater superficial petrosal and vidian nerves separately from the ganglion, leading to symptoms of unilateral dry eye without facial paralysis. The presence of a unilateral dry eye accompanied by facial pain (V_2), decreased corneal sensation (V_1), or a lateral rectus palsy (VI) suggests the possibility of a tumor of the middle cranial fossa or nasopharynx.[33,57]

As the facial nerve continues through the canal, it is susceptible to the effects of trauma, infiltration, and inflammation (mastoiditis). Depending on the position of the lesion, various seventh nerve functions may be preserved. Lesions past the geniculate ganglion will not affect lacrimation. Lesions past the stapedius branch do not cause hyperacusis. Lesions past the origin of the chorda tympani spare salivation and taste sensation, leaving only the facial musculature impaired.[56]

The extracranial portion of the nerve is particularly susceptible to trauma, especially surgical incisions or facial lacerations. The nerve also can be damaged by parotid tumors. Involvement of isolated branches of the facial nerve may produce regional facial paralysis and occasionally may produce sparing of the superior muscles, which is unrelated to the supranuclear innervation.

Despite the wide variety of intracranial pathology that can affect the facial nerve, the two most common causes of facial paralysis are trauma and idiopathic, or Bell's, palsy. As previously mentioned, traumatic injury can occur at any point in the nerve's course and may follow closed head trauma, fracture of the temporal bone, or facial laceration, or may develop as the result of surgical manipulation.

Bell's palsy is the most common cause of facial paralysis. Although a viral process has been theorized, the exact cause is unknown. Bell's palsy is usually acute and complete, and is not typically accompanied by other neurologic symptoms. It is critical that the clinician rule out the presence of infections (serous otitis, herpes zoster) or involvement of cranial nerves VI, V, and VIII before the diagnosis of a Bell's palsy is concluded.

Bell's palsy can occur at any age, but is most common between the ages of 15 and 45. It affects men and women equally. The hallmark of a Bell's palsy is the patient's ability to recover spontaneously, usually within 6 to 8 weeks. Lack of some degree of improvement in this period indicates the need for a more thorough workup to rule out intracranial disease.[44,56]

Recovery of facial paralysis also occurs through regeneration after cases of compressive injury and trauma, unless the nerve has been severed. The recovery of any facial palsy may be complete, partial, or may show misdirection. Aberrant regeneration may cause involuntary cocontraction of the facial muscles, or, if the parasympathetic fibers of the salivary gland innervate the lacrimal gland, the patient may develop tearing while eating (crocodile tears).

Vestibulocochlear Nerve

The vestibulocochlear nerve (VIII) is actually two separate sensory nerves that serve the structures of the inner ear. The vestibular portion communicates afferent stimulation from the semicircular canals and is responsible for the sense of orientation and balance. The cochlear division carries afferent information from the tympanic membrane and cochlea to provide auditory sensation.[58]

Anatomic Considerations

From their respective end organs, the two nerves unite to form a common trunk, which enters the posterior cranial fossa through the internal auditory meatus along with the facial nerve (VII) (Figure 1-7). After a short course, passing the cerebellopontine angle, the nerve enters the brain stem at the junction of the pons and the medulla (Figure 1-1). Within the brain stem the nerve separates into the cochlear and vestibular divisions, and each branch terminates in its associated nucleus. The nuclei of the eighth cranial nerves lie in the caudal end of the pons below the fourth ventricle.[58]

From the cochlear nucleus, auditory stimulus is transmitted to each temporal lobe through a network of both crossed and uncrossed pathways. Because of this bilateral projection, hearing is usually preserved in unilateral cerebral lesions or supranuclear lesions of the brain stem.

CLINICAL PEARL

Hearing is usually preserved in unilateral cerebral lesions or supranuclear lesions of the brain stem.

Vestibular fibers of the eighth nerve terminate in four separate nuclei and also project directly to the ipsilateral cerebellum. Neural impulses from the four nuclei proceed through a complex network of crossed and uncrossed pathways to innervate the spinal tract and contralateral cerebellum. Furthermore, vestibular information projects to the nuclei of cranial nerves III, IV, and VI through the medial longitudinal fasciculus to coordinate ocular movements with spatial orientation.[58]

Pathologic Considerations

The vestibulocochlear nerve may be affected at any point from the middle ear to the brain stem. The two divisions may be affected separately; however, because of their close anatomic relationship, they are frequently affected simultaneously.

Tinnitus is attributable to the cochlear portion of the eighth cranial nerve; it may be physiologic or it may be a manifestation of early nerve damage.[59]

Impaired hearing may be sensorineural in nature, or it may be secondary to a conduction defect in which the mechanics of the external or middle ear are abnormal. Gross testing of hearing can be done by comparing the volume of any soft sound in each ear (Figure 1-12). Conduction defects are commonly found in otitis media, obstruction of the external auditory canal or eustachian tube, and otosclerosis. Sensorineural deafness, which is more indicative of neural damage, can be distinguished from conduction deafness by the use of a tuning fork (Table 1-3 and Figure 1-13).[60]

 CLINICAL PEARL

Sensorineural deafness, which is more indicative of neural damage, can be distinguished from conduction deafness by the use of a tuning fork.

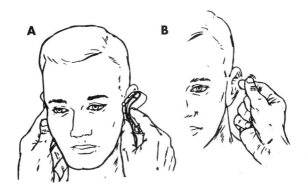

FIGURE 1-12 Gross testing of cranial nerve VIII, cochlear portion (hearing). **A,** The ticking of a watch. **B,** Rubbing the fingers together. (Modified from Rodnitzky RL: The basic neurologic examination. In Rodnitzky RL, ed: *Van Allen's pictorial manual of neurologic tests,* ed 3, Chicago, 1988, Mosby, 30. Reprinted by permission of Mosby, 1988.)

TABLE 1-3

Tuning Fork Tests to Distinguish between Conduction and Sensorineural Deafness (see Figure 1-13)

Test	Method	Results		
		Normal	Nerve damage	Conduction defect
Rinne	Base of vibrating tuning fork placed on mastoid process until subject no longer hears sound, then held in air next to ear	In air, vibration can still be detected	In air, vibration can still be detected	In air, vibration is not detected
Weber	Base of vibrating tuning fork placed on the vertex of the skull	Equal sound on both sides	Louder sound in normal ear	Louder sound in diseased ear

Damage to the vestibular portion of the eighth cranial nerve leads to symptoms of dizziness and disorientation (vertigo), and these symptoms are commonly associated with sensorineural deafness on the affected side.[58,59]

Impairment of both the vestibular and cochlear portions of the eighth nerve can be a presenting sign in acoustic neuroma or other tumors of the cerebellopontine angle. These tumors usually cause seventh nerve damage when they enlarge from the internal auditory meatus, and continued expansion can lead to involvement of the trigeminal nerve as well.[52,55] The resulting symptoms of vertigo, sensorineural hearing loss (VIII), unilateral facial paralysis (VII), and decreased corneal sensation with facial pain or numbness (V) are highly localizing and constitute a cerebellopontine angle syndrome (Table 1-2).

Lesions of the brain stem affecting the vestibulocochlear pathway within the medial longitudinal fasciculus frequently cause nystagmus but do not typically cause decreased hearing or vertigo.[58]

Glossopharyngeal and Vagus Nerves

The anatomic and pathologic characteristics of the glossopharyngeal (IX) and vagus (X) nerves are very similar; therefore the two nerves will be considered together. Clinically, the functions of the ninth and tenth cranial nerves are difficult to separate. The glossopharyngeal nerve is responsible for sensory innervation from the pharynx and soft palate, as well as taste sensation from the posterior one third of the tongue. The vagus nerve supplies motor function to the muscles of

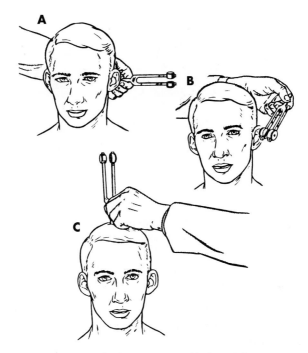

FIGURE 1-13 Tuning fork tests to distinguish nerve conduction defects from sensorineural damage. **A** and **B**, Rinne test. **C**, Weber test. See Table 1-3 also. (Modified from Rodnitzky RL: The basic neurologic examination. In Rodnitzky RL, ed: *Van Allen's pictorial manual of neurologic tests,* ed 3, Chicago, 1988, Mosby, 31. Reprinted by permission of Mosby, 1988.)

the larynx, pharynx, and soft palate, as well as enables visceral function of the organs of the thorax and abdomen. Furthermore, the two nerves help influence heart rate, respiration, and blood pressure.[44]

Patients with paralysis of the ninth and tenth cranial nerves may develop difficulty swallowing, hoarseness, and anesthesia of one side of the posterior pharynx.[44,59] Clinical evidence of paralysis of these nerves can be detected by observing the palate and by testing the patient's gag reflex. Unilateral paralysis of the soft palate will lead to deviation of the uvula toward the normal side. The gag reflex, which requires intact sensory impulses from the ninth nerve as well as intact motor impulse from the tenth nerve, can be tested by stimulating the posterior pharyngeal wall (Figure 1-14).[60]

Anatomic Considerations

The nuclei of the glossopharyngeal and vagus nerves lie in the medulla, and the nerves enter the brain stem at the lateral aspect in close association with the accessory nerve (XI). Together the glossopharyngeal, vagus, and accessory nerves exit the cranial cavity

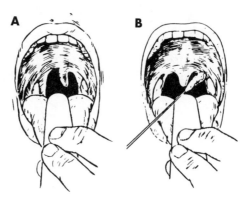

FIGURE 1-14 **A**, Paralysis of cranial nerves IX and X, and deviation of the uvula toward the normal side. **B**, Testing gag reflex of IX and XI. (Modified from Rodnitzky RL: Abnormal signs and symptoms: basis and interpretation. In Rodnitzky RL, ed: *Van Allen's pictorial manual of neurologic tests*, ed 3, Chicago, 1988, Mosby, 105. Reprinted by permission of Mosby, 1988.)

through the jugular foramen to innervate their respective organs (Figure 1-7).[59]

Pathologic Considerations

Lesions affecting the ninth and tenth cranial nerves are commonly posterior fossa tumors, vertebral artery aneurysms, or extracranial tumors that extend to the jugular foramen (Table 1-2). The ninth and tenth cranial nerves are particularly susceptible to nasopharyngeal carcinoma because of the jugular foramen's position above the nasopharynx.[33,44] Paralysis of these nerves may be seen in association with an ipsilateral Horner's syndrome in lesions that involve the descending sympathetic fibers within the spinal tract.[44]

Accessory Nerve

The accessory nerve (XI) is a purely motor nerve that innervates the sternocleidomastoid and trapezius muscles.[44] The trapezius muscle contracts to elevate the shoulder, whereas the sternocleidomastoid is responsible for rotation of the head.

CLINICAL PEARL

The accessory nerve is a purely motor nerve that innervates the sternocleidomastoid and trapezius muscles.

Patients with unilateral paralysis of the eleventh cranial nerve may exhibit a shoulder droop on the affected side, and clinical testing of the nerve consists of comparing the strength of each muscle group. This can be done by asking the patient to elevate both shoulders or to turn the head against the resistance of the examiner (Figure 1-15). Weakness of head turn to the right indicates a lesion involving the left nerve or muscle.[60]

Anatomic Considerations

The accessory nerve originates from the cervical portion of the spinal cord and actually enters the skull through the foramen magnum. It has a short intracranial course and promptly exits the cranial cavity through the jugular foramen in the company of the glossopharyngeal (IX) and vagus (X) nerves (Figures 1-1 and 1-7).[44]

Pathologic Considerations

Paralysis of the accessory nerve may be observed in tumors of the upper spinal cord; however, it is most commonly seen in pathology that also causes paralysis of the glossopharyngeal (IX) and vagus (X) nerves. The clinical significance of this combination is that it suggests involvement of the posterior clivus, particularly in the area of the jugular foramen (Vernet's syndrome) (Table 1-2).[44]

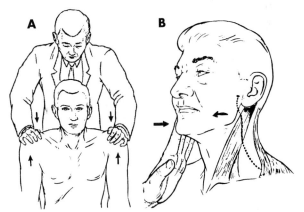

FIGURE 1-15 Testing cranial nerve XI. **A,** Trapezius muscles elevate the shoulders. **B,** Sternocleidomastoid muscles turn the head to the opposite side. (Modified from Rodnitzky RL: The basic neurologic examination. In Rodnitzky RL, ed: *Van Allen's pictorial manual of neurologic tests,* ed 3, Chicago, 1988, Mosby, 33. Reprinted by permission of Mosby, 1988.)

Hypoglossal Nerve

Similar to the accessory nerve (XI), the hypoglossal nerve (XII) is a purely motor nerve, and it innervates the muscles that control the movements of the tongue. The nerve can be tested clinically by asking the patient to protrude the tongue, move the tongue rapidly up and down, or push against the cheek with the tongue inside the mouth (Figure 1-16). Interruption of the hypoglossal nerve will result in ipsilateral weakness and a deviation of the tongue toward the affected side on protrusion.[60] Atrophy of the muscle will follow denervation (Figure 1-16, C).

Anatomic Considerations

The hypoglossal nerve originates in the lower medulla and exits the cranium through the hypoglossal foramen near the foramen magnum (Figures 1-1 and 1-7). It travels externally along the bases of the skull in close relation with the glossopharyngeal (IX), vagus (X), and accessory (XI) nerves as it proceeds to innervate the muscles of the tongue.[59]

Pathologic Considerations

Lesions affecting the hypoglossal nerve alone are uncommon; however, like the accessory nerve (XI), evidence of concurrent involve-

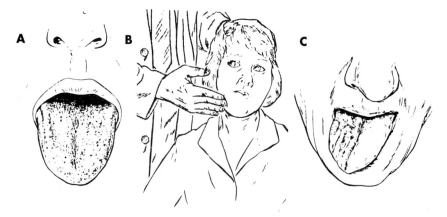

FIGURE 1-16 Testing cranial nerve XII. **A,** Protrusion of the tongue. **B,** Forcing the tongue to the cheek. **C,** Paralysis of XII on the right leads to deviation to the right and atrophy of the tongue. (Modified from Rodnitzky RL: Abnormal signs and symptoms: basis and interpretation. In Rodnitzky RL, ed: *Van Allen's pictorial manual of neurologic tests,* ed 3, Chicago, 1988, Mosby, 107. Reprinted by permission of Mosby, 1988.)

ment of the twelfth cranial nerve can provide information as to the extent and location of any suspected pathology.

References

1. Adams RD, Victor M: Disorders of smell and taste. In *Principles of neurology*, ed 4, New York, 1989, McGraw-Hill, 183-189.
2. Miller NR, ed: *Walsh and Hoyt's clinical neuro-ophthalmology*, ed 4, Baltimore, 1982, Williams & Wilkins, 1345.
3. Duke-Elder S, ed: *System of ophthalmology, vol II, the anatomy of the visual system*, St Louis, 1976, Mosby, 234.
4. Miller NR, ed: *Walsh and Hoyt's clinical neuro-ophthalmology*, ed 4, Baltimore, 1982, Williams & Wilkins, 41-53.
5. Glaser JS, Sadun AA: Anatomy of the visual sensory system. In Glaser JS, ed: *Neuro-ophthalmology*, ed 2, Philadelphia, 1990, JB Lippincott, 66-68.
6. Bergland RM, Ray BS, Torack RM: Anatomical variations in the pituitary gland and adjacent structures in 225 human autopsy cases, *J Comp Neurol* 28:93-99, 1968.
7. Sadun AA: Distinguishing between clinical impairments due to optic nerve or macular disease, *Metab Pediatr Syst Ophthalmol* 13:79-84, 1990.
8. Harrington D: Differential diagnosis of arcuate scotomas, *Invest Ophthalmol Vis Sci* 8:96-105, 1969.
9. Birchall C, Harris G, Drance S, Begg I: Visual field changes in branch retinal "vein" occlusion, *Arch Ophthalmol* 94:747-754, 1976.
10. Trobe JD, Glaser JS, LaFlamme P: Dysthyroid optic neuropathy. Clinical profile and rationale for management, *Arch Ophthalmol* 96:1199-1216, 1976.
11. Crane CG: The anatomical, pathological and clinical relationship of posterior sinuses to optic neuritis, *Ann Otol* 36:201-240, 1927.
12. Avery G, Tana RA, Close LG: Ophthalmic manifestations of mucoceles, *Ann Ophthalmol* 15:734-737, 1983.
13. Rush JA, Younge BR, Campbell RJ: Optic glioma: long-term follow up of 85 histopathologically verified cases, *Ophthalmology* 89:1213-1219, 1982.
14. Chutorian AM, Schwartz JF, Evans RA, Carter S: Optic gliomas in children, *Neurology* 14:82-95, 1964.
15. Glaser JS, Hoyt WF, Corbett J: Visual morbidity with chiasmal glioma: long-term studies of visual fields in untreated and irradiated cases, *Arch Ophthalmol* 85:3-12, 1971.
16. Wright JE, Call NB, Lairicos S: Primary optic nerve meningioma, *Br J Ophthalmol* 64:553-558, 1980.
17. Frisen L, Hoyt WF, Tengroth BM: Optociliary veins, disc pallor, and visual loss: a triad of signs indicating sphenoorbital meningioma, *Acta Ophthalmol* 51:241-249, 1973.
18. Miller NR, ed: *Walsh and Hoyt's clinical neuro-ophthalmology*, ed 4, Baltimore, 1982, Williams & Wilkins, 1347-1350.
19. Norwood EG, Kline LB, Chandra-Sekar B: Aneurysmal compression of the anterior visual pathways, *Neurology* 36:1035-1041, 1986.
20. Vinuela F, Fox A, Chang JK: Clinico-radiological spectrum of giant supraclinoid internal carotid artery aneurysms, *Neurology* 26:93-99, 1984.
21. Unsold R, Hoyt WF: Band atrophy of the optic nerve, *Arch Ophthalmol* 98:1637-1638, 1980.
22. Gartner S: Ocular pathology in chiasmal syndrome, *Am J Ophthalmol* 34:593-596, 1951.

23. Savino PJ, Paris M, Schatz NJ, Orr LS, Corbett JJ: Optic tract syndrome: a review of 21 patients, *Arch Ophthalmol* 96:656-663, 1978.

24. Bell RA, Thompson HS: Relative afferent pupillary defect in optic tract hemianopsias, *Am J Ophthalmol* 85:538-540, 1978.

25. Warwick R: Representation of the extra-ocular muscles in the oculomotor nuclei of the monkey, *J Comp Neurol* 98:449-503, 1953.

26. Duke-Elder S, ed: *System of ophthalmology, vol II, the anatomy of the visual system,* St Louis, 1976, Mosby, 480-497.

27. Glaser JS, ed: *Neuro-ophthalmology,* ed 2, Philadelphia, 1990, JB Lippincott, 372.

28. Miller NR, ed: *Walsh and Hoyt's clinical neuro-ophthalmology,* ed 4, Baltimore, 1982, Williams & Wilkins, 662-672.

29. Rucker CW: Paralysis of third, fourth, and sixth cranial nerves, *Am J Ophthalmol* 46:787-794, 1958.

30. Kissel JT, Burde RM, Klingele TG, Zeiger HE: Pupil-sparing oculomotor palsies with internal carotid and posterior communicating artery aneurysms, *Ann Neurol* 13:149-154, 1983.

31. Green WR, Hackett ER: Neuro-ophthalmological evaluation of oculomotor nerve paralysis, *Arch Ophthalmol* 72:154-167, 1964.

32. Swanson MW: Neuroanatomy of the cavernous sinus and clinical correlations, *Optom Vis Sci* 67:891-897, 1990.

33. Byers RM: Anatomic correlates in head and neck surgery. The lateral pharnygotomy. *Head Neck* 16(5):460-462, 1994.

34. Acers TE: Pseudo-orbital apex syndrome, *Am J Ophthalmol* 88:623-625, 1979.

35. Miller NR, ed: *Walsh and Hoyt's clinical neuro-ophthalmology,* ed 4, Baltimore, 1982, Williams & Wilkins, 680.

36. Miller NR, ed: *Walsh and Hoyt's clinical neuro-ophthalmology,* ed 4, Baltimore, 1982, Williams & Wilkins, 683.

37. Von Noorden GK, Murray E, Wong SY: Superior oblique paralysis. *Arch Ophthalmol* 104:1771-1776, 1986.

38. Flanders M, Draper J: Superior oblique palsy: diagnosis and treatment, *Can J Ophthalmol* 25:17-24, 1990.

39. Rush JA, Younge BR: Paralysis of cranial nerves III, IV, and V, causes and prognosis in 1000 cases, *Arch Ophthalmol* 99:76-79, 1981.

40. Carpenter MB, Batton RR: Abducens internuclear neurons and their role in conjugate horizontal gaze, *J Comp Neurol* 89:191-209, 1989.

41. Van Allen MW, Blodi FC: Neurologic aspects of Möbius syndrome, *Neurology* 10:249-259, 1960.

42. Hotchkiss MG, Miller NR, Clark AW, Green WR: Bilateral Duane's retraction syndrome. A clinical-pathological case report, *Arch Ophthalmol* 98:870-874, 1980.

43. Cogan DG, Victor M: Ocular signs of Wernicke's disease, *Arch Ophthalmol* 51:204-211, 1954.

44. Catalano PJ, Bergstein MJ, Biller HF: Comprehensive management of the eye in facial paralysis, *Arch Otolaryngol Head Neck Surg* 12(1):81-86, 1995.

45. Keane JR: Bilateral sixth nerve palsy, analysis of 125 cases, *Arch Neurol* 33:681-683, 1976.

46. Shrader EC, Schlezinger NS: Neuro-ophthalmological evaluation of abducens paralysis, *Arch Ophthalmol* 62:84-91, 1980.

47. Savino PJ, Hilliker JK, Casell GH, Schatz NJ: Chronic sixth nerve palsies. Are they really harbingers of serious intracranial disease? *Arch Ophthalmol* 120:1442-1444, 1982.

48. Galetta SL, Smith JL: Chronic isolated sixth nerve palsies, *Arch Neurol* 46:79-82, 1989.

49. Carpenter MB, Sutin J: *Human neuroanatomy,* ed 8, Baltimore, 1983, Williams & Wilkins, 385-401.

50. Parkinson D, Johnston J, Chaudhuri A: Sympathetic connections to the fifth and sixth cranial nerves, *Anat Rec* 191:221-226, 1978.

51. Miller NR, ed: *Walsh and Hoyt's clinical neuro-ophthalmology,* ed 4, Baltimore, 1982, Williams & Wilkins, 1061-1062.

52. Martuza RL, Parker SW, Nadol JB, Davis KR, Ojemann RG: Diagnosis of cerebellopontine angle tumors, *Clin Neurosurg* 32:177-213, 1985.

53. Horowitz SH: Isolated facial numbness: clinical significance and relation to trigeminal neuropathy, *Ann Intern Med* 80:49-53, 1974.

54. Miller NR, ed: *Walsh and Hoyt's clinical neuro-ophthalmology,* ed 4, Baltimore, 1982, Williams & Wilkins, 1057.

55. Perusse R: Acoustic neuroma presenting as orofacial anesthesia, *Int J Oral Maxillofac Surg* 23(3):156-160, 1994.

56. Shafshak TS, Essa AY, Bakey FA: The possible contributing factors for the success of steroid therapy in Bell's palsy: a clinical and electrophysiological study, *J Laryngol Otol* 108(11):940-943, 1994.

57. Chadwick D: The cranial nerves and special senses. In Walton J, ed: *Brain's diseases of the nervous system,* ed 10, New York, 1993, Oxford University Press, 76-126.

58. Adams RD, Victor M: Deafness, dizziness, and disorders of equilibrium. In *Principles of neurology,* ed 4, New York, 1989, McGraw-Hill, 226-245.

59. deGroot J, Chusid JG: *Correlative neuroanatomy,* ed 12, East Norwalk, Conn, 1988, Appleton & Lange, 155-166.

60. Rodnitzky RL: *Van Allen's pictorial manual of neurological tests,* ed 3, Chicago, 1988, Year Book Medical Publishers, 29-34, 101-107.

Acknowledgment

The author thanks Dr. Timothy I. Messer, VAMC, Fort Wayne, Indiana, for the design and production of Tables 1-1, 1-2, and 1-3.

2

Cavernous Sinus Disease

Joseph Sowka

Key Terms

trabeculated venous pool	cavernous sinus aneurysm	carotid-cavernous fistula
internal carotid artery	cavernous sinus meningioma	balloon angioplasty dural sinus fistula
cavernous sinus syndrome	aberrant third nerve regeneration	
pituitary adenoma		

The cavernous sinus (CS) is of paramount importance to the optometrist. A number of disease entities, including intracavernous carotid artery aneurysm, carotid and dural sinus fistula, primary neoplastic and metastatic disease, and inflammatory disease may involve the CS, resulting in visual deficits or abnormalities in neuroocular function. Indeed, many patients with CS disease are apt to present to the optometrist's office because of the following ocular sequelae: visual deficit, diplopia, orbital pain, pupillary abnormalities, proptosis, chemosis, and orbital congestion (see box on p. 45).

It is important for the clinician to carefully evaluate and workup the patient with suspected CS disease to establish the presumptive diagnosis and institute the appropriate management. Furthermore, neurologists, neurosurgeons, oncologists, and internists may rely on the optometrist's consultation and comanagement of any ophthalmic manifestations.

The key to understanding CS pathology and the subsequent ophthalmic sequelae is to appreciate CS morphology and to develop a conceptual understanding of the anatomic relationships of the structures within the sinus. Such knowledge allows the clinician to localize a disease process to the CS itself and to determine where the disease process is occurring within the sinus.

This chapter is divided into two parts. The first part delineates the anatomy of the CS with particular attention to the anatomic relationships of inclusive structures. The clinical correlates are stressed. The second part discusses the specific pathologies that can affect the CS along with their ocular ramifications. The optometric workup, necessary clinical and laboratory studies, and appropriate management strategies are emphasized.

Anatomy of the Cavernous Sinus

The reader is advised to refer repeatedly to Figures 2-1 and 2-2 as this portion is read. The CS should be envisioned as an architectural entity that has a defined configuration and houses certain structures.

Structure of the Sinus

The CS has traditionally been considered to be a trabeculated, largely unbroken, venous channel (Figure 2-1). The term "cavernous sinus" was originally applied descriptively to denote that the interior of the sinus is cavernous or plexiform. The unique appearance of the CS is

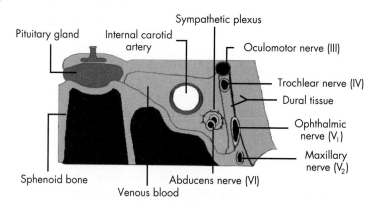

FIGURE 2-1 Diagrammatic representation of the anatomy of the left cavernous sinus. Cranial nerves III, IV, V_1, and V_2 are embedded in dural tissue while the CN VI, sympathetic plexus, and internal carotid artery are "free" within the venous blood of the cavern. The pituitary gland is dorsomedially located in the sella turcica. Inferiorly and inferomedially is the sphenoid bone and sinus.

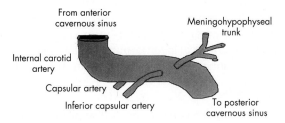

From anterior
cavernous sinus

Meningohypophyseal
trunk

Internal carotid
artery

Capsular artery

Inferior capsular artery

To posterior
cavernous sinus

FIGURE 2-2 Diagrammatic representation of the smaller branches of the intracavernous internal carotid artery (ICA).

due to the numerous filaments that subdivide the sinus. Some modern surgical studies imply that the CS is a plexus of various-sized veins rather than a trabeculated venous cavern. Most histologic reports, however, support the concept that the CS is indeed an unbroken venous channel, and this chapter embraces that traditional concept.[9-12]

Signs and Symptoms of Cavernous Sinus Disease

Visual deficit
Diplopia and ophthalmoplegia
Orbital or hemicranial pain
Pupil abnormalities
Proptosis
Chemosis
Orbital congestion
Ptosis
Orbital bruit

Note: Patients may present with some, all, or none of these signs and symptoms.

The paired CSs are approximately 1 cm wide and 2 mm long. They are located on each side of the sphenoid sinus, sella turcica, and pituitary gland just anterior to the trigeminal ganglion in Meckel's cave. They extend anteriorly from the superior orbital fissure to the apex of the petrous portion of the temporal bone, posteriorly. They are bordered medially by the sphenoid bone and laterally by dural tissue.[9,13,14]

The venous caverns of the CS are composed of dural tissue. The brain is enveloped by meninges composed of three membranes, the dura, arachnoid, and pia. The dura mater, from which the CS and all other intracranial venous sinuses originate, is a thick, collagenous membrane. This membrane is subdivided into two layers, the endosteal layer, which surrounds all bony structures, and the outer meningeal layer, which provides tubular sheaths for the cranial nerves as they pass through the cranium. The CS is formed by the separation of these layers, with the meningeal layer forming the lateral wall and the endosteal layer lining the sphenoid bone and forming the medial wall.[15]

Venous Components

The CS may be considered a trabeculated venous pool. The paired sinuses are interconnected via the intercavernous sinus (circular sinus). These interconnecting veins, which surround the sella and pituitary gland, explain why a vascular pathology in one sinus may cause affectations in the contralateral sinus.[9,13,14]

The CS receives most of its venous blood from the superior and inferior ophthalmic veins. The ophthalmic veins are valveless, and blood may flow retrograde in certain pathologic situations. These veins represent the venous drainage from the orbit, globe, extraocular muscles, and lid through the anterior ciliary, episcleral, subconjunctival, and conjunctival veins. Once the blood has pooled in the CS, the principal drainage is via the superior and inferior petrosal sinuses. The aqueous fluid percolates through the trabecular meshwork and proceeds along the same route.[15,16]

CLINICAL PEARL

The CS receives most of its venous blood from the superior and inferior ophthalmic veins.

Arterial Components

The arterial composition of the CS is entirely separate from its venous counterpart. The main arterial component is that part of the internal carotid artery (ICA) that traverses the interior of the CS. The ICA gives off smaller intracavernous branches, but completely retains its integrity within the sinus. There is no admixing of arterial and venous blood in the normal state.

The ICA enters the posterior aspect of the CS from the carotid canal and the foramen lacerum. It then ascends and turns abruptly to form an S-shape known as the carotid siphon. The ICA ascends to perforate and exit the CS superiorly, branching terminally into the middle and anterior cerebral arteries and the posterior communicating artery (Figure 2-2). Although the ICA can travel a somewhat variable intracavernous course, it is largely unhindered. Except for its entrance and exit, it is not encased in the dural sheath.[9,13,17]

The ICA has a variable relationship to the pituitary gland, which resides in the neighboring sella turcica (Figure 2-1). The ICA may be separated from the pituitary by as much as 7 mm or may be so close that the gland is indented. Because the pituitary gland is not spherical, a portion of the gland may actually overhang the ICA.[9]

The intracavernous ICA gives off several branches. Although the branching pattern is variable (Figure 2-2), the largest and most frequently encountered branch is the meningohypophyseal artery. This artery gives rise to the tentorial artery, inferior hypophyseal artery, and the dorsal meningeal artery, all of which supply the walls of the CS as well as the third, fourth, and sixth cranial nerves. These arteries supply the posterior pituitary capsule as well. The remaining branches of the intracavernous ICA are the inferior cavernous artery and McConnel's capsular artery.[9]

Neural Components

There are many important neural structures within the CS (see box below). Converging in the sinus are the oculomotor nerve (cranial nerve [CN] III), trochlear nerve (CN IV), ophthalmic division of the trigeminal nerve (CN V_1), maxillary division of the trigeminal nerve (CN V_2), abducens nerve (CN VI), and the sympathetic plexus (Figure 2-1). The oculomotor nerve innervates the superior rectus, inferior rectus, medial rectus, and inferior oblique as well as the levator of the upper lid. Its parasympathetic division subserves pupillary constriction. The trochlear nerve innervates the superior oblique, and subserves intorsion and depression. The abducens nerve subserves abduction. The trigeminal nerve provides sensation to the cornea, center and tip of the nose, forehead, and eyelid. The sympathetic plexus functions to innervate the pupillary dilator and the superior and inferior tarsal muscles. These muscles accessorize superior lid elevation and inferior lid depression, respectively.[9,15,18]

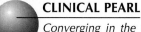 **Neural Structures Within the Cavernous Sinus**

Oculomotor nerve (CN III)
Trochlear nerve (CN IV)
Trigeminal nerve, ophthalmic division (CN V_1)
Trigeminal nerve, maxillary division (CN V_2)
Abducens nerve (CN VI)
Sympathetic plexus

CLINICAL PEARL

Converging in the sinus are the oculomotor nerve (cranial nerve [CN] III), trochlear nerve (CN IV), ophthalmic division of the trigeminal nerve (CN V_1), maxillary division of the trigeminal nerve (CN V_2), abducens nerve (CN VI), and the sympathetic plexus.

The maxillary division of the trigeminal nerve (CN V_2), although not technically a part of the CS, may rarely be affected by CS disease. The maxillary division of the trigeminal nerve lies in the dural tissue just inferior to the CS and is responsible for sensation to the lateral aspect of the nose and the lower lid.

Although there is some anatomic variability, the location of the neural components within the CS is generally consistent. CNs III, IV, and V_1 are embedded within the lateral sinus wall. CN VI and the sympathetic plexus course through the sinus itself. The proximity of CN VI to the sympathetic plexus and to the intracavernous ICA has the most variability.[9,13]

CNs III and IV are closely approximated, entering the sinus through the dural roof. This pairing is maintained within the lateral dural wall from the superior entrance to the exit anteriorly at the superior orbital fissure. Before exiting, CN III divides into a superior and inferior division. Thus the potential exists for isolated palsies of either the superior or inferior divisions of CN III, a situation that would localize to the anterior CS.[9,13] CN V_1 enters the CS posteriorly and inferiorly and courses upward within the lateral wall toward the superior orbital fissure. CN V_1 remains inferior to both CN III and CN IV.[13]

CN VI enters the sinus posteriorly after ascending the clivus. On entering the sinus, the nerve runs medially to CN V_1 and to the ICA. CN VI may not always be a single, continuous nerve. Rather, it may be split into multiple rootlets. There also may be fibrous attachments to the ICA.

The sympathetic plexus enters the sinus along with the ICA. The nerves cross over to CN VI before being distributed to CN V_1. The sympathetics do not share a relationship with either CN III or CN IV. The sympathetics exit the sinus with CN V_1 and pass through the ciliary ganglion without synapse.[9,13]

It is important for the clinician to fully understand the foregoing anatomic relationships before proceeding to the section on CS disease. For example, ophthalmoplegia of CNs III, IV, and VI along with deficits in V_1 and the sympathetic supply to the eye not only localize the disease process to the CS, but specifically localize the lesion to the posterior aspect of the sinus, where all of the neural structures enter. Multiple cranial nerve palsies combined with isolated superior or inferior divisional CN III palsies imply that the lesion is impacting the anterior CS. However, it is also important to remember that there is variability to the anatomic relationships of the structures within the CS. Patients rarely present with classic "textbook" signs and symptoms.

Disease Entities of the Cavernous Sinus

An ambiguity in ophthalmic literature requires clarification. The term "cavernous sinus syndrome" is often used when discussing CS pathology. The clinician may suspect that the term refers to a constellation of signs and symptoms that results from an independent disease entity. In fact, "cavernous sinus syndrome" does not relate to any single disease entity. Rather, the term is generic and connotes any disease process that affects the CS. Cavernous sinus syndrome implies a clinical picture that may include ophthalmoplegia, orbital congestion, vision loss, orbital or ocular pain, and exophthalmos. Thus any CS disease subsequently discussed may cause a CS syndrome.[19-23]

Entities Producing Cavernous Sinus Syndrome

A. Vascular disorders
  1. ICA aneurysm
  2. CS fistula
  3. Dural sinus fistula
  4. CS thrombosis
B. Neoplastic diseases
  1. Primary intracranial tumors
     a. Pituitary adenoma
     b. Meningioma
     c. Craniopharyngioma
     d. Sarcoma
     e. Neurofibroma
     f. Chordoma
     g. Chondroma
  2. Local metastasis
     a. Nasopharyngeal carcinoma
     b. Cyclindroma
     c. Squamous cell carcinoma
  3. Distant metastasis
     a. Lymphoma
     b. Myeloma
     c. Carcinoma
C. Inflammatory disease
  1. Bacterial sinusitis
  2. Mucocele
  3. Periostitis
  4. Herpes zoster
  5. Fungal mucormycosis
  6. *Treponema pallidum* (syphilis)
  7. Idiopathic
     a. Wegener's granulomatosis
     b. Sarcoidosis
     c. Tolosa-Hunt syndrome

CS: cavernous sinus; ICA: intracavernous carotid artery.

CLINICAL PEARL

Cavernous sinus syndrome implies a clinical picture that may include ophthalmoplegia, orbital congestion, vision loss, orbital or ocular pain, and exophthalmos.

Many disease processes affect the CS (see box on p. 49). A comprehensive list would include vascular disorders such as aneurysms, fistulas, and thromboses; neoplastic diseases such as pituitary adenomas, meningiomas, craniopharyngiomas, sarcomas, fibromas, chordomas, and chondromas; neoplastic diseases from metastases such as nasopharyngiomas, lymphomas, and myelomas; inflammation from sinusitis, mucoceles, syphilis, and mycobacteria; and idiopathic granulomatous inflammations. A detailed analysis of each of these entities is beyond the scope of this chapter. However, the more commonly encountered CS diseases are explored, and an attempt will be made to logically categorize these pathologies.[8]

Nonmetastatic Lesions

This section discusses the highly disparate entities of pituitary adenomas, intracavernous ICA aneurysms, and intracavernous meningiomas. All of these pathologies are nonmetastatic space-occupying lesions affecting the CS.

Pituitary Adenoma

The pituitary gland is a close anatomic neighbor of the CS. The gland lies in the pituitary fossa of the sella turcica (Figure 2-1). It is medial and slightly superior to the CS. Generally, the ICA is slightly inferior to the pituitary gland, but the two structures may make some contact.[9]

CLINICAL PEARL

The pituitary gland is a close anatomic neighbor of the CS.

A pituitary adenoma is a slow-growing, benign, nonmetastatic tumor of the pituitary gland. As the pituitary tumor expands, it tends to occupy intracranial space and may cause an increase in intracranial pressure. In addition, adjacent neural structures may be compressed. One is aware of the common sequelae of bitemporal hemianopsia as a result of compression on the optic chiasm from below. The pituitary adenoma may expand laterally and invade the CS, however. Although usually unilateral, bilateral asymmetric compression may occur with resultant bilateral, asymmetric cranial nerve palsies.[1,2,24-27]

The slow-growing nature of pituitary tumors may result in subtle cranial nerve defects because a cranial nerve is capable of detouring around a slow-growing mass. CN III is preferentially affected by the expanding pituitary adenoma because the nerve is at the same plane as the pituitary gland. CN VI is protected from the expanding mass because it is relatively shielded by the ICA.[27]

Although the CS sequelae of pituitary adenoma are typically insidious, an acute CS syndrome with single or multiple cranial nerve palsies can occur from pituitary apoplexy. Pituitary apoplexy is a sudden expansion of a preexisting pituitary adenoma due to an acute infarct and subsequent hemorrhage. The rapid growth in the pituitary tumor militates against the cranial nerves being able to compensate by altering their direction. In addition to the ophthalmoplegia, the patient experiences severe headache, nausea, vomiting, and visual deterioration.[26]

The diagnosis of pituitary tumor is made by using contrast-enhanced, thin-section, coronal computed tomography (CT) scanning that demonstrates the enlarged sella. Magnetic resonance imaging (MRI) better delineates the hemorrhage caused by pituitary apoplexy.[28]

Noncomplicated pituitary adenoma may be treated medically, radiologically, or surgically. Pituitary apoplexy can quickly evolve into a life-threatening situation, however, and is best treated by transsphenoidal resection of the mass.[26]

Cavernous Sinus Aneurysms

Aneurysms of the ICA within the CS are usually saccular (berry-shaped) outpouchings. These lesions are slowly progressive and sequentially involve CNs VI, III, V_1, and IV. CN VI is most prone to early compression because of its close proximity to the intracavernous ICA and its lack of structural support within the sinus.[24]

The clinical symptoms of intracavernous aneurysm are variable and include ophthalmoplegias, vision loss, exophthalmos, and interesting pupillary abnormalities. If CN III and the sympathetics are simultaneously compromised, the fixed, dilated pupil, associated with compression of CN III outside the CS, is usually not present. Rather, the pupil tends to be small, albeit nonresponsive to light and to near-effort. In fact, cranial nerve palsy in association with a ptosis and miosis (Horner's syndrome) suggests an intracavernous compressive lesion. The box on p. 52 summarizes the signs and symptoms of cavernous sinus ICA aneurysm.[24,29,30]

Signs and Symptoms of Cavernous Sinus ICA Aneurysm

Vision loss
Exophthalmos
Orbital or hemicranial pain
Diplopia
Single or multiple cranial nerve palsy
Horner's syndrome

Symptoms may be progressive, stable, or remitting

Note: Patients may present with some, none, or all of these features.

CLINICAL PEARL

Cranial nerve palsy in association with a ptosis and miosis (Horner's syndrome) suggests an intracavernous compressive lesion.

As the aneurysm expands anteriorly, the anterior clinoid, optic foramen, and superior orbital fissure may become eroded. Vision loss and exophthalmos may result. Posterior expansion erodes the petrous portion of the temporal bone, which may result in ipsilateral deafness and facial nerve palsy. Continued enlargement may cause a mass to form in the middle cranial fossa, resulting in compression of branches of the trigeminal nerve. Significant pain may result.[19,31]

The main concern with any intracranial aneurysm is rupture. When an intracranial artery ruptures, arterial blood may diffuse into the subarachnoid space, intraventricular space, or brain parenchyma. Coma, focal neurologic deficits, cerebral herniation, and death may ensue. Rupture of an intracavernous aneurysm is less apt to occur because the dural walls of the sinus provide a protective coat for the aneurysm. Should rupture occur, the results are usually less ominous because the arterial blood will be contained within the CS. The rupture, however, results in the admixing of arterial blood with the venous blood normally contained within the sinus.[31] The carotid-cavernous fistula results in characteristic signs and symptoms that will be described in a subsequent section.

Diagnosis of CS aneurysm is made on the basis of the clinical findings and confirmed on the basis of contrast-enhanced CT scans, MRI, or carotid angiography. Magnetic resonance imaging has largely replaced angiography because of the defined risks for morbidity or mortality of that invasive procedure (Figure 2-3).[31]

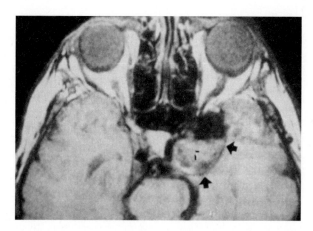

FIGURE 2-3 Magnetic resonance image (MRI) indicating left intra-cavernous ICA. (From Troost BT, Glaser JS: Aneurysms, arteriovenous communications, and related vascular malformations. In Tasman W, Jaeger EA, eds: *Duane's clinical ophthalmology.* Philadelphia, 1989, JB Lippincott, 3. Reprinted by permission of JB Lippincott, 1989.)

The treatment of CS aneurysms is surgical. Trapping and clipping of the aneurysm directly is very difficult to perform. Surgical ligation of the extracavernous portion of the ICA or aneurysmal occlusion with a detachable balloon has met with more success.[31] The morbidity and mortality of these procedures, however, are still quite high.[31,32]

Cavernous Sinus Meningioma

Cavernous sinus meningioma is a slowly growing, benign, nonmetastatic tumor. It may originate from the dura mater that makes up the walls of the CS or from the meninges covering the floor of the middle cranial fossa lateral to the sinus. As the tumor grows, it invades the sinus by lateral extension.[33-35] The cranial nerves within the lateral walls of the sinus are often involved, resulting in compressive neuropathies (Figure 2-4).

Like all disease entities that affect the CS, meningiomas have the potential of causing singular or multiple cranial nerve palsies of variable expression. A partial or total CN III palsy is most apt to occur because of its lateral position in the sinus. If the anterior portion of the CS is not involved, however, the inferior division of CN III, which carries the pupilomotor fibers, may be spared. Pupillary function may thus be normal. The pupil also may be quite small because of simultaneous involvement of the sympathetics. An isolated CN VI palsy may occur, with a resultant abduction deficit ipsilaterally. Isolated involvement of CN IV is uncommon with CS meningiomas.[33-36]

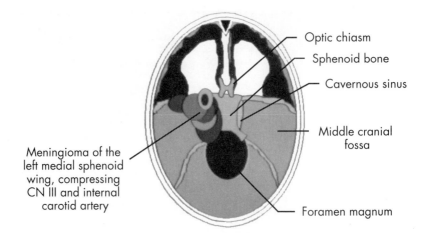

Optic chiasm

Sphenoid bone

Cavernous sinus

Middle cranial fossa

Meningioma of the left medial sphenoid wing, compressing CN III and internal carotid artery

Foramen magnum

FIGURE 2-4 Diagrammatic representation of a meningioma invading the left cavernous sinus and growing within the middle cranial fossa.

Diagnosis of CS meningioma is suspected when single or multiple cranial nerve palsies gradually evolve. Definitive diagnosis is made by contrast-enhanced CT or MRI. Computed tomography scans show tumor "blush" due to hypertrophied feeder vessels and an altered contour to the involved CS. Characteristically, the sinus is either compressed or distended, and the course of the ICA may be altered[28,34,37] (Figure 2-4).

Management of CS meningiomas is difficult because of the surgical inaccessibility of the CS and the risk of traumatizing the cranial nerves involved. Radiation has been only minimally effective. Because meningiomas are typically very slow-growing, surgical resection is not recommended unless the brain stem or vision is threatened or the patient suffers from intractable pain.

Primary Aberrant Third Nerve Regeneration

Aberrant regeneration of the CN III is a common sequela of acute injury to the nerve anywhere in its course. Common causes include trauma, compression from tumor or aneurysm, or inflammation. Presumably, regenerated axons, sprouting from the damaged nerve, go astray. As a result of their altered course, they do not innervate their original effectors. Clinical features include elevation of the upper lid on attempted adduction or depression (pseudo-Graefe's sign), adduction or retraction of the globe on attempted depression or elevation, absence of direct or indirect pupillary light reflex, and pupillary constriction on attempted adduction[38,39] (see box on p. 55).

Clinical Features of CN III Aberrant Regeneration

Elevation of the upper lid on attempted adduction or depression (pseudo von Graefe's sign)
Adduction or retraction of the globe on attempted depression or elevation
Absent pupillary light reaction with pupil constriction on attempted adduction
Often variable clinical features with pseudo von Graefe's sign most common and diagnostic

CLINICAL PEARL

Aberrant regeneration of the CN III is a common sequela of acute injury to the nerve anywhere in its course. Common causes include trauma, compression from tumor or aneurysm, or inflammation.

Primary aberrant third nerve regeneration is a special type of CN III regeneration without an obvious premonitory palsy. With the absence of an antecedent, acute palsy strongly implies the presence of a compressive lesion within the CS, such as an aneurysm or meningioma. Primary aberrant regeneration in a patient younger than 55 years of age is usually due to CS meningioma. Aneurysms are apt to cause the primary aberrant regeneration in patients over age 50 years.[33,34,38,40]

The presence of primary aberrant regeneration of CN III may be explained by the fact that aneurysms and meningiomas are very slow-growing. They may cause recurrent subclinical damage to the nerve, with resultant aberrant regeneration. The initial precipitant damage may never be recognized, but the resultant aberrant regeneration should not be missed.[38,41]

Cavernous Sinus Fistulas

A carotid-cavernous fistula is an abnormal communication between the ICA, or its branches, and the CS. Normally the ICA provides a closed conduit for arterial blood within the CS. Such an arrangement prevents the mixing of arterial and venous blood. In the event of a leak in the ICA or any of its branches, a fistula develops within the CS, resulting in the mixing of arterial and venous blood. Cavernous sinus fistulas may be classified etiologically (spontaneous or traumatic), angiographically (direct or dural), or hemodynamically (high-flow or low-flow).[29,42]

CLINICAL PEARL

A carotid-cavernous fistula is an abnormal communication between the ICA, or its branches, and the CS.

The classic carotid-cavernous fistula is a direct, high-flow vascular lesion that invariably results from trauma. The intracavernous ICA has formed a rent that allows the arterial blood to flow freely and vigorously into the CS (Figure 2-5). The large quantity of arterial blood filling the CS under high pressure produces a profound array of symptoms (see box below). The trapping of the arterial blood within the venous system, however, prevents a potentially fatal subarachnoid hemorrhage from occurring.[43]

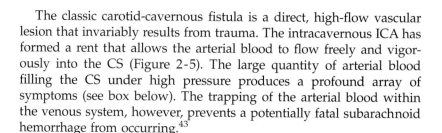

Clinical Features of Carotid–Cavernous Sinus Fistula

Diplopia and ophthalmoplegia
Orbital bruit
Arterialized conjunctival and episcleral vessels
Edema and chemosis of lid and conjunctiva
Elevated intraocular pressure

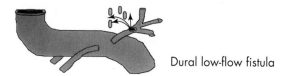

Dural low-flow fistula

Direct high-flow fistula
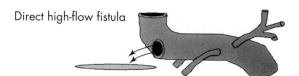

FIGURE 2-5 Diagrammatic representation of a direct high-flow fistula and a dural low-flow fistula resulting from tears in the ICA or branch, respectively.

The high-flow pool of mixed blood has two main potential avenues of egress: posteriorly through the inferior petrosal sinus and then into the jugular vein, or anteriorly through the superior ophthalmic vein and then into the eye and orbit. Posterior flow usually results in variable degrees of ophthalmoplegia. Anterior flow produces an astoundingly provocative clinical picture that is usually associated with the classic carotid-cavernous fistula (Figures 2-6, 2-7, and 2-8).

The primary result of retrograde flow through the valveless superior ophthalmic vein is a filling of the conjunctival and episcleral veins with arterial blood. This arterialization of the conjunctival and episcleral veins results in a dilated, tortuous, corkscrewlike appearance. Another sequela of the retrograde flow of arterial blood through the superior ophthalmic vein is the resulting venous stagnation and congestion that occurs when low-pressure venous blood encounters high-pressure arterial blood. Venous blood cannot adequately drain from the orbit and adnexa. The clinical picture of severe lid edema, chemosis, and orbital congestion results[7,22,44,45] (Figures 2-6 through 2-8).

Because the superior ophthalmic is engorged and distended by the back flow of the arterial blood, there may be a mass effect causing the vein to push the globe forward in the orbit, creating an exophthalmos. The exophthalmos may appear to pulsate as the systole of the heart is translated to the arterialized superior ophthalmic vein. The patient

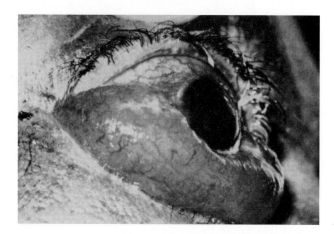

FIGURE 2-6 Severe conjunctival edema and vascular engorgement characteristic of a traumatic, direct, high-flow cavernous sinus fistula. (From Troost BT, Glaser JS: Aneurysms, arteriovenous communications, and related vascular malformations. In Tasman W, Jaeger EA, eds: *Duane's clinical ophthalmology*, Philadelphia, 1989, JB Lippincott, 19. Reprinted by permission of JB Lippincott, 1989.)

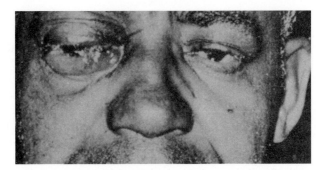

FIGURE 2-7 Severe conjunctival injection, chemosis, and lid edema characteristic of a traumatic carotid–cavernous sinus fistula. (From Troost BT, Glaser JS: Aneurysms, arteriovenous communications, and related vascular malformations. In Tasman W, Jaeger EA, eds: *Duane's clinical ophthalmology*, Philadelphia, 1989, JB Lippincott, 19. Reprinted by permission of JB Lippincott, 1989.)

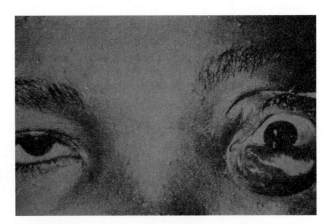

FIGURE 2-8 Severe lid and conjunctival vascular congestion and ophthalmoplegia associated with a high-flow carotid–cavernous sinus fistula. (From Troost BT, Glaser JS: Aneurysms, arteriovenous communications, and related vascular malformations. In Tasman W, Jaeger EA, eds: *Duane's clinical ophthalmology*, Philadelphia, 1989, JB Lippincott, 19. Reprinted by permission of JB Lippincott, 1989.)

may complain of an audible bruit, which the clinician may hear by auscultating the globe.[6,7]

Visual loss in high-flow carotid-cavernous fistulas may occur by several mechanisms. The prominent exophthalmos may result in prolonged corneal exposure and subsequent corneal scarring. Arterial insufficiency to the optic nerve can cause ischemic optic neuropathy. Venous stasis may lead to choroidal transudation, choroidal detachment, and subsequent angle closure glaucoma. Venous stasis also may lead to central vein occlusion with subsequent macular edema or macular cyst formation. Moreover, the central vein occlusion may lead to neovascularization of the iris and subsequent neovascular glaucoma.[5,46,47]

Diplopia after ophthalmoplegia is a frequent symptom of high-flow carotid-cavernous fistulas. Paresis of CN VI is the most common cause of the ophthalmoplegia, with involvement of CN III and CN IV occurring to a lesser degree. It is speculated that the posterior drainage of the fistula with subsequent distention of the inferior petrosal sinus compresses the CN VI against the petroclinoid ligament. Another cause of the diplopia is the engorgement of the extraocular muscles as a result of the failure of the muscular veins to drain adequately. A restrictive myopathy similar to thyroid ophthalmopathy ensues.[7,48-51]

The diagnosis of direct, high-flow carotid-cavernous fistula is usually made on the basis of clinical observation. Involvement of the contralateral side is explained on the basis of the intercavernous communications. Ultrasound scanning and neuroimaging show the engorgement of the superior ophthalmic vein, which is characteristic of carotid-cavernous fistula. Cerebral angiography provides the definitive diagnosis by demonstrating the rent in the intracavernous ICA[6,49,51-55] (Figure 2-9).

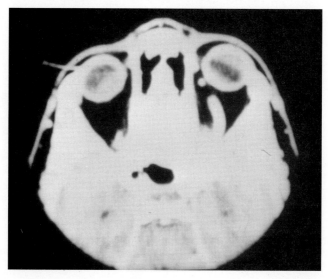

FIGURE 2-9 Contrast-enhanced CT scan showing engorged left superior ophthalmic vein from a low-flow dural sinus fistula. (From Sowka JW: Dural arteriovenous malformation, *J Am Optom Assoc* 60:846-848, 1989. Reprinted by permission of the Journal of the American Optometric Association, 1989.)

A direct, high-flow carotid-cavernous fistula, although not life threatening, is a neurosurgical urgency. The unpleasant cosmetic appearance, debilitating symptoms of bruit and diplopia, and the potential for profound visual loss mandate that an attempt be made to rectify the abnormality. An older approach involved direct microsurgical repair of the defective wall of the intracavernous ICA while maintaining its patency. This procedure was fraught with risk, however, because it involved opening the cranial vault, exposing the middle cranial fossa, and operating directly within the CS.[56,57]

Newer techniques involving thrombosis and embolization of the fistula have gained popularity because they result in a lower incidence of morbidity and mortality. One such procedure involves occluding the fistula by threading a catheter into the CS and placing embolic material, such as isobutyl-2-cyanoacrylate, into the ICA. A more popular procedure is to introduce a balloon into the intracavernous ICA through a catheter. The balloon is inflated and detached, and acts to seal the leak within the ICA. Finally, a balloon can be inflated and detached within the CS. This technique seals the leak from the venous side and is more apt to ensure patency of the ICA[58-60] (Figure 2-10).

The balloon catheter techniques are not without risks: inadvertent occlusion of the ICA may result in cerebral infarcts and neurologic stigmata. The balloon may deflate over time, resulting in fistula reformation. Overinflation of the balloon may compress some of the cranial nerves and exacerbate the diplopia. The CS wall may be perforated by the catheter, leading to subarachnoid hemorrhage and

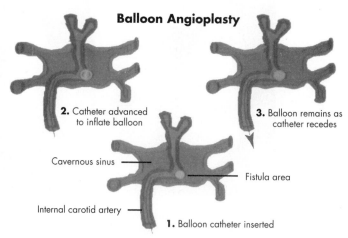

Balloon Angioplasty

2. Catheter advanced to inflate balloon

3. Balloon remains as catheter recedes

Cavernous sinus

Fistula area

Internal carotid artery

1. Balloon catheter inserted

FIGURE 2-10 Diagrammatic representation of repair of a carotid–cavernous sinus fistula via detachable balloon technique. A catheter with balloon is introduced into the ICA, inflated in the fistulous area, and remains while the catheter is removed.

death. Notwithstanding the obvious risks, however, successful occlusion of the fistula by any of the techniques mentioned previously usually results in reversal of most of the signs and symptoms and allows the patient to lead a normal life.[55,58-61]

The low-flow, dural sinus fistula (e.g., dural-CS arteriovenous malformation, dural arteriovenous malformation, spontaneous carotid-cavernous fistula, dural shunt syndrome, nontraumatic fistula, red-eyed shunt syndrome) represents a tear in one of the smaller branches of the intracavernous ICA (Figure 2-5). The meningohypophyseal artery is the most frequently involved branch, but the inferior artery of the CS, McConnel's capsular artery, or a subsequent branch of one of these smaller vessels also may tear. These branches are anatomically smaller than the ICA, and their intra-arterial perfusion pressure is much less. The fistula that results from a tear in their walls therefore is considered to be low-flow.

Dural sinus fistula is more prevalent in middle-aged or older females. It usually occurs spontaneously with no antecedent trauma. It is thought that the cause of these lesions is a rupture of a preexisting aneurysm or congenital arterial wall weakness from hypertension, atherosclerosis, collagen vascular disease, or childbirth.[22,44,45,62]

The dural sinus fistula usually produces a much less florid symptom complex than the high-flow, traumatic carotid-cavernous fistula. In fact, the signs and symptoms may be so subtle that the underlying condition is often misdiagnosed. These patients often present with a mildly injected eye because of the corkscrew appearance of the arterialized, episcleral vessels (Figure 2-11). They may relate that they have been undergoing treatment for a chronic conjunctivitis without any improvement. There may be minimal-to-no exophthalmos, orbital bruit, ophthalmoplegia, elevated intraocular pressure, or retinal vessel tortuosity. The ophthalmoplegia that does occur is usually secondary to CN VI palsy.[22,45,46,52,53]

Although the signs and symptoms of low-flow, dural sinus fistula are insidious, prolonged filling of the CS with arterial blood can cause an increase in signs and symptoms over time. Secondary open-angle glaucoma is a particular concern. The elevated pressure in the ophthalmic veins inhibits the aqueous from percolating through the trabecular meshwork, episcleral veins, anterior ciliary veins, and ophthalmic veins. For aqueous to circulate, the intraocular pressure must rise to exceed the elevated episcleral pressure.[62-64]

CLINICAL PEARL

Although the signs and symptoms of low-flow, dural sinus fistula are insidious, prolonged filling of the CS with arterial blood can cause an increase in signs and symptoms over time. Secondary open-angle glaucoma is a particular concern.

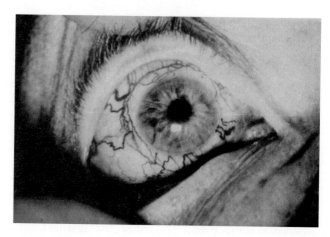

FIGURE 2-11   Arterialized conjunctival and episcleral veins from a low-flow dural sinus fistula. Note the 'corkscrew' appearance of the vessels under high vascular pressure. (From Sowka JW: Dural arteriovenous malformation, *J Am Optom Assoc* 60:846-848, 1989. Reprinted by permission of the Journal of the American Optometric Association, 1989.)

Management of secondary glaucoma in dural sinus fistula can be very challenging. Medications that enhance outflow, such as pilocarpine, are ineffective. Medications that decrease aqueous production, such as timolol or acetazolamide, may offer acceptable lowering of the intraocular pressure, but do nothing to reduce the episcleral resistance. It is generally advised that treatment should be directed at temporizing the glaucoma because spontaneous resolution of the dural sinus fistula frequently occurs.[63]

Interestingly, dural sinus fistula resolves spontaneously in 50% to 60% of cases.[22] It is thought that spontaneous thrombosis of the small arterial tear is the mechanism. Also, diagnostic angiography has been reported to have a therapeutic effect, with many lesions closing after this procedure. In view of the relatively benign nature of the condition, the dural sinus fistula generally should be managed conservatively. The risk of endovascular embolization techniques is greater than that which the patient would experience from the condition itself. In the absence of debilitating symptoms, the practitioner can be content with CT scans to confirm the diagnosis and with periodic monitoring for resolution or progression. Any worsening of the signs or symptoms may be due to a thrombosis of the superior ophthalmic vein.[22,44,46,52-54,62,63]

Cavernous Sinus Inflammation

Inflammations of the CS may be understood by examining the Tolosa-Hunt syndrome (THS) as a prototype. Tolosa-Hunt syndrome, also known as painful ophthalmoplegia, is an idiopathic granulomatous inflammation of the CS. There is no known association with any other systemic disease and there are no lesions outside the CS. Blood studies are essentially normal. The only test that has any diagnostic significance is the MRI, which may show the characteristic granulomatous soft tissue density.[3,4,21,65-67]

CLINICAL PEARL

Tolosa-Hunt syndrome, also known as painful ophthalmoplegia, is an idiopathic granulomatous inflammation of the CS.

The classic syndrome is characterized by ophthalmoplegia, due to involvement of either one or more of CNs III, IV, and V_1, and boring retroorbital or hemicranial pain. The pain component of THS may precede or follow the ocular muscle component, but it usually occurs concurrently with it. Occasionally, V_1 or the sympathetics are affected. If the latter nerves are involved, a Horner's syndrome will result. The optic nerve may be involved if the inflammation extends to the superior orbital fissure.[3,21,68]

Tolosa-Hunt syndrome may be either unilateral or bilateral and has no sexual predilection. The syndrome may present in patients between 3½ and 75 years, with the most prevalent onset being between the ages of 40 and 50 years.[4,21,67] The disease tends to wax and wane, with symptoms lasting from days to weeks. Spontaneous remissions occur, but symptoms may reappear. In addition, neurologic deficits from any one episode may remain.

When faced with painful ophthalmoplegia, the optometrist must consider many of the pathologic entities that have been previously discussed. In addition, diabetic ophthalmoplegia, aneurysm of the posterior cerebral artery, nasopharyngioma, and temporal arteritis must be part of the differential diagnosis.

Temporal arteritis, in particular, may mimic THS. However, the former condition usually occurs when the patients are between 60 and 70 years and has a strong female predilection. In addition, the visual loss in temporal arteritis is precipitous, and the erythrocyte sedimentation rate is quite elevated.

THS shows a dramatic response to high-dose systemic steroids. Smith and Taxdal[3] noted a complete resolution of all symptoms after 48 hours of steroid use and implied that a persistence of pain and ophthalmoplegia rules out a diagnosis of THS. The initial resolution of symptoms, however, does not necessarily guarantee the diagnosis of THS. Such entities as malignant lymphoma, intracavernous ICA aneurysm, posterior cerebral aneurysm, pituitary apoplexy, meningiomas, and other parasellar tumors initially may seem to remit on the usage of systemic steroids. The remission is not as complete as in the THS, and exacerbations occur on cessation of the therapy.[3,68-72]

CLINICAL PEARL

Tolosa-Hunt syndrome shows a dramatic response to high-dose systemic steroids.

After all other potential causes of painful ophthalmoplegia have been eliminated, the clinician may entertain the diagnosis of THS by exclusion. The presence of granulomatous soft tissue in the CS by MRI and the absolute response to systemic steroids confirm the diagnosis. The steroid dose should approximate 60 to 100 mg on a daily basis as a treatment regimen and should be continued for 1 week. After the pain and ophthalmoplegia have ceased, the steroids may be tapered rapidly.[73-75]

Metastatic Neoplastic Diseases

There are many metastatic processes that can invade the CS. The box below provides a partial list of these neoplasms. Rather than discussing each entity separately, this section addresses the group as a whole with some general comments as to pathogenicity, clinical course, diagnosis, and management.

Metastasis of malignant disease may constitute 23% of all parasellar lesions.[76] Cavernous sinus symptoms may be the first expression of an

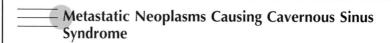

Metastatic Neoplasms Causing Cavernous Sinus Syndrome

Squamous cell carcinoma
Basosquamous cell carcinoma
Infiltrating ductal carcinoma of the breast
Malignant lymphoma
Adenocarcinoma
Neurotrophic malignant melanoma
Rhabdomyosarcoma
Nasopharyngeal carcinoma
Miscellaneous others

otherwise unknown malignancy or the first example of metastasis from a known primary site. The malignant cells can reach the CS in one of three ways: direct extension from adjacent structures, metastasis along regional neurovascular structures, and metastasis through blood or lymph.[76-82]

The most common malignancy to invade the CS by direct extension is nasopharyngeal carcinoma. This malignancy originates in the nasopharynx, erodes the neighboring bone, and infiltrates the CS to cause a CS syndrome. Nasopharyngeal carcinoma must always be considered when a patient presents with painful ophthalmoplegia, and biopsy of the nasopharynx should be performed.

CLINICAL PEARL

The most common malignancy to invade the CS by direct extension is nasopharyngeal carcinoma.

An example of a malignancy that metastasizes along neurovascular structures is a basosquamous cell carcinoma of the upper lip. This cancer infiltrates and grows along the maxillary division of CN V to invade the CS. Cancers that metastasize to the CS through the blood and lymph include cancers of the liver, lung, stomach, breast, prostate, face, and lymphatic system.[76,79,83]

The onset of symptoms from metastatic CS disease is usually very acute with rapid progression. Retroorbital and hemicranial pain with concomitant ophthalmoplegia are the most commonly reported symptoms.

Malignancy in the CS may proceed slowly and insidiously, however, and symptoms may improve temporarily with the use of steroids. As with other diseases of the CS, neuroradiology aids in diagnosis. Neuroimaging should be repeated at frequent intervals if the initial scans are negative but the patient continues to deteriorate. Magnetic resonance imaging may disclose masses in the CS and erosion of bony structures when malignancy is present. High-resolution, contrast-enhanced CT scan is the method of choice when CS malignancy is suspect. A mass that enhances with contrast, in association with bony erosion, is specifically pathognomonic of advancing malignancy.[77,79,84]

If CS malignancy is diagnosed or suspected, the patient should be referred to his or her general physician for a complete review of body systems to rule out a primary cancer site. Oncologic consultation will probably be sought, but the optometrist can be a valuable asset in the management of these patients if ocular sequelae are present.

The management of metastatic neoplasms of the CS involves direct radiation of the lesion and the sinus, as well as adjacent structures. Radiotherapy has proven efficacious in mitigating some of the clinical symptoms, although life expectancy is rarely prolonged.

Summary

The optometrist should consider CS disease in any patient who presents with any of the following: single or multiple cranial nerve palsies involving CNs III, IV, V_1, V_2, or VI; exophthalmos; retrobulbar or hemicranial pain; arterialized conjunctival and episcleral vessels; or a Horner's syndrome with an accompanying CN VI palsy. Subsequently, extensive blood studies should be performed in consultation with the general physician. The blood work should include a complete count with a differentiation of the blood cell types, an erythrocyte sedimentation rate, triiodothyronine, thyroxine, and thyroid-stimulating hormone levels for thyroid function, and an evaluation for syphilis (fluorescent treponemal antibody absorption test), Lyme disease, diabetes, and sarcoid angiotensin-converting enzyme (ACE). Finally, neuroimaging, including contrast-enhanced CT scans or MRI, should be ordered.

Once the diagnosis is made, the patient should be referred to his or her general physician for a review of all body systems. The general physician will refer the patient to the appropriate specialist. The optometrist should work in conjunction with the specialist to co-manage any ocular manifestations.

References

1. Rush JA, Younger BR: Paralysis of cranial nerves III, IV and VI. Cause and prognosis in 1,000 cases, *Arch Ophthalmol* 99:76-79, 1981.
2. Rucker CW: The causes of paralysis of the third, fourth, and sixth cranial nerves, *Am J Ophthalmol* 61:1293-1298, 1966.
3. Smith JL, Taxdal DSR: Painful ophthamoplegia: the Tolosa-Hunt syndrome, *Am J Ophthalmol* 61:1466-1472, 1966.
4. Roca PD: Painful ophthalmoplegia. The Tolosa-Hunt syndrome, *Ann Ophthalmol* 7:828-834, 1975.
5. Spencer WH, Thompson HS, Hoyt WE: Ischaemic ocular necrosis from carotid cavernous fistula, *Br J Ophthalmol* 57:145-152, 1973.
6. Bynke HG, Efsing HO: Carotid cavernous fistula with contralateral exophthalmos, *Acta Ophthalmol* 48:971-979, 1970.
7. Henderson JW, Schneider RC: The ocular findings in carotid cavernous fistula in a series of 17 cases, *Am J Ophthalmol* 48:585-596, 1959.
8. Bejandas FJ, Kline LB: Cavernous sinus syndrome. In Bajandas FJ, Kline LB, eds: *Neuroophthalmology review manual*, ed 3, Thorofare, NJ, 1988, Slack, 107-112.
9. Harris FS, Rhoton AL: Anatomy of the cavernous sinus. A microsurgical study, *J Neurosurg* 45: 169-180, 1976.
10. Winslow JB: In Bajandas FJ, Kline LB, eds: *Neuroophthalmology review manual*, ed 3, Thorofare, NJ, 1988, Slack, 107-112.

11. Parkinson D: Carotid cavernous fistula: direct repair with preservation of the carotid artery, *J Neurosurg* 38:99-106, 1973.

12. Wong A, Arnold R, Doran GA: A scanning electron microscopic investigation of the human cavernous sinus, *Aust Dent J* 39(4):266, 1994.

13. Swanson MW: Neuroanatomy of the cavernous sinus and clinical correlations, *Optom Vis Sci* 67(12):891-897, 1990.

14. Clemente CD, ed: *Gray's anatomy,* ed 30, Philadelphia, 1985, Lea & Febiger, 811-813.

15. Moore KL: *Clinically oriented anatomy,* ed 2 Baltimore, 1985, Williams & Wilkins, 853-855, 902-906, 821-825.

16. Bill A: Ocular circulation. In Moses RA, ed: *Adler's physiology of the eye,* St Louis, 1981, Mosby, 184-203.

17. Taptas JN: The so-called cavernous sinus: a review of the controversy and its implications for neurosurgeons, *Neurosurgery* 11:712-717, 1982.

18. Burde RM, Roper-Hall G: The extraocular muscles. In Moses RA, ed: *Adler's physiology of the eye,* St Louis, 1981, Mosby, 84-183.

19. Meadows SP: Intracavernous aneurysms of the internal carotid artery, *Arch Ophthalmol* 62: 566-574, 1959.

20. Glaser JS: Infranuclear disorders of eye movement. In Tasman W, Jaeger EA, eds: *Duane's clinical ophthalmology,* vol 2, Philadelphia, 1989, JB Lippincott, (12):21-31.

21. Kline LB: The Tolosa-Hunt syndrome, *Surv Ophthalmol* 27(2):79-95, 1982.

22. Keltner JL, Satterfield D, Dublin AB, Lee BCP: Dural and carotid cavernous sinus fistula: diagnosis, management, and complications, *Ophthalmology* 94:1585-1600, 1987.

23. Swanson M: Cavernous sinus syndrome from self-inflicted gunshot wound: case report and neuroanatomical correlation, *J Am Optom Assoc* 60(7):541-546, 1989.

24. Weinberger LM, Adler FH, Grant FC: Primary pituitary adenoma and the syndrome of the cavernous sinus: a clinical and anatomic study, *Arch Ophthalmol* 24:1197-1236, 1940.

25. Symonds CP: Oculomotor palsy as the presenting symptom of pituitary adenoma, *Bull Johns Hopkins Hosp* 111:72-82, 1962.

26. Robinson R, Toland J, Eustace P: Pituitary apoplexy: a cause for painful third nerve palsy, *Neuroophthalomology* 10(5):257-260, 1990.

27. Jefferson G: Extraseller extensions of pituitary adenomas, *Proc R Soc Med* 33:433-458, 1940.

28. Slamovits TL, Gardener TA: Neuroimaging in neuro-ophthalmology, *Ophthalmology* 96(4): 555-568, 1989.

29. Troost BT, Glaser JS: Aneurysms, arteriovenous communications, and related vascular malformations. In Glasser JS, eds: *Neuro-ophthalmology,* Philadelphia, 1990, JB Lippincott, 519-554.

30. Terry JE, Stout T: A pupil-sparing oculomotor palsy from a contralateral giant intracavernous carotid aneurysm, *J Am Optom Assoc* 61(8):640-645, 1990.

31. Barnett DW, Barrow DL, Joseph GJ: Combined extracranial-intercranial bypass and intraoperative balloon occlusion for the treatment of intracavernous and proximal carotid artery aneurysms, *Neurosurgery* 35(1):97-99, 1994.

32. Linskey ME, Sekhar LM, Hirsch WL, Yonas H, Horton JA: Aneurysms of the intracavernous carotid artery: natural history and indications for treatment, *Neurosurgery* 26:933-938, 1990.

33. Miller N: Tumors of the meninges and related tissues: meningiomas and sarcomas. In *Walsh and Hoyt's clinical neuro-ophthalmology,* ed 4, vol 3, Baltimore, 1988, Williams & Wilkins, 1325-1379.

34. Kotapka MJ, Kalia KK, Martinez AJ, Sekhar LN: Infiltration of the carotid artery by cavernous sinus meningioma, *J Neurosurg* 81(2):252-255, 1994.

35. Karp LA, Zimmerman LE, Borit A, Spencer W: Primary intraorbital meningiomas, *Arch Ophthalmol* 91:24-28, 1974.

36. Cogan DG: *Neurology of the ocular muscles,* Springfield, Ill, 1956, Charles C Thomas, 176.

37. Kline LB, Acker JD, Post JD: Computed tomographic evaluation of the cavernous sinus, *Ophthalmology* 89(4):374-385, 1982.
38. Cox TA, Worster JB, Godfrey WA: Primary aberrant oculomotor regeneration due to intracranial aneurysm, *Arch Neurol* 36:570-571, 1979.
39. Walsh FB: Third nerve regeneration: a clinical evaluation, *Br J Ophthalmol* 41:577-598, 1957.
40. Schatz NJ, Savino PJ, Corbett JJ: Primary aberrant oculomotor regeneration: a sign of intracavernous meningioma, *Arch Neurol* 34:29-32, 1977.
41. Levin PM: Intracranial aneurysms, *Arch Neurol Psychiatry* 67:771-786, 1952.
42. Spires R: Direct carotid-cavernous sinus fistulas, *Today's OR Nurse* 16(4):37-40, 1994.
43. Burde RM, Savino PJ, Trobe JD: Proptosis and adnexal masses. In *Clinical decisions in neuro-ophthalmology,* St Louis, 1985, Mosby, 275-302.
44. Keltner JL. A red eye and high intraocular pressure, *Surv Ophthalmol* 31(5):328-335, 1986.
45. Procope JA, Kidwell ED Jr, Copeland RA Jr, Perry AF: Dural cavernous-sinus fistula: an unusual presentation, *J Natl Med Assoc* 86(5):363-364, 1994.
46. Kupersmith MJ, Berenstein A, Choi IS, Warren F, Flamm E: Management of nontraumatic vascular shunts involving the cavernous sinus, *Ophthalmology* 95(1):121-130, 1988.
47. Buus DR, Tse DT, Parrish RK: Spontaneous carotid cavernous fistula presenting with acute angle-closure glaucoma, *Arch Ophthalmol* 107:596-597, 1989.
48. Leonard TJK, Mosley IF, Sanders MD: Ophthalmoplegia in carotid cavernous sinus fistula, *Br J Ophthalmol* 68:128-134, 1984.
49. Taniguchi RM, Gorge JA, Odom GL: Spontaneous carotid cavernous shunts presenting diagnostic problems, *J Neurosurg* 35:384-391, 1971.
50. Hawke SHB, Mullie MA, Hoyt WF, Hallinan JM, Halmogyi GM: Painful oculomotor nerve palsy due to dural-cavernous sinus shunt, *Arch Neurol* 46:1252-1255, 1989.
51. Newton TH, Hoyt WF: Dural arteriovenous shunts in the region of the cavernous sinus, *Neuroradiology* 1:71-81, 1970.
52. Sergott RC, Grossman RI, Savino PJ, Bosley TM, Schatz NJ: The syndrome of paradoxical worsening of dural cavernous sinus anteriovenous malformations, *Ophthalmology* 94(3):205-212, 1987.
53. Sowka JW: Dural arteriovenous malformation, *J Am Optom Assoc* 60(11):846-848, 1989.
54. Spector RH: Echographic diagnosis of dural carotid-cavernous sinus fistulas, *Am J Ophthalmol* 111:77-83, 1991.
55. Palestine AG, Younge BR, Piepgras DG: Visual prognosis in carotid-cavernous fistula, *Arch Ophthalmol* 99:1600-1603, 1981.
56. Dolenc V: Direct microsurgical repair of intracavernous vascular lesions, *J Neurosurg* 58:824-831, 1983.
57. Parkinson D, Downs AR, Whytehead LL, Syslak WB: Carotid cavernous fistula: direct repair with preservation of carotid, *Surgery* 76(6):882-889, 1974.
58. Mullan S: Treatment of carotid-cavernous fistulas by cavernous sinus occlusion, *J Neurosurg* 50:131-144, 1979.
59. Debrun G, Lacour P, Neneula F, et al: Treatment of 54 traumatic carotid cavernous fistulas, *J Neurosurg* 55:678-692, 1981.
60. Kupersmith MJ, Berenstein A, Flamm, E, Ransohoff J: Neuroophthalmologic abnormalities and intravascular therapy of traumatic carotid cavernous fistulas, *Opthalmology* 93:906-912, 1986.
61. Sabates FN, Tsai F, Sabated NR, Blitstein B: Transient cranial nerve palsies after cavernous sinus embolization, *Am J Ophthalmol* 111(6):771-773, 1991.
62. Phelps CD, Thompson HS, Ossoinig KC: The diagnosis and prognosis of atypical carotid-cavernous fistula (red-eyed shunt syndrome), *Am J Ophthalmol* 93:423-436, 1982.
63. Fiore PM, Latina MA, Shingleton BJ, et al: The dural shunt syndrome. I. Management of glaucoma, *Ophthalmology* 97:56-62, 1990.

64. Weekers R, Delmarcelle Y: Pathogenesis of intraocular hypertension in cases of arteriovenous aneurysm, *Arch Ophthalmol* 48:338-343, 1952.

65. Hunt WE, Meagher JN, LeFever HE, Zeman W: Painful ophthalmoplegia. Its relation to indolent inflammation of the cavernous sinus, *Neurology* 11:56-62, 1961.

66. Tolosa E: Periarteritic lesions of the carotid siphon with the clinical features of a carotid infraclinoid aneurysm, *J Neurol Neurosurg Psychiatry* 17:300-02, 1954.

67. Aron-Rosa D, Doyon D, Salamon G, Michotey P: Tolosa-Hunt syndrome, *Ann Ophthalmol* 10:1161-1168, 1978.

68. Andersson BI: Unusual course of painful ophthalmoplegia. Report of a case, *Acta Ophthalmol* 58:841-848, 1980.

69. Coppeto JR, Hoffman H: Tolosa-Hunt syndrome with proptosis mimicked by giant aneurysm of posterior cerebral artery, *Arch Neurol* 38:54-55, 1981.

70. Fowler TJ, Earl CJ, McAllister VL, McDonald WI: Tolosa-Hunt syndrome: the danger of an eponym, *Br J Ophthalmol* 59:149-154, 1975.

71. Koppel BS: Steroid-responsive painful ophthalmoplegia is not always Tolosa-Hunt, *Neurology* 37:544.

72. Spector RH, Fiandaca MS: The "sinister" Tolosa-Hunt syndrome, *Neurology* 36:198-203, 1986.

73. Goto Y, Hosokawa S, Goto I, Hirakata R, Hasuo K: Abnormality in the cavernous sinus in three patients with Tolosa-Hunt syndrome: MRI and CT findings, *J Neurol Neurosurg Psychiatry* 53:231-234, 1990.

74. Yousem DM, Atlas SW, Grossman RI, et al: MR imaging of Tolosa-Hunt syndrome, *AJR* 154:167-170, 1990.

75. Friedberg MA, Rapuano CJ: *Wills Eye Hospital office and emergency room diagnosis and treatment of eye disease,* Philadelphia, 1990, JB Lippincott, 251.

76. Ahmad K, Yamokoski C, Kim YH, Post MJD, Fayas JV: Involvement of cavernous sinus region by malignant neoplasms: report of 5 cases, *J Am Osteopath Assoc* 87(7):504-508, 1987.

77. Traserra J, Comas J, Conde C, Cuchi A, Cardesa A: Metastatic involvement of the cavernous sinus from primary pharyngolaryngeal tumors, *Head Neck* 12(5):426-429, 1990.

78. Godfredson E, Legerman M: Diagnostic and prognostic roles of ophthalmoneurologic signs and symptoms in malignant nasopharyngeal tumors, *Am J Ophthalmol* 59:1063-1069, 1965.

79. Post MJD, Mendez DR, Kline LB, Acker JD, Glaser JS: Metastatic disease to the cavernous sinus: clinical syndrome and CT diagnosis, *J Comput Assist Tomogr* 9(1):115-120, 1985.

80. Hufnagel TJ, Savino PJ, Zimmerman RA, Sergott RC: Painful ophthalmoplegia caused by neurotrophic malignant melanoma, *Am J Ophthalmol* 25(1):38-41, 1990.

81. Reynard M, Brinkley JR: Cavernous sinus syndrome caused by rhabdomyosarcoma, *Ann Ophthalmol* 15(1):94-97, 1983.

82. Thomas JE, Yoss RE: The parasellar syndrome: problems in determining etiology, *Mayo Clin Proc* 45:617-623, 1970.

83. Unsold R, Safran A, Safran E, Hoyt WF: Metastatic infiltration of nerves in the cavernous sinus, *Arch Neurol* 37:59-61, 1980.

84. Kline LB, Chandra-Sekar B: Pitfalls in computed tomographic elevation of the cavernous sinus, *Surv Ophthalmol* 29(4):293-296, 1985.

Acknowledgments

The author gratefully thanks Dr. Andrew Gurwood for his computer generated contributions of Figures 2-1, 2-2, 2-4, 2-5, and 2-10.

3

Pupillary Anomalies

Jeffrey S. Nyman

Key Terms

afferent pathway	relative afferent	Adie's tonic pupil
efferent pathway	pupillary defect	Horner's syndrome
sympathetic	light-near	hydroxyamphetamine
pathway	dissociation	dilation lag
anisocoria	Hutchinson's pupil	

Evaluation of the pupillary status is one of the most critical aspects of the ophthalmic examination. Through careful examination, one can gain important information regarding the anterior visual pathways, the efferent pupillary pathways, and the oculosympathetic pathways. This chapter serves as a guide to the clinical examination of the pupils, with emphasis placed on anatomic and pathophysiologic considerations. A thorough knowledge of these underlying principles is necessary for accurate diagnosis and appropriate management of patients with pupillary dysfunction.

CLINICAL PEARL

Through careful examination of the pupillary status, one can gain important information regarding the anterior visual pathways, the efferent pupillary pathways, and the oculosympathetic pathways.

Anatomic and Physiologic Considerations

The iris contains two types of smooth muscle fibers, the sphincter and the dilator, which serve to regulate the size of the pupil. The sphincter is a 1-mm circular band at the pupillary margin, whereas the dilator is a sheet of radially arranged smooth muscle fibers running from the iris root to the peripheral border of the sphincter.

The autonomic nervous system plays a major role in regulating the action of these muscles. The parasympathetic system exerts its influence by contracting the sphincter muscle, thereby constricting the pupil, in response to light or near reflex stimulation. A less important source of parasympathetic stimulation occurs in the orbicularis reflex (Piltz-Westphal reaction), in which forced closure of the lids results in miosis. This can be clinically useful in the evaluation of the efferent system in cases in which no reaction exists either to light or near reflex stimulation.

The sympathetic system dilates the pupils by contracting the radially arranged muscles. This is most commonly seen in the so-called psychosensory reflex, where dilation is a response to stimulation from the cerebral cortex. Stimulation of any sensory nerve also will cause pupillary dilation, although the mechanism is still controversial. Dilation may result from sympathetic stimulation or parasympathetic inhibition, or a combination of both.

Both the parasympathetic and sympathetic systems affect the size of the pupils at any given moment, and the balance between the two systems is in a constant state of flux. As a result, one normally can observe a small amount of fluctuation in pupillary size over time, even with no change in illumination or fixation. This is the phenomenon known as pupillary play, and it is important to recall when testing for the presence of a relative afferent pupillary defect (RAPD or Marcus Gunn[1] phenomenon) by using the swinging flashlight test of Levatin.[2] Active pupillary play can be the source of misdiagnosis in certain cases. Hippus has been termed by Adler[3] to be a pathologic exaggeration of the pupillary play phenomenon, but it is believed to be clinically insignificant by some neuro-ophthalmologists, including Lawton Smith.[4]

CLINICAL PEARL

Both the parasympathetic and sympathetic systems affect the size of the pupils at any given moment, and the balance between the two systems is in a constant state of flux.

Parasympathetic Pathways

The light reflex

The origin of the light reflex is generally thought to be any point in the retina that is stimulated by light. The reflex seems to be more easily elicited when light stimulates receptors in or near the macula. The most probable receptor organs are the rods and cones, as is the case for vision. The afferent pathway begins in the ganglion cell layer. Axons pass through the optic nerve, wherein slightly more than half decussate in the chiasm. Fibers originating in the nasal half of each retina cross, whereas those originating in the temporal half do not. Posterior to the chiasm, the afferent fibers pass into the optic tract. They separate from the tract in its posterior third, just anterior to the lateral geniculate body. They then enter the midbrain, reaching the pretectal nucleus by way of the superior brachium conjunctivum. Synapses occur in the pretectal nuclei, and the fibers then hemidecussate through the posterior commissure and proceed to terminate in the paired Edinger-Westphal nuclei (Figure 3-1).

The efferent pathway begins at the Edinger-Westphal nuclei. Parasympathetic fibers of the oculomotor nerve (CN III) course through the inferior division of the nerve when it bifurcates in the cavernous sinus. In the sinus, CN III is closely related to the first and second divisions of the trigeminal nerve (CN V). The oculomotor nerve enters the orbit through the superior orbital fissure to synapse

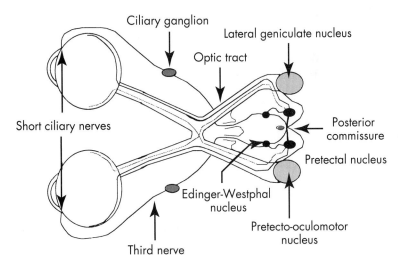

FIGURE 3-1 The light reflex pathway. Synapses occur in the pretectal nuclei, and the fibers then hemidecussate through the posterior commissure and terminate in the paired Edinger-Westphal nuclei. (Courtesy Andrew S. Gurwood, O.D.)

at the ciliary ganglion. The postganglionic fibers pass to the smooth muscle fibers of the iris sphincter through the short ciliary nerves. These nerves travel forward in the suprachoroidal space and release acetylcholine at the neuromuscular junction.

The near reflex

The near reflex is initiated by the attempt to fixate a near object. When gaze is shifted from distance to near fixation, a triad of responses occurs: convergence, accommodation, and pupillary constriction. The afferent path is probably similar to that of the light reflex back to the posterior third of the optic tract. From here fibers pass to the occipital cortex, then through the prestriate area to the premotor area of the frontal lobe. From here the fibers pass through the corona radiata and internal capsule to the oculomotor nucleus. The efferent pathway from the oculomotor nucleus is probably the same as in the light reflex, although it is possible that a separate path for near fibers may exist, and that these fibers do not form a synapse in the ciliary ganglion. The final path is through the third nerve directly, or through the ciliary ganglion to the ciliary and sphincter pupillae muscles.

Sympathetic Pathway

Pupillodilator pathway

The sympathetic pathway for pupillary dilation is well established in literature.[3,5] Afferent impulses from the cortex as well as other stimuli terminate in the hypothalamus. Sympathetic outflow then begins in the posterolateral area of the hypothalamus, and the preganglionic fibers pass uncrossed through the tegmentum of the midbrain and pons. These preganglionic fibers then pass through the lateral portion of the medulla and terminate in the dilator center of the spinal cord, lying in the lateral column of the cord at the junction of the thoracic and cervical regions, at the C8 to T2 cord level (the ciliospinal center of Budge). The fibers exit the cord in this region, through the white rami communicantes of the uppermost thoracic nerves, and pass up the cervical sympathetic trunk (closely related to the pleura of the lung apex). The fibers then reach the superior cervical ganglion (at the base of the skull), where the first synapse takes place. Postganglionic fibers run upward around the internal carotid artery and eventually join the trigeminal ganglion, passing into the orbit through the nasociliary nerve and entering the eye through the long ciliary nerves, eventually terminating at the dilator muscle (Figure 3-2).

Examination Techniques

The office examination of the pupils begins with careful observation of the size, shape, and position of the pupils under conditions of

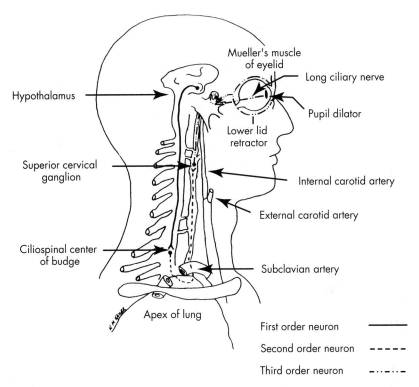

FIGURE 3-2 Pupillodilator pathway. Postganglionic fibers run upward around the internal carotid artery and eventually join the trigeminal ganglion. They pass into the orbit through the nasociliary nerve and enter the eye through the long ciliary nerves, eventually terminating at the dilator muscle.

normal illumination, which may vary from one doctor's office to another. What is of critical importance is that the individual practitioner be consistent in his or her use of room illumination, so that the "normal" illumination is the same each time the patient is examined.

In cases in which a pupillary anomaly is suspected, the patient should be tested in both dim and bright illumination. This helps differentiate a sympathetic defect from a parasympathetic one. In bright light, miosis due to a sympathetic weakness may be difficult to detect, because of the dominance of the parasympathetic system. In dim light, however, such a defect is readily apparent, showing increased anisocoria, the smaller pupil being on the affected side. Because the innervation will be intact in simple (essential) anisocoria, this technique also helps differentiate between this benign anisocoria and that caused by a Horner's syndrome. Here, the examiner should look for the presence of a dilation lag, a smaller pupil after 5 seconds of darkness than after 15 seconds[6] (see section on Horner's syndrome for further discussion). Conversely, the mydriasis found in parasympathetic paralysis, such as that found in third nerve disease, may be obvious in bright light, but difficult to detect in dim light.

The pupil size for both eyes should be measured while the patient is fixating a distant target situated slightly above the horizon, to avoid the possibility of near-reflex–induced miosis. It is recommended that pupillary size be measured using black circles or semicircles found on commercially available rulers or nearpoint cards. The maximum vertical size of the palpebral aperture should be measured and recorded at this time. In addition, close scrutiny of the pupils and surrounding structures may disclose the presence of iris atrophy, anterior or posterior synechiae, or other evidence of iris abnormality that may be helpful in making an appropriate diagnosis. The color of the irides should be recorded, as well as any anomalies of shape or position of either pupil.

Testing of the light reflexes (both direct and consensual) should be performed in a darkened room while the patient is fixating a nonaccommodative target, such as a muscle light. The stimulus for the test may be a penlight (with fresh batteries), a transilluminator, or another bright light source directed into the pupil from below the eye. A good alternative light source is the collimated beam of the binocular indirect ophthalmoscope. The light source should be directed directly into the pupil for a few seconds until maximum miosis occurs.

There has been some controversy regarding the optimal brightness of the light source necessary to best detect an afferent pupillary defect. Borchert and Sadun[7] have suggested that afferent pupillary defects are more obvious when testing with a relatively dim light source. This contention has been refuted in a 1990 study by Johnson,[8] which confirmed that brighter light sources will produce a greater, measured afferent pupillary defect. It also has been shown that a threshold level of illumination exists beyond which no further increase in afferent pupillary defect measurement occurs.[9] These studies support the continued use of a bright light source for testing the direct reflex, and for the detection of subtle afferent defects.

In cases where the light reflex is difficult to detect due to dark irides, a direct ophthalmoscope may be used by placing a +2.00-diopter lens in the scope and holding it 50 cm in front of the patient, using the large spot diaphragm. The pupil margin can be observed against the red fundus reflex, and the reaction can be detected.

Another important tool in the detection of the light reflexes in equivocal cases is the slit lamp biomicroscope. The light source is excellent, and the viewing system provides enough magnification and resolution to detect even the finest movements of the iris. The light source should be introduced obliquely so that the patient's distance fixation is not disturbed.

The presence and quality of the direct and consensual light reflex should be recorded for each eye. A useful approach would be to use a grading system of 0 to 4+, where 0 equals no response and 4+ equals a brisk response.

After testing for the light reflex and return of the pupils to normal size, the patient should be directed to fixate a near object of regard, and the presence or absence of pupillary constriction should be noted and recorded in a similar fashion as just described for the light reflex. The near reflex is best elicited in a semidarkened room. This response is often not as easy to elicit as the light reflex because of the voluntary control of accommodative vergence and the dependence on patient cooperation and convergence ability. In cases in which there is doubt as to the presence of this reaction, the patient should be asked to look at his or her own finger while the examiner taps the finger and brings it into the patient's line of sight. This allows for a summation of the visual, proprioceptive, and psychic elements of the near reflex to exert maximal influence.[4]

Types of Pupillary Anomalies

Simple, Central Anisocoria (Essential Anisocoria)

Loewenfeld[10] described the type of patient who presents with anisocoria with no associated neurologic or ophthalmic abnormalities, including normal pupillary reflexes. This kind of anisocoria is called "central" because it is probably caused by asymmetries of the supranuclear inhibitory control of the Edinger-Westphal nucleus. It is called "simple" for a number of reasons. First, it is simply an exaggeration of pupil behavior in normal subjects. Second, it may increase, decrease, or reverse sides within days or hours. Third, there is no pathologic significance to this condition.

Anisocoria is defined as a pupillary size difference of 0.4 mm or greater between the eyes.[11] The incidence of anisocoria in healthy subjects ranges from 1% to 90% in the literature,[10,12] depending on the criteria used. Loewenfeld[10] found an incidence of 21% in 425 patients under the age of 14 years. She also found that the incidence increases in older populations. Roarty and Keltner[13] found an incidence of significant anisocoria of 21% in a recent study of 88 healthy newborns.

Obviously, the incidence of anisocoria varies. It is worth emphasizing that normally reactive pupils without evidence of oculomotor dysfunction or lid abnormalities are most likely normal. Any anisocoria of 1.0 mm or less without associated neuro-ophthalmic signs should be considered of minimal significance.

CLINICAL PEARL

Any anisocoria of 1.0 mm or less without associated neuro-ophthalmic signs should be considered of minimal significance.

Some unusual cases of anisocoria have recently appeared in literature. Cheng and Catalano[14] presented the unusual cases of a father and daughter who developed unilateral mydriasis after a lack of sleep. There was no suggestion that this was caused by migraine, cyclic oculomotor paresis, or seizures, and the condition was hypothesized to be supranuclear in origin.

Four cases of pigment dispersion syndrome with the larger pupil on the side of greater iris transillumination also were reported in 1990.[15] These patients all had marked loss of pigment on the affected side, suggesting a likely mechanical cause for the anisocoria. One cannot assume a nonneurologic basis, however, just because of the coincidental finding of pigment dispersion syndrome.

Afferent Defects

Relative afferent pupillary defect

After testing the light and near reflexes, the swinging flashlight test should be employed to detect the presence of a relative afferent pupillary defect (Marcus Gunn phenomenon, RAPD). The patient is asked to fixate a nonaccommodative distance target. A bright light is introduced obliquely into one eye and held there for 2 to 3 seconds while the examiner observes the response in that eye. The light is then swung rapidly into the other eye while its response is observed. The light should be swung back and forth between the two eyes three or four times and then discontinued to avoid retinal bleaching. This swinging back and forth should be done in as rhythmic a fashion as possible.[16] If any doubt persists, the testing can be resumed after about 30 seconds.

If a lesion is present in one afferent visual pathway (anywhere from the retinal ganglion cell layer to the level of the lateral geniculate body on the affected side), the examiner will be able to detect a RAPD. The ease of detection is dependent on the magnitude of the defect. When a normal pupil is exposed to light in this manner, it is seen to constrict and then redilate somewhat, followed by some pupillary play (see above). This normal redilation and pupillary play should not be confused with a true RAPD.

In a marked RAPD, the pupils of both eyes are seen to dilate when the light source is swung into the affected eye. This is the phenomenon of pupillary escape described by Levatin.[2] Actually, what occurs is a relative decrease in pupillary constriction while under direct light stimulation of the affected eye. This relative decrease appears as a dilation when compared immediately with the intact consensual response from the unaffected eye.

In a subtle RAPD, the examiner needs to carefully observe the reactions in both eyes. In such a case, there actually may be an initial constriction when the light is swung into the involved eye. But as the light is held there for a few seconds, a pupillary dilation is seen that was not present when the other eye was stimulated. If escape is observed in both eyes, then the examiner should look for differences in the amount of redilation; in the eye with the conduction defect, the pupil consistently escapes to a wider dilation. This fact also emphasizes the need to be aware of any preexisting anisocoria, and to not be fooled into thinking that the larger pupil is dilating more than its fellow.

Cox[17] simulated an RAPD with neutral density filters and carefully studied the pupillary reactions by infrared pupillography. He concluded that the most sensitive criterion for detection of RAPD is not final size or redilation amplitude, but rather a difference in amplitude of initial consensual constriction versus the initial direct constriction. Relative afferent pupillary defect should be diagnosed when the consensual response is greater than the direct response.

CLINICAL PEARL

Relative afferent pupillary defect should be diagnosed when the consensual response is greater than the direct response.

Relative afferent pupillary defect can be arbitrarily graded on a scale of 1 to 4+, but a method has been described that allows for accurate and reliable measurement by holding neutral density filters in front of the better eye until the swinging light test is balanced.[18,19] This method has the advantage of providing a basis for comparisons at future visits, so that progression of disease may be assessed more accurately. The density of the filter needed to abolish the RAPD can be simply recorded in log units as a measure of the magnitude of the defect. Again, it is important to remember not to asymmetrically bleach the two retinas by holding the light longer on one eye than the other. The smallest defect that can be measured with confidence is 0.3 log, and 0.3 steps are used, up to 3.6 log units. The filters also can be helpful in determining the presence of a subtle defect. For example, if the clinician suspects a minimal RAPD in the left eye, a 0.3 filter placed over that eye should exaggerate the defect. If the same filter over the right eye eliminates the defect in the left eye, then a diagnosis of left RAPD is definitive.

If a positive RAPD is detected, then the patient usually has an ipsilateral optic neuropathy. The cause may be demyelination, ischemia, compression, or glaucoma. Supportive findings include reduced central acuity, color vision defects, central field defects, and abnormal visual-evoked potential in the involved eye.

If the involved eye has no light perception, then it will display no direct response to light, and its fellow will demonstrate no consensual response. Such a response has been labeled an amaurotic pupil.

Generally, a significant RAPD of about 1.0 log units is found in cases of recovered optic neuritis. Conversely, macular disease rarely produces a meaningful RAPD unless the vision is worse than 20/200. In retinal detachment, each quadrant of fresh bullous detachment produces about 0.3 log units RAPD. When the macula detaches, the RAPD increases to about 1.0 log units.[20]

In significant anisocoria, the eye with the smaller pupil has a relatively shaded retina. Thus, when doing the swinging flashlight test, one may see an apparent RAPD. This is especially so when the anisocoria approaches 2 mm, or when one pupil is very small. A slight RAPD may be seen in suppression amblyopia, but this is inconsistent with the degree of vision loss. Firth[21] pointed out in 1990 that RAPD is more likely to occur in anisometropic than in strabismic amblyopia, and that even patients with mild degrees of amblyopia may have an RAPD. Unilateral cataract generally produces no measurable RAPD, even when very dense. In an opaque white cataract, however, excess retinal stimulation may occur because of light scatter, thus producing a contralateral RAPD.[22]

Bell and Thompson[23] demonstrated that RAPD will be found in homonymous hemianopia of optic tract origin. The RAPD will be found in the eye contralateral to the side of the lesion because more than 50% of the nasal retinal fibers cross to the contralateral tract, and the nasal retina has a higher pupillomotor valence than the temporal retina. It should be noted that RAPD will not be present when the hemianopic lesions are beyond the lateral geniculate body, because the pupillary fibers are not involved. Moreover, a unilateral lesion in the pretectal nucleus or in the brachium of the superior colliculus will damage the pupillary fibers from the ipsilateral optic tract. A contralateral RAPD will result. Most often, the offending lesion is either an arteriovenous malformation or a pinealoma.

In 1946, Kestenbaum[24] reported that in patients with unilateral optic nerve disease, if one eye was covered while the other was exposed to bright light, the pupil of the affected eye would always settle at a larger diameter. He termed this pseudoanisocoria, and later implied that it might be an indicator of the difference in pupillomotor input between the two eyes. The difference in pupil size obtained in each eye in direct illumination while the other eye is occluded was studied recently by Jiang et al.[25] These authors termed this number

Kestenbaum's number and compared it with quantification of RAPD with neutral density filters. They found an excellent correlation between the two measurements. This may be especially helpful in patients with dark brown irides, because pupil diameter can be measured in bright light. The authors point out that this is a less precise measure of pupillomotor input asymmetry, but can be used when neutral density filters are not available.

Light-Near Dissociation and the Argyll Robertson Pupil

A review of the anatomy of the pupillary pathways shows that the near reflex fibers are more ventrally located than the light reflex fibers. As a result, a lesion may impact the afferent light reflex fibers and spare the near reflex fibers. If the near reaction is greater than the light reaction, light-near dissociation (LND) is said to exist. LND is a descriptive term that has replaced some older names such as "pseudo–Argyll Robertson pupil" and "Argyll Robertsonlike pupil."

CLINICAL PEARL

The near reflex fibers are more ventrally located than the light reflex fibers. As a result, a lesion may impact the afferent light reflex fibers and spare the near reflex fibers.

A special type of LND was first described by Argyll Robertson in 1869. All of his cases involved patients who had tabes dorsalis, a manifestation of neurosyphilis. According to the original criteria established by Argyll Robertson, the following conditions must be met:

1. Some degree of vision must be present.
2. There must be no reaction to light. If even a trace of light reaction is present, the Argyll Robertson criterion is not met. (This may have been true when early examiners observed pupillary reactions using candles or other relatively weak light sources. With today's bright light sources, however, and with the aid of magnification, many Argyll Robertson pupils that once were judged to have no light reaction might indeed show trace reactions.)
3. The near response must be normal.

Additional findings in the Argyll Robertson pupil include miosis and irregular shape, as well as difficulty dilating, either with mydriatics or sustained dark exposure. As a rule, the condition is bilateral, although often it is asymmetric. It may be unilateral, however, depending on the location of the lesion.

The site of the lesion responsible for the Argyll Robertson pupil has been debated since the initial description over 120 years ago. Argyll

Robertson believed the lesion was located in the cervical spinal cord, but anatomic evidence of a focal lesion (in the cord or elsewhere) has not been demonstrated. Other sites that have been suggested include the afferent light reflex pathway, the ciliary ganglion, the ciliary nerves, the iris, the efferent third nerve, the oculomotor nucleus, and the pretectal-oculomotor fibers. The latter site is the most likely location for the lesion, and would account for the sparing of the near reflex fibers.

Any patient presenting with pupillary findings suggestive of those described by Argyll Robertson should undergo a fluorescent treponemal antibody absorption test (FTA-ABS) to rule out the likelihood of neurosyphilis. The differential diagnosis includes many other entities, including diabetes mellitus, multiple sclerosis, encephalitis, degenerative central nervous system disease, mid-brain neoplasm, and many other conditions.[26]

CLINICAL PEARL

Any patient presenting with pupillary findings suggestive of those described by Argyll Robertson should undergo a fluorescent treponemal antibody absorption test (FTA-ABS) to rule out the likelihood of neurosyphilis.

Light-near dissociation is actually a generic term that includes not only Argyll Robertson pupils, but pupils that have a diminished (not necessarily absent) light response in the presence of a normal near response. Syphilis is the most common cause of LND, so FTA-ABS testing is always indicated. Other causes of LND include the following:

- Advanced diabetes mellitus
- Pituitary tumors
- Midbrain lesions
- Myotonic dystrophy
- Adie's tonic pupil
- Familial amyloidosis
- Aberrant regeneration of CN III

Midbrain lesions in the pretectal area produce LND and are often neoplastic in origin. Pinealomas produce a constellation of signs and symptoms known as Parinaud's syndrome (Sylvian aqueduct syndrome, dorsal midbrain syndrome). In these cases, there is bilateral LND, but the pupils are mid-dilated, often unequal in size, and oval-shaped.[27] Other neurologic signs that assist in making the appropriate diagnosis are decreased convergence and retraction nystagmus in attempted upgaze. Finally, tumors, such as gliomas of the quadrigeminal plate and vascular occlusive lesions, can produce LND.[5]

Efferent Defects

It is generally accepted that the efferent pathway of the parasympathetic system begins in the cells of the Edinger-Westphal nucleus and other portions of the oculomotor nucleus involved in the pupillary response to near stimulation. Nuclear lesions therefore are considered in this section.

Oculomotor nerve (cranial nerve III) palsy

Efferent pupillary defects of neurologic origin are either part of the clinical presentation of an oculomotor (CN III) palsy or an isolated internal ophthalmoplegia. Lesions affecting the parasympathetic pupillomotor fibers in the midbrain or in their peripheral course to the sphincter muscle can produce a paralysis of pupillary constriction, resulting in a fixed, dilated pupil. In peripheral lesions, unilaterality is more common than in pure nuclear lesions. If the parasympathetic nerves to the ciliary muscle are simultaneously affected, accommodation is paralyzed, and internal ophthalmoplegia is said to exist.

If a nuclear lesion occurs, the result is a true internal ophthalmoplegia consisting of absence of light reaction, both direct and consensual, as well as loss of the near and orbicularis reflexes. The condition may be unilateral or bilateral, but is usually the latter. The presence of such a lesion is usually indicative of serious disease and is a common finding in pineal tumors. Other possible causes include vascular accidents, infections, demyelinating disease, and trauma. Vascular disease and demyelination in this area often produce associated signs, such as nuclear ophthalmoplegia, paralysis of upward gaze, loss of convergence, exotropia, and other defects of ocular movement.[28]

Hutchinson's pupil

Hutchinson's pupil is a fixed, dilated pupil that results from a traumatic compression of the oculomotor nerve. The pupillomotor parasympathetic fibers run in the superficial portion of the oculomotor nerve as it exits from the interpeduncular fossa. Because of their superficial location in this area, these fibers are quite susceptible to external compression. Such compression occurs most often as a result of an aneurysm of the posterior communicating artery at its junction with the posterior cerebral artery.[29] The nerve, however, may also be compressed as a consequence of traumatic transtentorial herniation of the hippocampal gyrus, yielding the classical unilateral dilated, fixed pupil. Thus evaluation for

Hutchinson's pupil is extremely important in the comatose patient who has sustained a head injury.

It should be noted that vasculopathic oculomotor disease caused by diabetes or arteriosclerosis does not usually compromise the pupillary fibers. These ischemic pathologies affect the central core of the nerve as opposed to its peripheral coats.

Aberrant regeneration of the third nerve

Lesions resulting in total third nerve paralysis are usually of sudden onset and are the result of carotid aneurysm or head trauma. They result in total ptosis, a fixed and dilated pupil, and an eye turned down and out. These lesions are characterized pathologically by degeneration of oculomotor and preganglionic pupillomotor axons. Because of scar formation in the affected nerve, regeneration of these axons is often disorganized, and may result in the motor fibers extending peripherally and making contact with different effectors than the ones they originally served. This situation has been termed *aberrant regeneration of the third nerve,* and produces a number of interesting clinical signs, including pupillary anomalies in the pseudo–Argyll Robertson pupil[30] and in Czarnecki's sign[31] (discussion to follow). The nonpupillary and pupillary findings of aberrant regeneration of CN III are listed in the box on p. 85.

CLINICAL PEARL

Lesions resulting in total third nerve paralysis are usually of sudden onset and are the result of carotid aneurysm or head trauma. They result in total ptosis, a fixed and dilated pupil, and an eye turned down and out.

The pseudo–Argyll Robertson pupil consists of an apparently fixed and dilated pupil, which on close scrutiny does not react to light, but does modestly constrict on convergence. The pupil also constricts on adduction, but this is most easily noted when the patient is asked to fixate a distant target in such a way that the affected eye adducts. When he or she is asked to return to primary distance gaze, the pupil is seen to dilate slightly. The constriction of the pupil on convergence or adduction is due to misdirection of fibers from the medial rectus to the pupil; Czarnecki's sign may be present. Czarnecki and Thompson[31] described sector contractions of the iris sphincter in response to light, sector contractions associated with eye movements, and abnormal "hippus" in patients with no light reaction, which remains present in the dark and is not synchronous with the normal pupillary play in the normal eye.

Clinical Signs in Aberrant Regeneration of CN III

Nonpupillary signs
  Upper lid retraction on downgaze (pseudo von Graefe's sign)
  Lid retraction and depression in horizontal gaze maneuvers (lid synkinesis)
  Retraction and adduction of the globe on attempted upgaze
  Monocular vertical optokinetic responses
Pupillary signs
  The pupil may remain fixed and dilated
  The pupil may return to normal
  A pseudo–Argyll Robertson pupil may develop
  Czarnecki's sign

Aberrant regeneration is important clinically in the differential diagnosis of the original third nerve lesion. Its presence strongly suggests that more than 3 months have passed since the onset of the palsy.[4] Aberrant regeneration is not seen in oculomotor paresis of ischemic origin because the direction of the degenerating axoplasm has not been disturbed by external compression. Thus it is not seen in diabetic or arteriosclerotic third nerve palsies.

CLINICAL PEARL

Aberrant regeneration is important clinically in the differential diagnosis of the original third nerve lesion. Its presence strongly suggests that more than 3 months have passed since the onset of the palsy.

The tonic pupil

The tonic pupil is the result of a lesion involving the ciliary ganglion and the postganglionic fibers. Characteristic findings include a very poor or absent reaction to light and a very slow reaction to near. Careful observation of the pupillary responses and attention to other clinically relevant data is necessary for early diagnosis and effective management (see the box on p. 86).

Thompson[32] classified tonic pupils etiologically as either local, neuropathic, or idiopathic (Adie's). The most common type is Adie's tonic pupil, which occurs most commonly in young women between the ages of 20 and 40 years. They usually present with unilateral blurred near vision and asymptomatic anisocoria.[33] These patients often report an antecedent mild upper respiratory infection.

In the early stage, an Adie's pupil is dilated and reacts poorly to light and near effort. Misdiagnosis is possible at this point in the examination. It is important to note that the pupil will constrict after continued exposure to light, but this reaction is very slow and may not be observed without the aid of the biomicroscope. In addition, the response is usually present in some segments of the pupil and absent in others (segmental palsy). This has been termed "vermiform" or wormlike movement in the early neuro-ophthalmic literature.[34] Thompson[35] studied these movements in great detail, and recommends that the best way to observe them is to open the beam of the slit lamp wide and bring it in from the side so that all the iris detail is visible. A dim light should be used so that the patient can tolerate it, and the lamp should be turned alternately on and off. This allows observation of large sectors of the sphincter that fail to constrict but are dragged in passively by adjacent reactive segments. This results in a misshaped (oval) pupil, with flatter margins in palsied sectors, and tighter curvature in the active sectors. "Stromal streaming" occurs in the pupillary zone and collarette, with radial stromal markings streaming toward the active areas and away from the paretic areas.

Characteristic Findings in Adie's Tonic Pupil

Occurs commonly in young women between age 20 to 40 years
Unilateral blurred vision
Asymptomatic anisocoria
Antecedent mild upper respiratory infection
Dilated pupil with poor reactions to light and near effort
Segmental pupil response with oval pupil shape
"Stromal streaming"
Slow and tonic near response that is greater than the light response
Tonic redilation as gaze shifts from near to distance
Random changes in pupil size
Variable effect on accommodation
Pupil becomes smaller with passage of time
Involvement of second eye more likely with passage of time
Diminished deep tendon reflexes of the knee and ankle
Diminished corneal sensation in affected eye

The near response in Adie's pupil is slow and tonic, but is generally greater than the light response. Often, Adie's pupil is misdiagnosed as an Argyll Robertson pupil. The near effort response is best observed after prolonged near fixation, a situation that causes the pupil to slowly constrict and remain constricted for a long time. This reaction is often segmental and in the same sectors as in the light response. The enhanced near effort response is thought to be due to the fact that accommodative synapses in the ciliary ganglion outnumber pupillomotor synapses by about 30 to 1.[36]

Perhaps the most distinguishing feature of an Adie's pupil is the tonic redilation as the patient shifts gaze from near to distance. Because redilation is so sluggish, the affected pupil may be the smaller one for some time.

CLINICAL PEARL

Perhaps the most distinguishing feature of an Adie's pupil is the tonic redilation as the patient shifts gaze from near to distance. Because redilation is so sluggish, the affected pupil may be the smaller one for some time.

Random changes in size also may be seen in the tonic pupil. The pupil may be larger in the morning and smaller in the afternoon, or it may vary irregularly during the day.[37] The tonic pupil may be dilated in a darkened room, but it dilates so poorly that it actually may be smaller than its normal fellow, as in the above-mentioned circumstance.

Accommodation is often affected in the acute stage of tonic pupil, but to a variable degree. The most disturbing effect to the patient is a tonicity of accommodation, where the patient has difficulty shifting gaze from distance to near, or vice versa.[38]

Approximately half of patients with Adie's pupils recover accommodation within 2 years. The pupil tends to become smaller as time passes, and may even be smaller than its fellow, contributing to misdiagnosis. The tonic pupil retains its poor light response and its segmental nature, however. Involvement of the second eye is not unusual, and occurs at the rate of approximately 5% per year. Deep tendon reflexes of the knee and ankle are diminished in most cases, although the relationship of this phenomenon to the pupillomotor lesion remains unclear. It is not unusual to find diminished corneal sensation in the affected eye, because sensory corneal nerves pass through the ciliary ganglion.[39]

Differential diagnosis in tonic pupil is aided by pharmacologic testing, using the principle of denervation supersensitivity developed by Cannon.[40] Adler and Scheie[41] found that the tonic pupil in Adie's patients was supersensitive to dilute methacholine chloride (Mecholyl, Gordon Laboratories, Upper Darby, PA). Methacholine eye drops are no longer commercially available, so dilute pilocarpine has been substituted in concentrations of 0.125% or 0.1%. Application of such solutions causes constriction of the tonic pupil, with no noticeable effect on the normal pupil. Ciliary muscle supersensitivity also occurs using 0.25% pilocarpine, but the diagnostic response here consists of an increase in dioptric power of at least 1 diopter, and a brow ache, ½-hour after administration of the drops.[42]

Pharmacologic mydriasis

Perhaps the most common cause of a fixed, dilated pupil in clinical practice is inadvertent self-administration with mydriatic/cycloplegic drops. This is most often seen in health care workers such as optometrists, ophthalmologists, technicians, nurses, and pharmacists. The mechanism of action with parasympatholytic drugs is paralysis of the sphincter by receptor blockage at the neuromuscular junction. With sympathetic drugs, the mechanism is alpha-receptor stimulation of the dilator muscle. To differentiate pharmacologic dilation from neurologic dilation, the principle of denervation supersensitivity can be used. As previously stated, damaged pupillomotor fibers cause a denervated iris sphincter to constrict to weak concentrations of pilocarpine, whereas normal or pharmacologically dilated pupils do not constrict to weak miotic drops.[43]

Sympathetic System Lesions

Inhibition (Horner's syndrome)

Horner's syndrome generally refers to clinical triad of miosis, ptosis, and facial anhidrosis (reduced sweating). It occurs as a result of decreased sympathetic innervation to the ocular structures. Its expression is variable and can range from mild paresis to complete paralysis of the system (see the box below). Asymptomatic cases may be missed without careful observation and adherence to proper examination technique.

Clinical Findings in Horner's Syndrome

Classical clinical triad:
  Ptosis
  Miosis
  Facial anhidrosis
Other possible findings:
  Ocular hypotony
  Increased amplitude of accommodation
  Heterochromia

Complete Horner's syndrome results in the previously described clinical triad and also may cause ocular hypotony, increased amplitude of accommodation, and pigmentary changes (heterochromia). Pupillary reactions to light and near are unimpaired. Therefore, testing in a brightly lit room decreases the anisocoria, and may prevent accurate diagnosis; testing in dim illumination yields the best chance of revealing a Horner's miotic pupil. Other factors contribute to the amount of anisocoria in patients with Horner's syndrome (see the box below).

Factors Contributing to the Amount of Anisocoria in Horner's Syndrome[28]

Brightness of the examiner's light (greater anisocoria in dim light)
Completeness of the injury
Alertness of the patient
Extent of reinnervation of the dilator muscle
Degree of denervation supersensitivity
Fixation of the patient at distance or near
Concentration of circulating adrenergic substances in the blood

---

Many different lesions may impact the sympathetic pathway as it proceeds along its circuitous pathway. Lesions may occur in the brain stem and spinal cord, in the cervical sympathetic chain, at the base of the skull, and in the carotid canal and middle ear. The lesions can be classified as either central (first-order neuron), preganglionic (second-order neuron), or postganglionic (third-order neuron) (see the box below and on p. 90).

Classification of Lesions by Location in Horner's Syndrome

Central (first-order) neuron
  Lateral medullary infarction
  Other brain stem infarction
  Cerebral infarction
  Intracranial tumor
  Trauma (including surgical)
  Multiple sclerosis
  Syrinx
  Transverse myelopathy
  Other/unknown

> ### Classification of Lesions by Location in Horner's Syndrome—cont'd
>
> Preganglionic (second-order) neuron
>   Thoracic and neck tumor
>   Trauma (including surgical)
>   Other/unknown
> Postganglionic (third-order) neuron
>   Intracranial tumor (cavernous sinus)
>   Trauma (including surgical)
>   Vascular headache syndrome
>   Other/unknown

Specific localization of the site of the lesion is best indicated by noting the presence of associated neurologic signs and symptoms. The pupillary abnormalities are similar regardless of the location of the lesion. For instance, in Wallenberg's lateral medullary syndrome, there are enough characteristic associated neurologic findings to make pharmacologic pupillary testing unnecessary. Horner's syndrome in association with a sixth nerve palsy and hypesthesia strongly suggests cavernous sinus involvement. Most cases of isolated postganglionic Horner's syndrome have a benign origin, most commonly vascular headache syndrome. Localization also can be supported by the distribution of the facial anhidrosis (Table 3-1).

Pharmacologic testing may be useful in ascertaining whether the lesion involves the first, second, or third division of the pathway. Cocaine only dilates the pupil if norepinephrine is being released at postganglionic nerve endings in the dilator muscle. This does not occur in Horner's pupils, and locally applied cocaine (2% to 10%) fails to cause pupillary dilation if any part of the sympathetic pathway is disrupted.[44] It has been demonstrated that a postcocaine anisocoria value of at least 1.0 mm is required to make the diagnosis

TABLE 3-1

Localizing Value of Distribution of Anhidrosis in Horner's Syndrome

Location of lesion	Distribution of anhidrosis
Brain stem	Variable, but may include entire ipsilateral half of body
Ventral roots of cervicothoracic cord (or sympathetic chain in neck)	Ipsilateral side of face and neck; sometimes upper extremity
Postganglionic neuron at base of skull or in the orbit	Part of the forehead

of Horner's syndrome.[45,46] These authors point out that the cocaine test is just one indicator of Horner's syndrome. In the absence of other characteristic signs, a given amount of postcocaine anisocoria does not make a definitive diagnosis. The cocaine test is useful to confirm the presence of a sympathetic pupillary defect, but it does not indicate the location of the lesion.

Hydroxyamphetamine testing can assist in such localization.[47] This drug applied topically fails to cause pupillary dilation if the postganglionic pathway is disrupted. At least 2 days should pass after performing the cocaine test, because cocaine blocks the nerve terminal's uptake of hydroxyamphetamine, as well as norepinephrine. Hydroxyamphetamine is an indirect-acting sympathomimetic agent that causes release of norepinephrine from the normal presynaptic sympathetic nerve terminal and dilates only those pupils whose postganglionic sympathetic neuron is intact. The amount of dilation is dependent on the site of the lesion and the residual norepinephrine at the nerve terminal. A minimal or absent dilation suggests a postsuperior cervical ganglion lesion, whereas a normal response as compared with the fellow eye suggests a presuperior cervical ganglion lesion. Hydroxyamphetamine has been very difficult to obtain, as lamented in an editorial by Burde and Thompson.[48] Allergan Pharmaceuticals (Irvine, CA), however, has recently made arrangements to make the drug available for pupillary testing.[49]

Locally applied dilute epinephrine or phenylephrine has been reported to demonstrate sympathetic supersensitivity at the dilator muscle in postganglionic lesions. Although dilute concentrations may dilate a Horner's pupil, this may not be evident unless the eye has been pretreated with 2% cocaine; therefore, epinephrine testing alone is not useful in the topical diagnosis of Horner's syndrome. In addition, such denervation sensitivity varies with the completeness of the lesion and with its distance from the iris. Therefore, a partial postganglionic Horner's pupil may be less supersensitive than a complete preganglionic one.

As previously discussed, the phenomenon known as dilation lag[6] can be very useful in diagnosing Horner's syndrome. Because of the lack of active radial pull of the dilator muscle, there is a slow and delayed dilation in darkness in a Horner's pupil. Polaroid flash photographs taken in light, after 4 to 5 seconds of darkness, and after 10 to 12 seconds of darkness, demonstrate this phenomenon, and allow diagnosis of a Horner's pupil by physiologic methods.

CLINICAL PEARL

Because of the lack of active radial pull of the dilator muscle, there is a slow and delayed dilation in darkness in a Horner's pupil.

As stated, associated neurologic signs and symptoms are most critical in establishing the site of the lesion. Age of onset also may help point the clinician toward the location and likely cause. Trauma is the most common cause in patients up to the age of 20, whereas the odds of a neoplastic lesion increase in each decade after the age of 30.

References

1. Anderson B: Marcus Gunn pupil (letter), *Neurology* 44(12):2422, 1994.
2. Levatin P: Pupillary escape in diseases of the optic nerve, *Arch Ophthalmol* 62:768-779, 1959.
3. Adler FH: *Physiology of the eye,* ed 4, St Louis, 1965, Mosby, 203.
4. Smith JL: *Neuro-ophthalmology tapes, The Pupil,* 9820 SW 62 Ct, Miami, Fla, 1974.
5. Thompson HS: Pupillary light-near dissociation: a classification, *Surv Ophthalmol* 19:290-292, 1975.
6. Pilley SF, Thompson JS: Dilation lag in Horner's syndrome, *Br J Ophthalmol* 59:731-735, 1975.
7. Borchert M, Sadun AA: Bright light stimuli as a mask of relative afferent pupillary defects, *Am J Ophthalmol* 106:98-99, 1988.
8. Johnson LN: The effect of light intensity on measurement of the relative afferent pupillary defect, *Am J Ophthalmol* 109:481-482, 1990.
9. Browning DJ, Tiedeman JS: The test light affects quantitation of the afferent pupillary defect, *Ophthalmology* 94:53, 1987.
10. Loewenfeld IE: "Simple, central" anisocoria: a common condition, seldom recognized, *Trans Am Acad Ophthalmol Otolaryngol* 83:832-839, 1977.
11. Thompson HS: The pupils. In Moses RA, ed: *Adler's physiology of the eye,* ed 7, St Louis, 1981, Mosby, 326-356.
12. Toulemont PJ, Urvoy M, Coscas G, Lecallonnec A, et al: Association of congenital microcoria with myopia and glaucoma. A study of 23 patients with congenital microcoria, *Ophthalmology* 102 (2):193-198, 1995.
13. Roarty JD, Keltner JL: Normal pupil size and anisocoria in newborn infants, *Arch Ophthalmol* 108:94-95, 1990.
14. Cheng MMP, Catalano RA: Fatigue-induced familial anisocoria, *Am J Ophthalmol* 109:480-481, 1990.
15. Feibel RM, Perlmutter JC: Anisocoria in the pigment dispersion syndrome, *Am J Ophthalmol* 110:657-660, 1990.
16. Thompson HS, Jiang MQ: Letter to the editor, *Ophthalmology* 94:1360, 1987.
17. Cox TA: Pupillographic characteristics of simulated relative afferent pupillary defects, *Invest Ophthalmol Vis Sci* 30:1127-1131, 1989.
18. Fineberg E, Thompson HS: Quantitation of the afferent pupillary defect. In Smith JL ed: *Neuro-ophthalmology Focus 1980,* New York, 1979, Masson, 25-29.
19. Thompson HS, Corbett JJ, Cox TA: How to measure the relative afferent pupillary defect, *Surv Ophthalmol* 26:39-42, 1981.
20. Thompson HS, Corbett JJ: Swinging flashlight test (letter), *Neurology* 38:154-156, 1989.
21. Firth AY: Pupillary responses in amblyopia, *Br J Ophthalmol* 74:676-680, 1990.
22. Lam BL, Thompson HS: A unilateral cataract produces a relative afferent pupillary defect in the contralateral eye, *Ophthalmology* 97:334-338, 1990.
23. Bell RA, Thompson HS: Relative afferent pupillary defect in optic tract hemianopia, *Am J Ophthalmol* 85:538-540, 1978.
24. Kestenbaum A: *Clinical methods of neuro-ophthalmological examination,* New York, 1946, Grune & Stratton, 290.
25. Jiang MQ, Thompson HS, Lam BL: Kestenbaum's number as an indicator of pupillomotor input asymmetry, *Am J Ophthalmol* 107:528-530, 1989.

26. Loewenfeld IE: The Argyll Robertson pupil, 1869-1969, a critical survey of the literature, *Surv Ophthalmol* 14:199-299, 1969.

27. Seybold ME, Yoss RE, Hollenhorst RW, Moyer NJ: Pupillary abnormalities associated with tumors of the pineal region, *Neurology* 21:232-237, 1971.

28. Walsh FB, Hoyt WF: *Clinical neuro-ophthalmology,* ed 3, Baltimore, 1979, Williams & Wilkins, 464-534.

29. Weinstein JM: Pupillary disorders, *Current Opinion Ophthalmol* 1:453-462, 1990.

30. Ford FR, Walsh FB, King A: Clinical observations on the pupillary phenomena resulting from regeneration of the third nerve with special reference to the Argyll Robertson pupil, *Bull Johns Hopkins Hosp* 68:309-318, 1941.

31. Czarnecki JSC, Thompson HS: The iris sphincter in aberrant regeneration of the third nerve, *Arch Ophthalmol* 96:1606-1610, 1978.

32. Thompson HS: A classification of tonic pupils. In Thompson HS, ed: *Topics in neuro-ophthalmology,* Baltimore, 1979, Williams & Wilkins, 95-96.

33. Thompson HS: Adie's syndrome: some new observations, *Trans Am Ophthalmol Soc* 75:587-626, 1977.

34. Sattler CH: Ueber wurmförmige Zuckungen des Sphincter iridis, *Klin Monatsbl Augenheilkd* 49:739-745, 1911.

35. Thompson HS: Segmental palsy of the iris sphincter in Adie's syndrome, *Arch Ophthalmol* 96:1615-1620, 1978.

36. Warwick R: The ocular parasympathetic nerve supply and its mesencephalic sources, *J Anat* 88:71-93, 1954.

37. Chadwick D: The cranial nerves and special senses. In Walton J, ed: *Brain's diseases of the nervous system,* ed 10, New York, 1993, Oxford University Press, 89-91.

38. Moore RF: Physiology and pathology of the pupil reactions, Cases, *Trans Ophthal Soc UK* 44:38-43, 1924.

39. Purcell JJ, Krachmer JH, Thompson HS: Corneal sensation in Adie's syndrome, *Am J Ophthalmol* 84:496-500, 1977.

40. Cannon WB: A law of denervation, *Am J Med Sci* 198:737-743, 1939.

41. Adler FH, Scheie H: The site of the disturbance in tonic pupils, *Trans Am Ophthalmol Soc* 38:183-192, 1940.

42. Bell RA, Thompson HS: Ciliary muscle dysfunction in Adie's syndrome, *Arch Ophthalmol* 96:638-642, 1978.

43. Jacobson DM: A prospective evaluation of cholinergic supersensitivity of the iris sphincter in patients with oculomotor nerve palsies, *A J Ophthalmol* 118(3):377-383, 1994.

44. Thompson HS: Diagnostic pupillary drug tests. In *Current concepts in ophthalmology,* vol 3, St Louis, 1972, Mosby, 76-90.

45. Van der Wiel HL, Van Gijn J: The diagnosis of Horner's syndrome: use and limitations of the cocaine test, *J Neurol Sci* 73:311-316, 1986.

46. Kardon RH, Denison CE, Brown CK, Thompson HS: Critical evaluation of the cocaine test in the diagnosis of Horner's syndrome, *Arch Ophthalmol* 108:384-387, 1990.

47. Thompson HS, Mensher JH: Adrenergic mydriasis in Horner's syndrome. The hydroxyamphetamine test for diagnosis of postganglionic defects, *Am J Ophthalmol* 72:472-480, 1971.

48. Burde RM, Thompson HS: Hydroxyamphetamine: a good drug lost? [editorial], *Am J Ophthalmol* 111:100-102, 1991.

49. Levi L: Ocular motor nerves and the pupil, *Current Opinion Ophthalmol* 2:544-559, 1991.

Acknowledgments

The author thanks Drs. Helene Kaiser and Andrew Gurwood for the illustrations.

4

Ocular Motility Dysfunction*

Bruce G. Muchnick

Key Terms

supranuclear gaze centers	saccadic disorders	aberrant regeneration
paramedian pontine reticular formation (PPRF)	medial longitudinal fasciculus	Bielschowski head tilt test
	skew deviation	Duane's retraction syndrome
pursuit disorders	internuclear ophthalmoplegia	
vestibular nystagmus	Parinaud's syndrome	

A critical development in the course of human evolution has been the refinement of binocular vision. This ability to place an image of interest on both foveas simultaneously and in all positions of gaze, must occur in spite of head movement or object motion. Without a means to counteract even the subtlest of head movements, images would sweep across the retina, causing degradation of visual acuity. Even the tiniest of head vibrations due to the cardiac pulsation would blur vision if there were no compensatory mechanism.

This chapter is divided into two sections. The first section deals with the supranuclear motility system and its anatomy, examination, and disease processes. The second section reviews the infranuclear motility system, comprising eye movements generated by the third, fourth, and sixth cranial nerves.

---

*Illustrations in this chapter were created by the author.

Supranuclear Motility System

There are four general classes of eye movements known as supra-nuclear ocular motility systems. Each acts to stabilize retinal images and is defined by the specific stimulus needed to initiate the given movement, and a description of the type of movement elicited.

The first of these eye movements, the smooth pursuit system, acts to hold the image of a moving target on the fovea. Another one, the saccadic system, directs both foveas toward the image of regard. The vestibular-optokinetic movements act to hold the images of the visualized world steady on the retina during head rotation. Finally, the vergence system acts to move the eyes in opposite directions so that images of a single object in space are placed simultaneously on the fovea.[1]

These complex supranuclear eye movements take the coordinated efforts of whole muscle groups. No one muscle is involved and so disorders of the supranuclear system cause a loss of one or more of these gaze functions, rarely producing the complaint of diplopia.

When patients experience two different images seeming to occupy the same location in space, they may complain of "double vision." It must not be assumed, however, that these complaints of diplopia always represent a misalignment of the eyes. For example, a patient with monocular diplopia may have normal eye posture. Furthermore, because a patient may suppress the vision in the nonfixating eye, the lack of a diplopic complaint in no way negates the presence of strabismus.

Misalignment of the two visual axes with complaints of diplopia rarely occur as a result of disorders of the supranuclear, internuclear, or nuclear areas for cranial nerves III, IV, and VI. More commonly, ocular misalignment is due to disease processes in the infranuclear structures, including the fascicle, the nerve, the myoneural junction, or the extraocular muscles, (see section on Infranuclear Motility System p. 111).

The supranuclear gaze centers are responsible for the eye movements involving vestibular, optokinetic, saccadic, smooth pursuit, and vergence systems. Each of these are presented with their anatomic substrates described. The significant pathologic processes commonly affecting each system are presented, along with the relevant differential diagnosis and treatment modalities.

Pursuit System

This system allows for smooth, slow (40°/sec) eye movement, which enables the viewer to track targets by keeping the image-of-regard on the fovea. This response is stimulated by movement of an image on

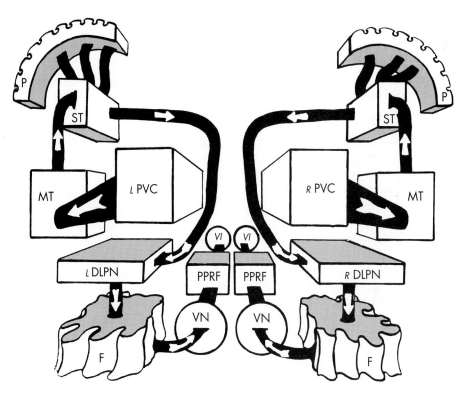

FIGURE 4-1 Pursuit pathway. *RPVC:* right posterior visual cortex; *LPVC:* left posterior visual cortex; *MT:* middle temporal visual area; *ST:* medial superior temporal visual area; *LDLPN:* left dorso-lateral pontine nuclei; *RDLPN:* right dorsolateral pontine nuclei; *F:* flocculus; *VN:* vestibular nuclei; *PPRF:* paramedian pontine nuclei; *VI:* sixth nerve nuclei.

the retina, usually near the fovea. The anatomic substrate for the pursuit system is found in the occipitoparietal junction.[1]

Neural Pathway of the Pursuit System

Cortical control of the smooth pursuit system arises from the parieto-occipito-temporal junction (POT) and is known as the parieto-occipito-temporal-mesencephalic pathway. There is ipsilateral control of the pathway, so that the left POT controls smooth pursuits to the left and the right POT controls smooth pursuits to the right.[2] It should be stated that the exact neural pathway is not yet known, although the signal to begin a pursuit movement begins in the paramedian pontine reticular formation (PPRF; Figure 4-1).[3,4]

Clinical Examination of the Pursuit System

Patients with smooth pursuit disorders rarely have visual complaints because they can use a series of saccades to track moving objects.

Test patients by having them keep their heads still while tracking a slowly moving target with their eyes. An optokinetic nystagmus flag may be passed in front of the patients to elicit pursuit movements (slow phases of the nystagmus).

The abnormal pursuit movement will be replaced by a series of saccades while the patients follow the target.

Pursuit Disorders

Disorders of the smooth pursuit system are caused by lesions in the occipitoparietal junction, the PPRF (although the PPRF is not a major part of the pursuit pathway), and the brain stem. The disorders are typified by a series of small saccades replacing the long pursuit movement. This may be due to disorders of the cerebellum, such as multiple sclerosis (MS), aging, medications (e.g., tranquilizers), and progressive supranuclear palsy.[5,6]

It is important to realize that lesions of the optic tract, temporal lobe, or occipital lobe that produce a homonymous hemianopsia will not usually affect the smooth pursuit system. A deep posterior hemispheric lesion with hemianopsia, however, will produce an abnormal pursuit away from the hemianopsia.[4]

Disorders of the pursuit system are divided into unilateral and bilateral dysfunction. Unilateral pursuit paresis, as described above, arises from deep occipital lesions, causing a hemianopsia and a "saccadic" pursuit in the direction of the lesion.[11] Bilateral dysfunction manifests itself as a reduction in pursuit velocity when a patient attempts to follow a target. A number of small saccades replace the one long pursuit movement. This may be due to sedative drug use, fatigue, or cerebral, cerebellar, and brain stem disease.[5]

Saccadic System

These most rapid of eye movements (500°/sec) allow the visual system to move to accurately pinpoint the image of an object on the fovea.[1]

The quick phases of vestibular nystagmus are considered saccades, as are involuntary and voluntary fixation changes.

Saccadic movements may be stimulated by conscious command of the observer toward a visual or auditory point of interest, or by unconscious random eye movements or rapid eye movement sleep.

Anatomically, nonfoveal saccadic initiation most likely begins in the contralateral frontal eye fields (specifically Brodman's Area 8) and superior colliculi, and foveal saccades are initiated at the occipito-parietal junction. The major pathway of the saccadic projections arrives at the PPRF at the level of the abducens nucleus. The PPRF is responsible for conjugate ipsilateral horizontal gaze movements. Vertical saccadic movements require bilateral cortical mediation.[1]

Neural Pathway of the Saccadic System

Horizontal saccades begin in the contralateral frontal lobe. The descending, polysynaptic saccadic fibers decussate at the midbrain–pontine junction and terminate in the contralateral PPRF (Figure 4-2).[7]

The reticular formation in the pons generates saccades of all types by inputs to the ocular motor nuclei. Stimulation of the left Brodman's Area 8 causes a conjugate saccade to the right, and stimulating the right Brodman's Area 8 causes movement to the left.

Clinical Examination of Saccadic Disorders

To clinically evaluate saccadic eye movements, have the patient alternate vision between two objects, both horizontally and vertically in all positions of gaze. Look for saccadic slowing, lack of accuracy,

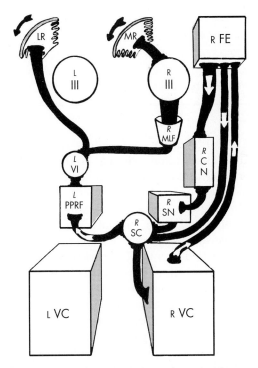

FIGURE 4-2 Saccadic pathway. *rVC:* right visual cortex; *lVC:* left visual cortex; *rFE:* right frontal eyefield; *rCN:* right caudate nucleus; *rSN:* right substantia nigra; *rSC:* right superior colliculus; *lPPRF:* left paramedian pontine reticular formation; *l VI:* left sixth nerve nuclei; *rMLF:* right medial longitudinal fasciculus; *r III:* right third nerve nucleus; *l III:* left third nerve nucleus; *MR:* right medial rectus; *LR:* left lateral rectus.

lag of initiation, and inappropriate saccades. Saccadic slowing can best be demonstrated by having the patient fixate between two widely spaced targets. Note any saccadic lag by timing the initiating of the saccade.

If a saccadic disorder is noted, then further neurologic evaluation is needed to localize the lesion based on the anatomic organization of the saccadic system.

Saccadic Disorders

Disorders that affect saccades may be classified by their effect on saccadic characteristics. Thus we see pathology of saccadic speed, accuracy, initiation, and inappropriateness.[8]

Slow saccades occur in patients with extraocular muscle dysfunction, ocular motor nerve paresis, or medial longitudinal fasciculus (MLF) lesions, causing internuclear ophthalmoplegia (INO). Internuclear ophthalmoplegia is characterized by slow saccadic adduction (see section on Horizontal Gaze Palsies p. 107).

CLINICAL PEARL

Slow saccades occur in patients with extraocular muscle dysfunction, ocular motor nerve paresis, or medial longitudinal fasciculus (MLF) lesions, causing internuclear ophthalmoplegia (INO).

Central neurologic disorders causing slow saccadic movements include Huntington's chorea, lipid storage disorders, and progressive supranuclear palsy. In addition, slow saccades are expected in sleepy, intoxicated, or aged patients.

Huntington's chorea is an autosomally dominant genetic disease with slow onset in the late 30s. The face and distal extremities demonstrate inappropriate movements. Mental deterioration eventually leads to dementia. The early eye sign is a loss of saccadic velocity. Saccades are often slow, particularly in the vertical direction, most likely because of lesions in the MLF.[9]

Inaccurate saccades are primarily due to cerebellar disease, although they can occur in patients with brain stem disorders and visual field hemianopsias.

Inappropriate saccades that interfere with vision may be caused by progressive supranuclear palsy, cerebellar disease, Huntington's chorea, and MS.

Supranuclear palsy is a degeneration of the central nervous system in elderly patients, first showing loss of downgaze along with immobility of the neck. Loss of upgaze, then horizontal gaze, and finally pursuits follows. A loss of facial expression and dementia is inevitable.

Death usually will follow within a decade of onset. The first eye movement to be affected is downward gaze, with horizontal and upward eye movements lost later in the course of the disease. Saccades become slowed and are of reduced size. All movements eventually are extinguished. The administering of dopaminergic drugs helps locomotion but not eye movements.[10]

Like pursuit disorders, saccadic disorders may be caused by unilateral or bilateral lesions. An acute, unilateral frontal lesion with preservation of the contralateral hemisphere usually produces a transient saccadic palsy, which improves and eventually resolves with time. This rarely occurs with a chronic process such as neoplasm. The pursuit system is not affected.[1]

Bilateral frontal lesions cause saccadic paresis in both directions. Again, the pursuit system is unaffected. Oculomotor apraxia, or the inability to initiate normal horizontal saccades, occurs because of such bilateral frontal lesions.[11] Delayed initiation of saccades may be observed in the elderly, inattentive, and intoxicated patients. If it occurs in the alert patient, it causes ocular motor apraxia and may be due to bilateral parietal lobe lesions. Another cause of delayed saccadic initiation is Parkinson's disease.[12]

Parkinson's disease is a degeneration of the extrapyramidal system and may cause a loss of upward gaze, followed by downward gaze, and finally horizontal eye movements. Convergence may fail, producing diplopia at near. Involuntary head motions and drooling may occur. The disease is characterized by tremor, muscular rigidity, and progressive supranuclear palsy with decreased convergence, superior gaze immobility, and saccadic initiation delays.[12]

Vestibular-Optokinetic System

The vestibulo-ocular reflex acts to steady retinal images during head movement. It is driven by sensory cells within the semicircular canals. These sensory cells detect motion, whether due to gravity or acceleration, in their given plane.

CLINICAL PEARL

The vestibulo-ocular reflex acts to steady retinal images during head movement. It is driven by sensory cells within the semicircular canals, which detect motion.

The vestibulo-ocular reflex acts to produce an eye movement that is equal and opposite to quick, short-lived head motions. The optokinetic system stabilizes the image during a prolonged rotation of the head (such as an ice-skater spinning for 30 seconds).[13]

Neural Pathway of the Vestibular-Optokinetic System

The semicircular canals are stimulated by transient head motion, which causes mechanical shearing effects on specialized hair cells within the canals. These cells transduce endolymph movement into neural impulses that are sent to the contralateral horizontal gaze center. Information sent from the right semicircular canal travels to the left horizontal gaze center, resulting in slow eye movement to the left. The optokinetic neural pathway is as yet unknown (Figure 4-3).[1,13]

Clinical Examination of Vestibular Disease

When a patient has complaints of dizziness, vertigo, or imbalance, you must consider vestibular disease. A patient who reports a sensation of

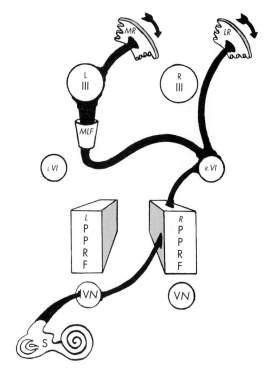

FIGURE 4-3 Neural pathway for vestibular eye movements: vestibular and cochlear testing. *S:* right semicircular canal; *VN:* vestibular nuclei; *rPPRF:* right paramedian pontine reticular formation; *lPPRF:* left paramedian pontine reticular formation; *R VI:* right sixth nerve nuclei; *L VI:* left sixth nerve nuclei; *MLF:* medial longitudinal fasciculus; *R III:* right third nerve nuclei; *L III:* left third nerve nuclei; *LR:* right lateral rectus muscle; *MR:* left medial rectus muscle.

rotation of one side may have peripheral vestibular disease affecting the opposite side. On examination the slow phase of the nystagmus will be away from the affected side.

To examine for vestibular imbalance, hold the patient's head still and have him or her fixate a distant target. Look for any nystagmus-type movements. Small movements may be discerned by using ophthalmoscopy to visualize a retinal structure (e.g., the nerve head) minutely quivering.

Vestibular nystagmus is accentuated when fixation is removed, so the patient may be fogged with high plus lenses in a trial frame. If still no nystagmus is noted, have the patient shake his or her head horizontally for 10 seconds and then stop. Look for a residual jerk nystagmus. Then repeat this test in the vertical plane.

CLINICAL PEARL

Vestibular nystagmus is accentuated when fixation is removed.

Finally, caloric testing can adequately evaluate the integrity of the labyrinthine apparatus. To test the horizontal canal, the patient is placed in a supine position with the head raised 30°. This places the horizontal canal into a vertical position. Introduction of cold water into the external auditory canal produces convection currents in the endolymph, which causes a jerk nystagmus whose fast phase is opposite the ear tested. If warm water is introduced, then the fast component is toward the same ear being tested. To remember this test, use the mnemonic COWS, which stands for Cold, Opposite; Warm, Same (Figure 4-3).[1,13]

Vestibular Disease

Vestibular disease causes a "saw-tooth" nystagmus, characterized by slow-phase drifts of constant velocity with corrective quick phases.

Peripheral vestibular disease should be differentiated from central lesions. Peripheral disease affecting primarily the labyrinthine apparatus generally causes an acute sensation of severe vertigo and deafness. It is usually caused by toxic reactions, infections, and inflammatory processes.

Central vestibular disease usually presents with chronic mild vertigo and no deafness. This is usually due to ischemia, acoustic neuroma, or demyelinating disease.[14]

Unilateral peripheral disorders of the vestibular system typically produce nystagmus due to differences in the neural activity between the left and right vestibular nuclei. Recovery usually occurs unless there has been some destruction of a single canal that causes a residual permanent nystagmus.

A bilateral peripheral vestibular loss of semicircular function causes image movement across the retina with every head movement. Eventually the patient will adapt to this condition.[15]

Wallenberg's Syndrome and the Vestibular System

Wallenberg's syndrome is caused by a lateral medullary infarction secondary to an occlusion of the posterior-inferior cerebellar artery, causing a disorder of the central vestibular connections. The patient will exhibit nystagmus with the slow-phase toward the side of the lesion. There also will be ipsilateral hypotropia, causing a skew deviation (vertical misalignment) and a hemifacial ipsilateral loss of pain and temperature sensation. A loss of pain and temperature sensation also will occur in the contralateral body and limbs. An ipsilateral Horner's syndrome may be noted. These clinical signs and symptoms will vary greatly, depending on the amount of brain stem and cerebellar damage.[15]

Vergence System

When a viewed object changes its distance from the observer, disparate retinal images stimulate the vergence system to either diverge or converge to reestablish bifoveal vision. This system, unlike the others, causes the eyes to move in opposite directions. The higher supranuclear pathways responsible for convergence and divergence remain largely unknown, although we know that convergence motor cells are located in the midbrain reticular formation dorsal to the oculomotor nucleus.

There are two stimuli that cause the vergence response. One is caused by the disparity of the two retinal images and causes a fusional vergence movement. The other stimuli is the retinal blur that occurs when an object changes its distance to the observer. This causes an accommodative vergence response, as part of the near triad along with lens accommodation and pupil miosis.

Vergence Disorders

Those disorders affecting the vergence system may best be divided into congenital and acquired defects of either convergence or divergence. Although the symptom of diplopia is rare in the other classes of eye movements, it is often reported in cases of divergence or convergence paralysis.

Clinical Examination of Vergence Disorders

It is first essential to determine if the presenting strabismus is an inborn defect, which is usually due to systemically benign visual system "miswiring" (or a lack of cortical fusional ability), or an acquired defect with significant neurologic implications. This is not an uncommon diagnostic dilemma.

First, a complete history is essential. If the patient reports a childhood history of "squint" or "crossed-eyes," then, unless additional significant neurologic signs and symptoms are present, the history has settled the issue. Typically, a lack of diplopia in these cases is due to suppression or amblyopia. In this case the patient may report a "lazy eye," which possibly was treated with patching therapy as an infant.

Uncommonly, a case of anomalous retinal correspondence may be uncovered, which also permits vision without diplopia. In this case a peripheral retinal area of the strabismic eye somehow acquires an anomalous common direction with the fovea of the fixating eye. This is clearly a sensory adaptation to chronic strabismus.

If the history fails to settle the matter, then an examination is crucial to rule out significant neurologic disease and to confirm long-standing strabismus.

The ocular misalignment must be measured in all positions of gaze. If the amount of deviation is equal in all positions of gaze no matter which eye is fixating, then this is a strabismus of long standing, because the ocular system has had a long time to adjust to the misalignment of the eyes. It is termed a concomitant strabismus, which is nonparetic in nature, and rarely has significant neurologic ramifications. By far the most common cause of comitant deviations is childhood strabismus, which is usually congenital, but may be acquired as in cases of vergence paresis and skew deviation.

Many patients have benign comitant phorias when tested with the alternate-cover or prism tests. These usually present no significant disturbance to the visual system, although some have proposed that these small deviations may be responsible for headaches, asthenopia, and reading complaints.

True concomitant strabismus exists if the fusional mechanism of the visual system cannot overcome the amount of deviation. Nonparalytic strabismus may be due to orbital disease, refractive error, or error of accommodative-convergence synkinesis.

If childhood strabismus is not determined by history, but is still suspected, it may be helpful to find amblyopia of long standing. Also, the presence of large fusional amplitudes points to childhood deviation, particularly if a decompensating phoria in an adult is suspected.

If childhood strabismus is ruled out, then acquired comitant deviation, including vergence paresis or skew deviation, should be considered.

Vergence Paresis

Vergence paresis, an acquired form of comitant deviation, includes both divergence and convergence paresis. Unlike childhood strabismus, divergence and convergence paralysis causes symptoms of diplopia.[16]

In divergence paralysis, a supranuclear paresis causes esotropia equal in all positions of gaze. Although simulating a mild bilateral sixth nerve palsy, divergence paralysis is considered by most to be a separate entity from sixth nerve palsies and divergence insufficiencies. If no other signs are present, then no other testing need be performed. The condition tends to be benign and self-limiting. Its cause may be head trauma, lumbar puncture, presumed viral infection, or idiopathic.[14]

Convergence paralysis is also an acquired comitant supranuclear gaze disorder that has a deviation equal in all positions of gaze. Full adduction is present during conjugate eye movements. This condition is difficult to differentiate from convergence insufficiency. It can be due to demyelinating disease, ischemia, or influenza infection.[14]

Skew Deviation

Skew deviation is a comitant or noncomitant (paralytic) vertical deviation and is invariably present with other neurologic signs. Skew deviation is associated with posterior fossa disease. Internuclear ophthalmoplegia often presents with a unilateral hypertropia, causing a skew deviation.[17]

Differential Diagnosis of Gaze Abnormalities

Gaze palsies result in an inability to produce saccadic or pursuit eye movements, and are caused by lesions anywhere from the cerebral cortex to the PPRF.

CLINICAL PEARL

Gaze palsies result in an inability to produce saccadic or pursuit eye movements, and are caused by lesions anywhere from the cerebral cortex to the PPRF.

Gaze palsies can be divided into horizontal and vertical gaze palsies. Horizontal gaze deficits may occur because of developmental anomalies in the motor neurons of the abducens nuclei, in intrinsic brain stem disease as in internuclear ophthalmoplegia, or in PPRF lesions causing pontine gaze paralysis.[18]

Vertical gaze palsies occur in pretectal disease (loss of downgaze), aqueductal stenosis, tumors of the pineal gland, and MS causing Parinaud's syndrome (loss of upgaze). Progressive supranuclear palsy, Parkinson's disease, and chronic progressive supranuclear palsy (CPEO) may demonstrate combination losses of upgaze and downgaze.

Horizontal Gaze Palsies

Congenital absence of all horizontal conjugate eye movements occurs in familial paralysis of horizontal gaze. This is a rare condition and is theorized to be due to a developmental anomaly of the abducens motor nuclei.[1]

An example of a more common horizontal gaze palsy is INO caused by a lesion in the MLF between the abducens and oculomotor nuclei. The hallmark sign of INO is a lag of the ipsilateral medial rectus muscle when adducting. The contralateral eye exhibits an abducting nystagmus, although the origin of this nystagmus is unknown (Figure 4-4).[19]

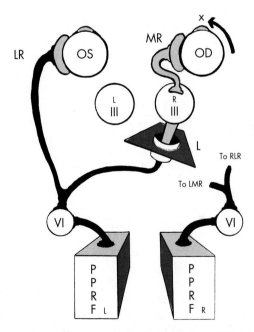

FIGURE 4-4 Internuclear ophthalmoplegia. *RPPRF:* right paramedian pontine reticular formation; *LPPRF:* left paramedian pontine reticular formation; *VI:* sixth nerve nucleus; *RLR:* right lateral rectus muscle; *LMR:* left medial rectus muscle; *L:* lesion of right medial rectus muscle; *R III:* right third nerve nucleus; *L III:* left third nerve nucleus; *MR:* right medial rectus muscle; *LR:* left lateral rectus muscle; *OD:* right eye; *OS:* left eye; *X:* adduction deficit of OD.

Multiple sclerosis is the most likely cause of an INO in a young adult. If the INO patient is older than 50 years of age, then brain stem vascular occlusive disease should be considered.[20]

CLINICAL PEARL

Multiple sclerosis is the most likely cause of an INO in a young adult. If the INO patient is older than 50 years of age, then brain stem vascular occlusive disease should be considered.

If the INO is produced by a midbrain lesion, it is usually bilateral (called a BINO), is characterized by an absence of convergence, and is called an anterior INO. There will be a bilateral abduction nystagmus. If the patient is exotropic (called a WEBINO), the medial rectus nuclei or MLF may be involved. A posterior INO is due to a lesion in the sixth nerve nuclei in the pons and produces an abduction deficit.[21-23]

A horizontal gaze paresis may occur in lesions of the PPRF, which produces an ipsilateral conjugate horizontal gaze palsy. If the ipsilateral PPRF (or abducens nuclei) and the parabducens nuclei are involved, this will produce a total horizontal gaze paralysis of both eyes toward the side of the lesion. If a lesion of the ipisilateral MLF also occurs, then the ipsilateral eye also fails to make a contralateral gaze motion. This is called a one-and-a-half syndrome. These patients will usually appear exotropic. In this syndrome, the eye ipsilateral to the lesion will be totally immobile during attempted horizontal gaze motions, and the contralateral eye will only be able to abduct (Figure 4-5).[1,24]

Vertical Gaze Palsies

Isolated upgaze and downgaze palsies remain rare disorders. Pretectal disease causes isolated downgaze palsies, and lesions of the posterior commissure produce isolated upgaze palsies.[25]

Parinaud's syndrome usually presents as a paresis of saccadic upgaze. Patients usually first notice this when playing sports. They may lose the ability to upward gaze to shoot basketball or serve a tennis ball. Clinically, on attempted superior gaze, the eyes will converge and retract into their orbits. This is due to stimulation of both medial recti muscles by the third nerve nucleus. Other findings in Parinaud's syndrome include partial third, fourth, or sixth nerve palsies, skew deviations, papilledema, mid-dilated light-near dissociation pupils, and lid retraction (Collier's sign). Causes of Parinaud's syndrome include trauma, stroke, MS, neurosyphilis, aqueductal stenosis, and pineal gland tumors.[26]

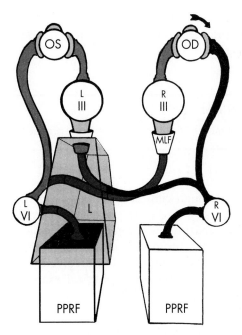

FIGURE 4-5 One-and-a-half syndrome. *PPRF:* paramedian pontine reticular formation; *R VI:* right sixth nerve nuclei; *L VI:* left sixth nerve nuclei; *L:* lesion of the left MLF and PPRF; *MLF:* medial longitudinal fasciculus; *R III:* right third nerve nucleus; *L III:* left third nerve nucleus; *OD:* right eye; *OS:* left eye.

Combination Upgaze and Downgaze Palsies

Three disorders that may have a combined upgaze and downgaze paresis are progressive supranuclear palsy (PSP), Parkinson's disease, and chronic progressive external ophthalmoplegia. These are caused by supranuclear lesions, although the ocular motor nuclei may be involved. Progressive supranuclear palsy and Parkinson's disease have been discussed previously in this chapter.

Chronic progressive external ophthalmoplegia (CPEO) actually refers to a number of clinical symptoms marked by the development of slowly progressing external ophthalmoplegia. It appears clinically similar to progressive supranuclear palsy. Chronic progressive external ophthalmoplegia has been classified by Rowland into ocular myopathies (i.e., Graves' disease, orbital pseudotumor), neuromuscular junction disorders (i.e., myasthenia gravis), neural myopathies, and uncertain origins. There is debate as to whether CPEO is neurologic or myopathic in nature.[14,15]

Summary

- Supranuclear motility disorders rarely produce the complaint of diplopia.

CLINICAL PEARL

Supranuclear motility disorders rarely produce the complaint of diplopia.

- A thorough clinical examination of the patient, combined with an understanding of the relevant neuroanatomy, should approximate the area involved and perhaps generate a differential diagnosis. Further neuroinvestigative techniques, such as radiologic examination, should pinpoint the involved area and, when combined with laboratory and other physical examination findings, pinpoint the cause of the disorder.

Clinical Examination of the Supranuclear System

History

1. Disorders of the supranuclear system rarely present with complaints of diplopia.
   Is the patient complaining of any significant neurologic problems, such as headache, paresthesias, anesthesias, amnesias, loss of vision?
2. Preliminary examination
   a. Visual acuity
   b. Visual fields
   c. Color vision
   d. Stereopsis testing
   e. Contrast sensitivity
3. Range of motions
   a. Ductions
   b. Versions
4. Alignment of visual axis
   a. Red glass test
   b. Maddox rod test
   c. Cover-uncover
   d. Alternate cover
5. Saccades and nystagmus
   a. Rule out nystagmus and inappropriate saccades in primary gaze
   b. Note latency, velocity, and accuracy of saccades

   6. Vestibular testing
       a. Visual acuity during head shaking
       b. Ophthalmoscopy of retinal structures to detect micronystagmus
       c. Caloric testing
   7. Smooth pursuit tests
       a. Patient to track small object
   8. Vergence testing
       a. Test fusional amplitudes
       b. Near point of convergence

Infranuclear Motility System

Most cases of paralytic strabismus, if not restrictive in nature or secondary to myasthenia gravis, are due to lesions affecting the ocular motor cranial nerves, their fascicles, or their nuclei. The recognition that a problem exists will begin either with symptomatic complaints by the patient of diplopia, or with objective clinical signs of ocular motor paresis on ductions, versions, red glass, Maddox rod, cover–uncover, and alternate cover testing. Also, if the patient exhibits a head tilt or turn, no matter how subtle, this may be another indication of a potential ocular misalignment.

Once you have determined that a potential ocular motor palsy exists, it is essential to isolate the nerve or nerves involved, based on the affected motility pattern. Having pinpointed the nerve or nerve group involved, the location of the lesion—whether in the nucleus, fascicle, nerve, neuromuscular junction, or muscle—can be predicted based on the history, age of the patient, motility pattern, and concurrent neurologic signs. Finally, based on the above factors, a differential diagnosis is developed. Accurate diagnosis and pinpointing of the lesion's location requires consultation with such medical specialties as radiology, neurology, and endocrinology.

There are three cranial nerves controlling ocular motor motility. These are the oculomotor nerve (cranial nerve III), the trochlear nerve (cranial nerve IV), and the abducens nerve (cranial nerve VI) (see Chapter 1).

Higher cortical centers in the brain control the nuclei of each nerve to allow precise alignment and movement of the eyes. Lesions of these supranuclear centers, as previously discussed, cause gaze palsies due to a combinational loss of muscle groups. This rarely produces the complaint of diplopia.

Lesions of the infranuclear areas, including the nerve nuclei, fascicles, nerve, neuromuscular junction, or muscle, may produce single or combinational ocular motor palsies. If a lesion occurs in isolation, and only one nerve is affected, then a distinctive pattern of motility deficit is usually readily recognizable. More complicated nerve combinational losses may produce a variety of abnormal motility patterns requiring an extensive diagnostic workup. By determining which ocular motor nerves are affected and understanding the significant neuroanatomy, the location of the lesion may be approximated, and then a differential diagnosis may be generated based on location of the lesion and the significant epidemiology of the case. Actual diagnosis usually requires radiologic imaging and neurologic consultations.

Oculomotor Nerve Palsy

Functional Anatomy of the Third Cranial Nerve

The third cranial nerve supplies somatic motor fibers to the medial rectus for adduction, inferior rectus for downgaze, inferior oblique and contralateral superior rectus for upgaze, and both of the levator palpebrae superioris muscles for elevation of both lids. It also provides parasympathetic input to the constrictor pupillae of the pupillary miosis, and the ciliary muscles of the ciliary body for accommodation.

The nuclei of the somatic motor component lie near the midline of the midbrain at the level of the superior colliculus. Just lateral and inferior to the third nerve nuclei is the MLF. The oculomotor nuclear complex contains subnuclei that supply individual muscles (see Chapter 1).

After the lower motor neurons leave the oculomotor complex, they course through the red nucleus and emerge in the interpeduncular fossa between the pons and the midbrain. Near here, these motor fibers combine with parasympathetic fibers from the Edinger-Westphal nucleus. Together they form the oculomotor nerve, which passes anteriorly through the dura and enters the cavernous sinus. The third nerve courses through the cavernous sinus superior to the trochlear nerve, passes through the superior orbital fissure, where it branches into a superior and inferior division, and then enters the orbit. The inferior division innervates the medial rectus, inferior oblique, and inferior rectus muscles. The superior division innervates the levator palpebrae superioris and superior rectus muscles. The parasympathetic fibers branch off the inferior division to terminate in the ciliary ganglion.[28]

Diagnosis of Oculomotor Nerve Palsy

Diagnosis of third nerve palsy is best approached anatomically, because a characteristic pattern of functional loss is dependent on the location of the lesion along the path of the nerve.

Nuclear Third Nerve Lesions

We can predict what would happen in a hypothetical patient with a complete nuclear third nerve lesion. There would be a unilateral third nerve palsy with the eye appearing "down-and-out" and unable to accommodate. There would be paralysis of the contralateral superior rectus muscle, as well as a bilateral ptosis (because the levator is bilaterally innervated). Also, the ipsilateral pupil would be dilated and unreactive to direct or consensual stimuli.

Isolated complete lesions of the oculomotor nuclei are virtually unheard of. This is because infarcts affecting these nuclei would also involve surrounding areas, causing vertical gaze palsies. There are reported cases of single third nerve muscle paresis involving just a few muscles and the pupil, but there were always concurrent neurologic signs. Specific mesencephalon lesions were postulated (by Waring et al.[1]) to explain these cases. Also, there may be cases of congenital third nerve palsies, but these tend to be incomplete and unilateral.

Fascicular Third Nerve Lesions

As the fascicles of the oculomotor nerve leave the nuclear area and pass through the midbrain, they may be subjected to lesions whose location may be inferred by concurrent neurologic deficits. The adjacent structures most commonly affected include the red nucleus, cerebral peduncle, and the entire brain stem.

If a third nerve palsy presents with a contralateral cerebellar ataxia and slow tremor, this implies involvement of the third nerve and the adjacent red nucleus. This is called Claude syndrome.

A lesion affecting the cerebral peduncle along with the adjacent third nerve produces a third nerve palsy with contralateral hemiparesis and is called Weber syndrome.

If a large lesion, usually produced by an infarct or tumor, involves the third nerve, red nucleus, and cerebral peduncle, then Benedikt's syndrome is produced. If this is accompanied by a vertical gaze palsy, then Nothnagel's syndrome results.

Precavernous Third Nerve Palsies

Lesions affecting the oculomotor nerve as it passes from the brain stem to the cavernous sinus arise from aneurysm, infection, blood problems, and tumor. Differentiation of these causes in the office is helped by the presence or absence of the concurrent symptoms and clinical signs of pain and pupillary involvement. A third nerve presenting with orbital and facial pain may be due to compression of the oculomotor neural bundles as they pass by an aneurysm of the posterior communicating artery. Furthermore, the aneurysm typically produces a dilated pupil and ptosis in conjunction with the third nerve palsy.

During cerebral herniation, the uncus of the temporal lobe may compress the third nerve against the clivus or the temporal edge, first producing mydriasis, followed by external ophthalmoplegia.

Cavernous Sinus Third Nerve Palsies

As the third nerve passes through the cavernous sinus, it is susceptible to aneurysm, thrombosis, tumor, infection, and inflammation (see Chapter 2). Usually the fourth and sixth nerves also become involved, producing a combinational nerve palsy.

A patient presenting with a third nerve palsy with ptosis, diplopia, and facial pain along with trochlear and abducens nerve involvement may have a compressional effect from an aneurysm.

Intraorbital Third Nerve Palsies

Isolated lesions of either the superior or inferior branches of the third nerve have been known to occur. It is rare to have an isolated lesion to an individual muscle. All cases of isolated inferior branch palsies (presumed to be viral) have recovered spontaneously.[27] Isolated inferior rectus muscle palsies likewise recovered spontaneously.[28]

Other Cases of Third Nerve Palsies

Infarction of the oculomotor nerve may result from diabetes, collagen-vascular disease, and hypertension. Along with aneurysm, vascular disease due to diabetes mellitus and hypertension were the most common causes of third nerve palsies. The lesion in diabetes has been found on pathologic sectioning to be present in the cavernous sinus or subarachnoid areas.

The presenting feature in diabetic third nerve palsy may be facial pain, followed by diplopia or ptosis. The pain then abates. The pupil is usually spared in diabetic third nerve, unlike aneurysmal third nerve involvement. Third nerve palsy may be the presenting symptom of diabetes.

Severe head trauma causing bone fracture and unconsciousness may cause an oculomotor palsy. Traumatic injury to the nerve may occur as it exits the brain stem, in its subarachnoid portion, or as it enters the supraorbital fissure. Twelve percent of patients with giant cell arteritis present with third nerve palsy, requiring an erythrocyte sedimentation rate and possible temporal artery biopsy for positive confirmation of the disorder.[29]

Aberrant Regeneration

After oculomotor palsy due to aneurysm, trauma, and migraine, the third nerve fibers may resprout and innervate different muscles. This causes anomalous synkinesis effects such as lid elevation and miosis during adduction or downgaze, lid depression or abduction, and absence of pupil response. Aberrant regeneration in the absence of a third nerve palsy may indicate a mass lesion of the cavernous sinus.

Pupil Involvement in Third Nerve Palsies

If a third nerve presents with orbital pain, it may be due to either an aneurysm or vascular-occlusive disease such as diabetes. If it is due to aneurysm, arteriography is essential for diagnosis. But this technique has an inherent risk of significant morbidity and is thus a procedure not to be performed unless an aneurysm is highly suspected and vascular-occlusive disease has been ruled out.

It was Goldstein and Cogan[30] who, in 1960, showed that pupillary sparing occurs in 80% of patients with vascular-occlusive third nerve palsy, but in less than 10% in patients with aneurysmal third nerve. Therefore, a third nerve palsy with pupil involvement may be due to aneurysm and may require an arteriography. A third nerve with pupil sparing is usually due to vascular-occlusive disease, although it may be found to be spared in early aneurysmal cases, and arteriography should only be considered if additional signs point to a vascular abnormality.

The explanation for pupil-sparing third nerve palsies may be found in the anatomic location of the pupillary fibers. They lie superficially on the nerve, so they are susceptible to compressional lesions like aneurysm. Vascular-occlusive diseases infarct the central nerve while sparing most of the superficial pupil fibers, however, and so the pupil is relatively spared.

Third Nerve Palsies in Children

Almost half of the cases of oculomotor palsies in children are congenital, whereas a fourth are traumatic. Neoplasms and aneurysms account for most of the remaining cases. Most cases of congenital third nerve palsy exhibit aberrant regeneration. Birth trauma is assumed to be the likely cause.

Management of Third Nerve Palsies

Patients under the age of 40 who present with isolated third nerve palsies require a computed tomography (CT) scan, cerebrospinal fluid study, and cerebral angiography, whether or not the pupil is spared. Patients over the age of 40 with pupil-sparing oculomotor palsies are assumed to have vascular-occlusive disease, and are therefore just observed weekly for 1 month, and then every month for 6 months. These patients should have a blood pressure and diabetes workup. Any sign of pupil involvement in these older patients requires an immediate arteriography, CT scan, and cerebrospinal fluid examination.

CLINICAL PEARL

Patients under the age of 40 who present with isolated third nerve palsies require a computed tomography (CT) scan and cerebrospinal fluid study.

Trochlear Nerve Palsy

Functional Anatomy of the Fourth Cranial Nerve

The fourth, and smallest, of all cranial nerves supplies somatic motor fibers to the superior oblique muscle of the eye. The nucleus of the trochlear nerve is located in the midbrain at the level of the inferior colliculus, near the midline, at the caudal end of the third nerve complex.

As the axons leave the nucleus dorsally, they decussate (the only cranial nerve that does so) to eventually innervate the contralateral superior oblique muscle.

After decussation, the axons proceed ventrally as they curve forward and around the cerebral peduncle, piercing the dura anteriorly with the third nerve.

The fourth nerve then enters the cavernous sinus, running along its lateral wall, through the superior orbital fissure to enter the eye. This represents the longest intracranial course of any cranial nerve. The tendon of the muscle then courses through the trochlea and is contiguous with the superior oblique. Stimulation of the fourth nerve causes contraction of the superior oblique muscle, thus depressing, abducting, and intorting the eye (see Chapter 1).

Diagnosis of Trochlear Nerve Palsy

Any patient presenting with a vertical muscle weakness must be worked up for trochlear nerve palsy. If a palsy exists, the affected eye will exhibit a hyperdeviation and a weakness to lateral and downward gaze. This is best diagnosed by a four-step procedure including the Bielschowski head tilt test.

To isolate which muscle is causing the vertical deviation, proceed with the following four steps.

1. Determine which eye is hypertropic or hyperphoric: Have the patient stare straight ahead in primary gaze. The hypertropia may be obvious, or Maddox rod with or without cover-uncover or alternate cover testing may be necessary. A vertical prism bar is employed to measure the vertical component.

2. Determine if the vertical deviation is greatest to left or right gaze: Have patients follow a target to their left and then to their right. You may be able to see which direction or gaze causes a worsening hypertropia. If not, red lens or Maddox rod testing with a vertical prism bar can measure the hyperdeviation to left or right gaze.

3. Determine if the deviation is greatest on upgaze or downgaze when the patient is looking to the affected side: Once you have determined the horizontal gaze that causes the greatest deviation, have the patient look in that direction, and then attempt to elevate and depress the eyes. You may see an obvious worsening of the

vertical deviation to either superior or inferior gaze, or you may have to employ the red lens or Maddox rod/vertical prism bar test.

4. Determine if the hyperdeviation is greatest in left head tilt or right head tilt: While patients are staring straight ahead in primary gaze, have them tilt their head to the left and then the right. You may see which head tilt worsens the vertical deviation (this will be opposite the head tilt the patient prefers), or you may have to employ the Maddox rod/vertical prism bar test.

To better understand the testing procedures for the diagnosis of vertical ocular motor deviation, we will present a case example (Figure 4-6, *A* to *D*).

A patient presents with complaints of sudden onset of diplopia. In questioning the patient, you find that the diplopia is vertical in nature. The following represents a typical testing procedure for this vertical deviation.

1. In primary gaze: With a Maddox rod oriented vertically (to produce a horizontal red line image) in front of the right eye, hold a white light at 24 inches from the patient. The patient staring straight ahead at the two images notes that the red line is below the white light. Therefore the right eye is the hyperdeviated eye. This may be due to a weakness in the depressors of the right eye (the right inferior rectus [RIR] or right superior oblique [RSO]), or a weakness in the elevators of the left eye (the left superior rectus [LSR] or left inferior oblique [LIO]). The diagnosis has been narrowed from eight muscles affected to four (Figure 4-6, *A*).

2. In horizontal gaze: Now the patient is asked to look left and right through the Maddox rod and prism bar. He or she notes that on right gaze the white light is almost touching the red line. Therefore, there is no hyperdeviation in this position of gaze. But on left gaze, the red line is well below the white light, even further than when looking straight ahead. Because the weakness is worse to left gaze, it may be due to a weakness in the muscle that helps the right eye

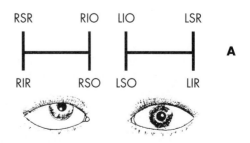

FIGURE 4-6. **A,** Primary gaze. *Continued*

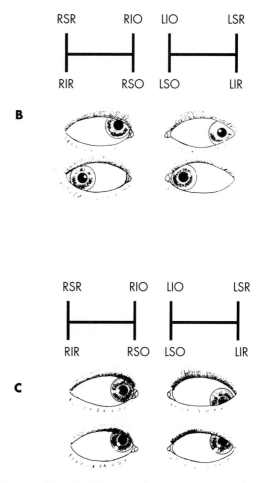

FIGURE 4-6—cont'd. B, Horizontal gaze. **C**, Vertical gaze.

depress when adducting (RSO), or may be due to a weakness of the muscle that helps the left eye elevate when abducting (LSR). The field of possible muscles has been narrowed to two (Figure 4-6, *B*).

3. In vertical gaze: Finally, while this patient is looking toward the horizontal direction that causes the greatest vertical deviation (in this case, the left), the target light is lifted upward, above horizontal. In this position, the patient notes little separation of the white light from the red line. Therefore the elevator of the left eye in this position (LSR) is not affected. But as the light is brought down below the horizontal meridian, the patient notes increasing separation. This implicates the depressor muscle of the right eye in this position (RSO) as being the muscle involved (Figure 4-6, *C*).

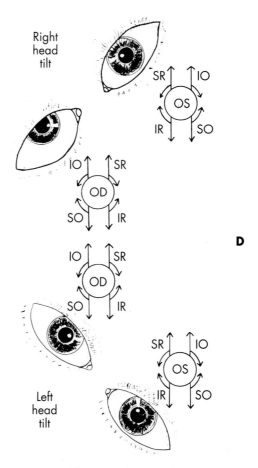

Right
head
tilt

Left
head
tilt

D

FIGURE 4-6—cont'd D, Bielschowski head tilt test.

These three steps will diagnose most acute muscle palsies, but with time there is a "spread-of-concomitance" so that the deviations become equal in all directions of gaze. This spread-of-concomitance makes the three-step diagnosis equivocal, because the patient may, with time, fixate with the affected eye. The Bielschowski head tilt test can be effective in diagnosing the affected occular muscle when the spread of concomitance has occurred.

4. Bielschowski head tilt test: The patient looks through the Maddox rod in front of the right eye and the vertical prism bar in front of the left eye. This patient then tilts his or her head first to the left. When performing this maneuver, the right eye must extort by stimulation of the RIR and the RIO, and the left eye must intort by stimulation of the LSR and the LSO. The patient notices no increase in the separation of light from the bar, so there is no increase in hyperdeviation when tilting to the left.

However, when the patient tilts his or her head to the right, he or she sees the white light move well above the red line. This implies an increasing right hyperdeviation. To decide what muscle is involved, look at what happens as the head is tilted to the right. The right eye must now intort, using stimulation of the RSO and the RSR. The left eye must extort using the LIR and the LIO. But, because it is a right hyperdeviation, it must be either the right depressor and intorter (RSO) or the left elevator and extorter (LIO). It cannot be the LIO because, back when the patient looked to the right in horizontal gaze testing (step 2), there was no vertical deviation. If there was an LIO palsy, step 2 would have shown a vertical deviation to the right as opposed to left gaze (as in this case). Therefore the Bielschowski head tilt test has shown the affected muscle to be the RSO, independent of whether there has been a spread-of-concomitance (Figure 4-6, *D*).

The diagnostic approach should be anatomic, ruling out nuclear, fascicular, subarachnoid, cavernous sinus, superior orbital fissure, and orbital causes.

Nuclear and Fascicular Fourth Nerve Palsy

Nuclear and fascicular fourth nerve palsies are rare. The fourth nucleus may be absent or congenitally hypoplastic. The nucleus also may be affected by neurosurgical intervention, trauma, brain stem tumors, hemorrhage, infarction, or demyelinating disease.

Subarachnoid Fourth Nerve Palsy

Head trauma is the most common cause of trochlear nerve palsy, because frontal head injury can cause a contrecoup shock wave to disrupt one or both fourth nerves as they emerge together in the anterior medullary velum (anterior roof of the fourth ventricle). This produces a unilateral or bilateral fourth nerve palsy.

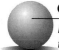

CLINICAL PEARL

Head trauma is the most common cause of trochlear nerve palsy, because frontal head injury can cause a contrecoup shock wave to disrupt one or both fourth nerves as they emerge together in the anterior medullary velum (anterior roof of the fourth ventricle).

Bilateral trochlear nerve palsy produces an alternating hyperdeviation that depends on the direction of horizontal gaze. Other causes of subarachnoid trochlear involvement include posterior communicating or basilar artery aneurysm, infarction due to diabetes, tumor, or meningitis.

Cavernous Sinus and Superior Orbital Fissure Fourth Nerve Palsy

After trauma, infarction due to diabetes is the most common cause of fourth nerve palsies, and accounts for one fifth of all cases. The prognosis for recovery is better than in traumatic injury. If the palsy occurs in the fourth to fifth decades, almost all cases improve spontaneously within 6 months. Other causes of cavernous sinus fourth nerve palsy include aneurysm, tumor, herpes zoster, and carotid-cavernous fistula.

Orbital Fourth Nerve Palsy

If a patient presents with normal eye posture in the primary position of gaze, but on adduction the eye depresses and cannot elevate well, then Brown's superior oblique tendon syndrome must be suspected. The affected eye elevates well in the abducted position.

This syndrome may be congenital or acquired. It is due to a shortened superior oblique muscle tendon, so when adducting, the sheath is taut, thus limiting elevation of the eye. When abducting, the sheath is looser, allowing elevation. Surgical intervention is necessary for correction of this syndrome.[29]

Fourth Cranial Nerve Palsy in Children

Most cases of childhood fourth nerve palsy are congenital, although one third may be from trauma. If a sudden onset of vertical diplopia is found in a patient in the first to third decade of life, with no history of trauma or with no concurrent neurologic signs, then most likely this patient has a decompensating phoria. The presence of large fusional amplitudes will help in this diagnosis. Symptoms of diplopia or headache may be relieved by prescribing vertical prisms.[1]

Management of Fourth Nerve Palsies

Most cases of fourth nerve palsies are traumatic in origin or decompensating phorias. Any patient, regardless of age, with an atraumatic sudden onset of trochlear palsy who has large vertical fusional amplitudes needs no extensive neurologic workup, because it is congenital in nature. If there are no significant fusional amplitudes, then a Tensilon test is mandatory to rule out myasthenia gravis, and radiologic tests must be used to rule out a compressive tectal lesion. If the Tensilon test is negative, the patient should have a general systemic workup to rule out diabetes or hypertension as a possible cause of infarct.

Because isolated nonischemic fourth nerve palsies are rare, in-depth neurologic investigations should only proceed if there is a progression of clinical signs and symptoms. These cases require a CT scan and cerebral angiography.

Abducens Nerve Palsy

Functional Anatomy of the Sixth Cranial Nerve

The abducens nerve is a somatic motor nerve that innervates the lateral rectus of the eye. When contracted, the lateral rectus muscle acts to abduct the eye.

The nuclei of the abducens nerve is close to the midline, ventral to the fourth nerve, in the pontine tegmentum. Axons from the nuclei project ventrally, emerging at the ventral surface of the brain stem between pons and medulla. Running ventrally, the abducens nerve pierces the dura, bends around the petrous portion of the temporal bone, and enters the cavernous sinus. It runs lateral to the internal carotid artery and medial to the other nerves of the cavernous sinus, and enters the eye in the medial superior orbital fissure. Once entering the orbit, it innervates the lateral recti muscle (see Chapter 1).

Diagnosis of Abducens Nerve Palsy

Even though sixth nerve involvement is the most commonly reported of the ocular muscle palsies, no definitive diagnosis is made in about one quarter of the cases. The most common cause of abducens nerve palsies is most likely ischemia to the nerve secondary to diabetes or hypertension. As in third and fourth nerve palsies, restoration of nerve function occurs in 3 to 6 months.

CLINICAL PEARL

The most common cause of abducens nerve palsies is most likely ischemia to the nerve secondary to diabetes or hypertension.

As with the other ocular motor nerves, diagnosis should be consistent with the location of the lesion along the path of the sixth nerve, from nucleus to orbit.

Nuclear and Fascicular Abducens Nerve Palsies

Nuclear sixth nerve palsies are usually due to developmental abnormalities, injury, or tumor, and are typically characterized by horizontal gaze palsy.

As the fascicles of the sixth nerve pass the pyramidal tract (through medial pons), they are susceptible to infarction of the medial inferior pons, producing ipsilateral abducens palsy and facial weakness with contralateral hemiplegia. This is known as Millard-Gubler syndrome. Demyelinating disease also may affect the fascicular sixth nerve area.[31]

Subarachnoid Sixth Nerve Palsy

In its subarachnoid region, the sixth nerve may be compressed by berry aneurysm or tumor, disrupted by trauma or meningitis, or lesioned during neurosurgical intervention.

Petrous Sixth Nerve Palsy

As the sixth nerve courses over the petrous portion of the temporal bone, it may be disrupted by temporal bone fractures secondary to trauma.

It is also susceptible to infection from the mastoid process, which, if also affecting the nearby fifth (trigeminal) cranial nerve, causes an abducens palsy, facial pain, and possible deafness. This is known as Gradenigo's syndrome. If not caused by tumor, the prognosis in most cases of Gradenigo's syndrome is for full and spontaneous recovery.[30]

Cavernous Sinus and Orbital Abducens Nerve Palsy

As with other ocular motor nerves, the sixth cranial nerve is susceptible to internal carotid artery aneurysm, carotid-cavernous fistula, tumor, and herpes zoster while in the cavernous sinus. Tumors, such as nasopharyngeal carcinoma, may affect the sixth as it passes into the orbit.

Sixth Nerve Palsies in Children

Tumor should be suspected in all cases of abduction weakness in children. It is essential to look for any cerebellar signs, papilledema, or worsening of the palsy over time, which would indicate an expanding space-occupying lesion. Trauma is another common cause of abducens nerve palsy in childhood (40% of cases in one study).[1] All cases of ocular motor palsy in children should be evaluated for battered child syndrome.

Virus also may cause sixth nerve palsies in children. Neurologic examination (with CT scan, cerebrospinal fluid study, and Tensilon test) will be negative and most cases recover spontaneously.

Duane's Retraction Syndrome

There are three forms of Duane's retraction syndrome, although all are associated with narrowing of the palpebral fissure (apparent globe retraction) on adduction. This syndrome is more common in women and girls, and may be unilateral or bilateral, although the left eye is affected more than the right.

Type 1 Duane's has limited abduction but normal adduction, type 2 is characterized by normal abduction but poor adduction, and type 3 exhibits limited abduction and adduction. There is no treatment necessary in cases of Duane's syndrome because these patients rarely complain of diplopia, and maintain good stereopsis in primary gaze.[29]

Bilateral Sixth Nerve Palsies

Most cases of bilateral abducens palsy are caused by neoplasm. The second most common cause is demyelinating disease.[1] It is important to know that bilateral sixth nerve palsies are never caused by infarction, so an atraumatic patient presenting with this disorder requires a workup to rule out space-occupying lesions, multiple sclerosis, subarachnoid hemorrhage, and infection.[30]

CLINICAL PEARL

Most cases of bilateral abducens palsy are caused by neoplasm. The second most common cause is demyelinating disease.

Management of Sixth Nerve Palsies

A sixth nerve palsy in a child with no history of trauma should be observed every few weeks. If there is any progression of the paresis, then a neurologic workup to rule out neoplasm is warranted. Usually young patients who do not improve in 6 months receive cranial imaging, but in most cases, no lesions are found. Surgery may eventually help these patients.

Those patients in the second to fourth decade who present with acute isolated sixth nerve paresis should have a medical examination to rule out diabetes mellitus, hypertension, and collagen-vascular disease, and have a neurologic evaluation to rule out myasthenia gravis. Usually patients are just observed until improvement is noted (usually in 6 months).

Over the age of 40, patients with sixth nerve palsy due to infarction usually present with orbital pain. These patients should be examined for diabetes mellitus and hypertension, plus an erythrocyte sedimentation rate to rule out giant cell arteritis.

Any sixth nerve palsy with ipsilateral facial pain must have a CT scan of the mastoid to rule out Gradenigo's syndrome secondary to inflammation, infection, or a tumor of the tip of the petrous pyramid.

All bilateral sixth nerve patients must have a neuroradiologic examination to rule out a tumor causing increased intracranial pressure. Also, papilledema should be ruled out in these cases.

Combination Ocular Motor Palsies

Multiple ocular palsies may arise from lesions anywhere from their nuclear areas to the orbit. Many occur where the nerves lie close together in the cavernous sinus, and a number of conditions can cause combinational losses. These include aneurysm, tumor, diabetic-induced infarction, and herpes zoster. If other signs are present, such as orbital pain due to trigeminal involvement, this further supports a cavernous sinus location. If visual loss is a concurrent sign, then the lesion is more likely near the orbit where the second (optic) cranial nerve is closest to the ocular motor bundles.

Trauma is a significant cause of multiple ocular motor nerve palsies. Injury can occur in the subarachnoid and orbital regions. The trauma usually must be severe to cause multiple loss.

Exposure to toxic environmental poisons also may cause ocular motor combined palsies. The location of the lesion remains uncertain.

References

1. Leigh RJ, Zee DS: The neurology of eye movement. In *Contemporary neurology series*, Philadelphia, 1983, FA Davis, 3-116.
2. Glaser JS: Neuro-ophthalmology. In Glaser JS, ed: *Neuro-ophthalmology*, Philadelphia, 1990, JB Lippincott, 279-406.
3. Eckmiller R: The neural control of pursuit eye movements, *Physiol Rev* 67:797, 1987.
4. Lynch JO, Mountcastle VB, Talbot WH, et al: Parietal lobe mechanisms for directed visual attention, *J Neurophysiol* 40:364-379, 1977.
5. Troost BT, Abel LA: Pursuit disorders, In Lennerstrand G, Zee DS, Keller EL, eds: *Functional basis of ocular motility disorders*, New York, 1982, Pergamon Press, 511-576.
6. Zee DS, Yamazaki A, Butler PH, Gucer G: Effects of ablation of flocculus and paraflocculus on eye movements in primates, *J Neurophysiol* 46:888-899, 1981.
7. Troost BT, Dell'Osso LF: Fast eye movements (saccades): basic science and clinical correlations. In Thompson HS, ed: *Topics in neuro-ophthalmology*, Baltimore, 1979, Williams & Wilkins, 250-262.
8. Bahill AT, Troost BT: Types of saccadic eye movements, *Neurology* 29:1150, 1979.
9. Collewish H, Went LN, Tamminga EP, et al: Oculomotor defects in patients with Huntington's disease and their offspring, *J Neurol Sci* 86:307, 1988.
10. Steale JO, Richardson JO, Olszeluski J: Progressive supranuclear palsy, *Arch Neurol* 10:333-352, 1968.
11. Cogan DG, Chu FC, Reingold D, et al: A long-term follow-up of congenital ocular motor apraxia: case report, *Neuro Ophthalmol* 1:145-147, 1980.
12. White DB, Saint-Cyrja, Tomlinson RD, et al: Ocular motor deficits in Parkinson's disease. III: Coordination of eye and head movements, *Brain* 111:115, 1988.
13. Troost BT: An overview of ocular motility neurophysiology, *Ann Otol Rhinol Laryngol* (suppl 86):29, 1981.
14. Marsden CO, Kahn S, eds: *Movement disorders*, Boston, 1987, Butterworths.
15. Zee DS: Brainstem and cerebellar deficits in eye movement control, *Trans Ophthal Soc UK* 105:599, 1986.
16. Daroff RB, Hoyt WF: Supranuclear disorders of ocular control systems in man: clinical, anatomical and physiological correlations. In Bach-Y-Rita P, Collins CC, Hyde JE, eds: *The control of eye movements*, New York, 1971, Academic Press, 222-247.
17. Keane JR: Ocular skew deviation: analysis of 100 cases, *Arch Neurol* 32:186-188, 1975.
18. Zackon DH, Sharpe JA: Midbrain paresis of horizontal gaze, *Ann Neurol* 16:495-499, 1984.
19. Cogan DG: Internuclear ophthalmoplegia: typical and atypical, *Arch Ophthalmol* 40:587-588, 1970.

20. Muri RM, Meienberg O: The clinical spectrum of internuclear ophthalmoplegia in multiple sclerosis, *Arch Neurol* 42:851-853, 1985.
21. Crane JB, Yee RD, Baloh RW, Hapler R: Analysis of characteristic eye movement abnormalities in internuclear ophthalmoplegia, *Arch Ophthalmol* 101:209-210, 1983.
22. McGaitrick P, Eustace P: The WEBINO syndrome, *Neuro Ophthalmol* 5:109-111, 1985.
23. Zee DS, Hain TO, Carl JR: Abduction deficit in internuclear ophthalmoplegia, *Ann Neurol* 21:383-385, 1967.
24. Wall M, Wrat SH: The one-and-one-half syndrome: a unilateral disorder of the pontine tegmentum—a study of 20 cases and a review of the literature, *Neurology* 33:971-980, 1983.
25. Buttner-Ennever JA, Buttner U, Cohen B, Baumgartner G: Vertical gaze paralysis and the rostral interstitial nucleus of the medial longitudinal fasciculus, *Brain* 105:125-143, 1982.
26. Piernot-Dessilligny CH, Chain F, Gray F, et al: Parinaud's syndrome, *Brain* 105:667-668, 1982.
27. Susac JO, Hoyt WF: Inferior branch palsy of the ocular motor nerve, *Ann Neurol* 2(4):336-339, 1977.
28. Wilson-Pauwals L, Akesson EJ, Stewart PA. In *Cranial nerves—anatomy and clinical comments,* Philadelphia, 1988, BC Decker, 6-58.
29. Miller NR: *Walsh and Hoyt's clinical neuro-opthalmology,* Baltimore, 1985, Williams & Wilkins, 559-784.
30. Goldstein J, Cogan D: Diabetic ophthalmoplegia with special reference to the pupil, *Arch Ophthalmol* 64:592-596, 1960.
31. Raulen JPH, Sanders EACM, Hogenhuis LAH: Eye movement disorders in multiple sclerosis and optic neuritis, *Brain* 106:127-140, 1983.

5

The Eyelid and Neuro-ocular Disease

Andrew S. Gurwood

Key Terms

orbicularis oculi	neurogenic ptosis	Graves'
muscles of Müller	blepharospasm	ophthalmopathy
Marcus Gunn	apraxia of lid	Dalrymple's sign
jaw-winking	opening	von Graefe's sign
myogenic ptosis	lid retraction	Collier's sign
chronic progressive		
external		
ophthalmoplegia		

The eyelid, with its complicated anatomic structure and plethora of integrated neurologic connections, can serve as an indicator of impending, beginning, or advancing neurologic disease. Patients who present with eyelid dysfunction, whether by symptomatology or by clinical observation, warrant special attention.

This chapter explores eyelid dysfunction as it relates to neurologic disease and begins by discussing the pertinent eyelid anatomy relevant to normal neurologic function. Subsequently, a selection of neurologic and neuro-ocular diseases that manifest in the eyelid is presented. The disease entities are categorized in a logical fashion so that the clinician can integrate eyelid neuropathy with other aspects of neuro-ocular disease. Data collection and laboratory testing are

127

stressed so that the optometrist can establish the differential diagnosis and participate in the management of these entities.

Neuroanatomy of the Eyelid

The muscles of the eyelid consist of the orbicularis oculi, the aponeurosis of the levator palpebrae superioris (levator), and the palpebral muscles of Müller. The neural innervation consists of the facial nerve (CN VII), the oculomotor nerve (CN III), the sympathetics, and the sensory branches of the trigeminal nerve (CN V).

CLINICAL PEARL

The muscles of the eyelid consist of the orbicularis oculi, the aponeurosis of the levator palpebrae superioris (levator), and the palpebral muscles of Müller.

The orbicularis oculi is an oval sheet of concentric muscle fibers that covers the lids and the regions of the forehead and face around the orbital margin (Figure 5-1). The muscle mass is divided anatomically and functionally into an orbital part and a palpebral part. The orbital portion surrounds the orbital margin and the contiguous regions of the eyebrows, temple, and cheek. The palpebral portion forms two half-ellipses, one on each lid. This palpebral portion of the orbicularis oculi is further divided into a preseptal part, which overlies the orbital septum of the upper and lower lids, and a pretarsal part, which overlies the upper and lower tarsal plates. The pretarsal portion of the orbicularis oculi has four specialized components: the anterior lacrimal muscle (muscle of Gerlach), the pars lacrimalis (tensor tarsi muscle), the pars ciliaris (muscle of Riolan), and the pars subtarsalis.[1-4]

The overall function of the orbicularis oculi muscle is to close the eyelids. Its specific actions are variable, however, depending on which portion of the muscle is specifically brought into play. For example, the orbital portion of the orbicularis oculi functions to forcibly close the lids. The action is voluntary and purposive. The palpebral portion of the muscle functions alone in gentle eyelid closure as in sleeping or blinking. Its action is largely involuntary. The upper portion of the preseptal orbicularis oculi is the main depressor of the upper lid, whereas the lower portion is the main elevator of the lower lid. Contraction of the upper and lower preseptal muscles expands the lacrimal sac. Contraction of the upper and lower pretarsal muscles narrows the lacrimal ampullae and shortens the canaliculi. The

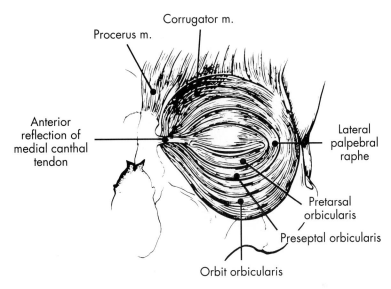

Procerus m.

Corrugator m.

Anterior
reflection of
medial canthal
tendon

Lateral
palpebral
raphe

Pretarsal
orbicularis

Preseptal orbicularis

Orbit orbicularis

FIGURE 5-1 The orbital portion of the orbicularis oculi surrounds the orbital margin and the contiguous regions of the eyebrows, temple, and cheek. The palpebral portion forms two half-ellipses, one on each lid. (From McCord CD Jr: Surgery of the eyelids. In Tasman W, Jaeger EA, eds: *Duane's clinical ophthalmology,* vol 5, chap 5, Philadelphia, 1990, JB Lippincott. Reprinted by permission of JB Lippincott, 1990.)

marginal muscle of Riolan keeps the lids in close apposition to the globe in all its movements.[1-4]

The levator muscle originates from the apex of the orbit above the annulus of Zinn. It runs forward under the roof of the orbit lying on the superior rectus. A short distance behind the orbital septum, the levator assumes the form of an expanded aponeurosis. The tendinous sheet of the levator courses forward between the superior orbital margin and the globe and enters the lid above the tarsal plate (Figure 5-2). The essential function of the levator muscle is to elevate the upper lid. The eyelid may be indirectly elevated by the frontalis muscle, however. This muscle covers the frontal surface of the scalp, inserts into the skin of the eyebrow, and interdigitates with the superior orbital portions of the orbicularis oculi. The frontalis elevates the eyebrow, an action that subsequently elevates the upper eyelid.[1-4]

The palpebral muscles of Müller consist of two small sheets of smooth muscle fibers, one in each lid. The superior palpebral muscle arises from the under surface of the levator. It courses downward and forward between the levator and the conjunctiva and inserts onto the upper margin of the tarsal plate. The inferior palpebral muscle arises from the fascial sheet of the inferior rectus. It courses upward toward

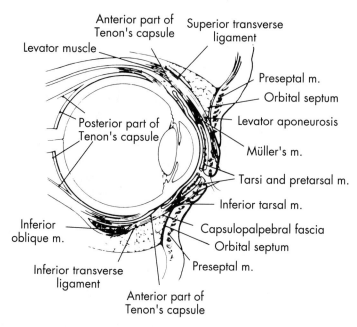

Anterior part of
Tenon's capsule

Superior transverse
ligament

Levator muscle

Preseptal m.

Orbital septum

Levator aponeurosis

Posterior part of
Tenon's capsule

Müller's m.

Tarsi and pretarsal m.

Inferior tarsal m.

Inferior
oblique m.

Capsulopalpebral fascia

Orbital septum

Preseptal m.

Inferior transverse
ligament

Anterior part of
Tenon's capsule

FIGURE 5-2 The tendinous sheet of the levator courses forward between the superior orbital margin and the globe and enters the lid above the tarsal plate. (From McCord CD Jr: Surgery of the eyelids. In Tasman W, Jaeger EA, eds: *Duane's clinical ophthalmology,* vol 5, chap 5, Philadelphia, 1990, JB Lippincott. Reprinted by permission of JB Lippincott, 1990.)

the lower fornix and inserts onto the bulbar conjunctiva and, along with the sheath of the inferior rectus, onto the tarsal plate. The superior palpebral muscle accessorizes the levator in initiating lid elevation and maintaining upper lid tonus. The inferior palpebral muscle is thought to assist the inferior rectus muscle in retracting the lower lid.[1-4]

The orbicularis oculi is innervated by the temporal and zygomatic branches of the facial nerve (CN VII). The frontalis is innervated by the temporal branch of CN VII. The levator is innervated by the superior branch of the oculomotor nerve (CN III). The palpebral muscles of Müller are innervated by the sympathetics derived from the cavernous plexus. The sensory innervation to the upper lid is derived from the supraorbital branch of the ophthalmic division of the CN V. The sensory innervation to the lower lid is by the infraorbital branch of the maxillary division of CN V.[1-4]

The vertical height of the palpebral aperture averages 10 mm. The width of the palpebral aperture measures approximately 32 mm. The upper lid margin usually lies 1 to 2 mm below the superior limbus. The normal position of the globe within the socket measures from 15 to 24 mm by Hertel exophthalmometry.[5-8]

Anatomic Variations

Anatomic variations in the bony structure of the orbit can result in variations in the configuration of the lids and palpebral apertures. Race-related, upward displacement of the temporal canthi (mongoloid obliquity) is a normal anatomic variation with no pathologic significance.[9] Downward displacement of the temporal canthi (antimongoloid obliquity) is another nonpathologic anomaly that is often observed in African-Americans. Mongoloid and antimongoloid obliquities may be noted in certain hereditary systemic syndromes, however, such as Jacob's syndrome, Laurence-Moon-Biedl syndrome, Down syndrome, craniofacial dysotosis, cri du chat syndrome, and Turner's syndrome.[9,10]

Eyelid Neuropathies

When considering neuro-ocular disease that affects the eyelids, one must remember that the fundamental motor actions of the lids alter their position. Thus the lids may be opened, causing a widening of the palpebral fissure, or closed, causing a narrowing of the palpebral fissure. Any lesion that affects the salient lid musculature, whether directly or through the myoneural junction, or impinges on CN III, CN VII, or the sympathetics, influences these motor functions and affects the position of the eyelids. Moreover, lesions in the brain stem or cavernous sinus that result in eyelid neuropathies also might impact other neural structures. Analyzing the signs and symptoms associated with eyelid dysfunction may serve to localize the site of the lesion.

Ptosis

Ptosis (blepharoptosis) is defined as a drooping of the upper eyelid. This downward displacement may be caused by a dysfunction of the lid elevators or by a weighting of the lid by extra mass added to its substance. Ptosis may be broadly classified into two categories, congenital and acquired.

Congenital Ptosis

Congenital ptosis is usually unilateral and results from a developmental dystrophy of the levator.[11,12] Patients with congenital ptosis may have other associated signs such as oculomotor dysfunctions, Marcus Gunn jaw-winking, aberrant connection of CN III to the lateral rectus muscle (Duane's retraction syndrome), strabismus, and rarely, Horner's syndrome (see the box on p. 132). Congenital ptosis also may be transient. Children born of mothers who have myasthenia gravis (MG) may have a congenital ptosis that only lasts for several weeks.[13] This temporary ptosis occurs because of the passage of antibodies across the placenta against acetylcholine (ACh) receptors. Myasthenia gravis is discussed in greater detail in another section.

CLINICAL PEARL

Children born of mothers who have myasthenia gravis (MG) may have a congenital ptosis that only lasts for several weeks. This temporary ptosis occurs because of the passage of antibodies across the placenta against acetylcholine (ACh) receptors.

Congenital Ptosis and Its Associated Signs

Unilateral as a rule
Usually from developmental dystrophy of levator
Patients often present with oculomotor dysfunctions
Rule out Marcus Gunn jaw-winking phenomenon
Rule out aberrant cranial nerve III connection to lateral rectus (Duane's retraction syndrome)
May result from strabismus
Horner's syndrome (rare)
Transient congenital ptosis of infants born to mothers with MG

The jaw-wink phenomenon is a particularly curious but benign congenital affectation. First described by Marcus Gunn as maxillo-palpebral synkinesis in 1883, the jaw-wink phenomenon represents an anomalous innervation of the motor component of the CN V.[14] This motor nerve normally innervates the muscles of mastication. In certain patients, however, the nerve also sends fascicles to the ipsilateral levator. In the typical situation, the patient presents with a congenital ptosis. As the patient opens his or her mouth, the lid tends to elevate. As the patient moves his or her jaw to the opposite side, the lid elevates to a greater degree. When the patient closes his or her mouth, the lid returns to its ptotic position (Figure 5-3). Atypical presentations include elevation of the lid on protrusion of the jaw or tongue, or on sucking, smiling, or clenching of the teeth.

Acquired Ptosis

Acquired ptosis is usually subdivided into four categories: mechanical, myogenic, neurogenic, and traumatic. The clinician should understand that any acquired ptosis may result from more than one condition.

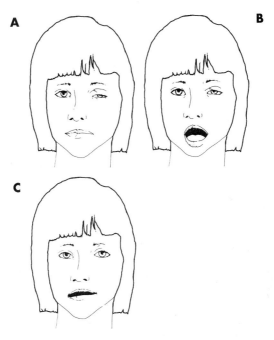

FIGURE 5-3 Marcus Gunn jaw-winking. **A**, Note ptosis. **B**, As patient opens her mouth, the lid elevates. **C**, As the patient moves her jaw to the opposite side, the lid elevates to a greater degree.

CLINICAL PEARL

Acquired ptosis is usually subdivided into four categories: mechanical, myogenic, neurogenic, and traumatic.

Mechanical ptosis

Mechanical ptosis was described by Beard[15] as being secondary to conditions that add mass to the lid and increase its weight or interrupt the lid motility as a result of scarring. Generally, the elements that cause mechanical ptosis result in a lid deformity.[16] This sign can aid the clinician in establishing the diagnosis.

Benign lid tumors such as hordeola, chalazia, and neurofibromas, or malignant neoplasms such as squamous cell carcinoma, basal cell carcinoma, and malignant melanomas are examples of weight-producing lid lesions. Lid edema secondary to a focal allergic reaction from a contact allergen also may produce a mechanical ptosis due to an increase in lid mass. Infectious processes such as preseptal cellulitis may thicken the lid or cause scarring, which interferes with its motility. Other causes of mechanical ptosis include dermatochalasis, blepharochalasis, and cicatrix. Dermatochalasis occurs in older adults and involves the herniation of orbital fat into the lids through a dehiscence in the orbital septum. Blepharochalasis occurs in children and manifests as a loss of elasticity and tone of the levator aponeurosis as well as a redundancy of lid tissue from repeated lid swellings. Cicatricial ptosis results from an ocular pemphigoid scar or a scar from lid surgery.[17,18] The box below summarizes the causes of mechanical ptosis.

Summary of Causes for Mechanical Ptosis

1. May be secondary to any condition adding mass to the upper eyelid
   Hordeola
   Chalazia
   Neurofibroma
   Neoplasm
   Squamous, basal cell, or other malignant melanoma
2. Lid edema
   Focal allergic response
   Infectious mass, i.e., preseptal cellulitis
3. Lid anomalies or deformities
   Blepharochalasis
   Cicatricial ptosis, i.e., from pemphigoid scarring
   Scarring from eyelid surgery

The clinician may be able to eliminate a mechanical ptosis by dealing with the underlying cause. Removal of the offending allergen usually results in the diminution of the lid edema in a focal allergic reaction. Hot compresses and topical antibiotics most often result in complete resolution of an internal hordeolum. If a chalazion does not shrink with a regimen of hot compresses, intralesional injections with triamcinolone or surgical excision will eliminate the mass. Preseptal cellulitis is best managed by systemic antibiotics such as penicillin or erythromycin.[19]

Neurofibromas are benign, soft lesions that represent sequelae of von Recklinghausen's disease. They are often associated with yellow-tan spots on the skin known as café-au-lait spots.[20] Surgical excision usually is successful in restoring normal lid configuration and function. The malignant tumors usually are found in adults. The potentially extensive nature of these lesions mandates referral to an oculoplastics specialist for surgical removal. Dermatochalasis, blepharochalasis, and cicatricial ptosis are also best managed by the oculoplastics surgeon.

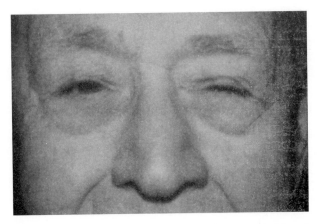

FIGURE 5-4 Senile ptosis. This defect probably is due to a dehiscence of the levator aponeurosis.

Myogenic ptosis

Myogenic ptosis most often is caused by defects within the levator or its tendon. Loss of tone within the superior palpebral muscle of Müller, however, may be contributory.

Senile involutional ptosis is the most common cause of isolated, nonmyasthenic myogenic ptosis.[15,17,21] This defect is thought to be due to a disinsertion or dehiscence of the levator aponeurosis that occurs with age (Figure 5-4). The lid droop is exacerbated by a loss of tone of the superior Müller's muscle. This type of ptosis may range from being very mild to being severe enough to cause a functional or cosmetic disturbance. Surgical correction may have to be considered.

In the presence of normal pupils, MG is always suspect as the cause of acquired myogenic ptosis. Myasthenia gravis is a disorder of skeletal muscle rather than smooth muscle, a fact that explains the sparing of the pupil in this disorder. Specifically, the ACh receptors on the motor end plate of the skeletal muscle receptor are blocked or degraded by circulating antibodies. Some studies have shown a reduction in functional receptor sites of as much as 60%.[22,23] Myasthenia gravis and thyroid disease are often associated together because of the immunologic origin common to both disorders. Circulating antithyroid antibodies have been found in 30% to 40% of all patients with MG, and thyroid function tests should be performed on these patients.[22-24]

CLINICAL PEARL

In the presence of normal pupils, MG is always suspect as the cause of acquired myogenic ptosis. Myasthenia gravis is a disorder of skeletal muscle rather than smooth muscle, a fact that explains the sparing of the pupil in this disorder.

TABLE 5-1
Myasthenia Reference Table

Classification	Incidence	Onset	Signs/symptoms
1. Pediatric			
A. Neonatal	10% to 20% (+)* monitor MG	At birth	Resolution in 6 weeks
B. Congenital/juvenile	—	Birth through life	Severe ocular signs Mild generalized disease
2. Adult			
A. Ocular myasthenia	15% to 20% of all patients	Variable	Mild signs; good prognosis
B. Mild and generalized	—	Slow onset	Gradual skeletal muscle weakness Moderate response to medicines
C. Moderate and generalized	—	Slow onset	Slowly progressive; respiratory distress possible
D. Acute fulminating	—	Rapid onset	Severe generalized disease Severe signs occur in 6 months; high mortality; poor response to drugs
E. Late severe	—	Slow onset (>2 years)	Sudden onset of severe myasthenic symptoms

*In neonates whose mothers have a positive history for myasthenia gravis.
MG: myasthenia gravis.
Modified from Rodgin, SG: Ocular myasthenia gravis, *J Am Optom Assoc* 61:384-389, 1990.

Myasthenia gravis has an incidence of 2:20,000 in the general population, with a slight predilection for women when occurring before the age of 40. In women, it usually becomes manifest during the second decade. In men, the onset usually occurs after the age of 50. Ninety percent of all MG patients present with some ocular manifestation during the course of their disease. Ptosis is the initial sign in 75% of such patients. If the ocular signs remain isolated for longer than 2 years, it is unlikely that systemic MG will develop. Indeed, 20% of all MG patients only manifest ocular signs or symptoms.[23] These ocular myasthenics can be divided into pediatric and adult varieties (Table 5-1).

The reduction in functional receptor sites explains the abnormal fatigability of the extraocular muscles and skeletal muscles within the lid. The ocular motility defects that occur in MG may mimic an isolated extraocular muscle palsy or a supranuclear motility defect. The patient may complain of intermittent diplopia due to involvement of the medial rectus or superior rectus muscles, exhibit an apparent convergence or gaze defect, or manifest nystagmus. In addition to the levator weakness, which results in a variable and fatigable ptosis, the orbicularis oculi muscle may manifest intermittent weakness. A variable lagophthalmos may occur. These motility and lid phenomena may be minimal or absent when the patient awakens. As the day progresses, the muscular dysfunctions become more pronounced.

CLINICAL PEARL

In MG, the reduction in functional receptor sites explains the abnormal fatigability of the extraocular muscles and skeletal muscles within the lid.

In addition to ptosis, the patient may exhibit a contralateral lid retraction.[4,6,23,24] This apparently paradoxical lid retraction may be understood by the following explanation: The patient with a bilateral ptosis that is asymmetric may attempt to elevate the lids by using increased neurologic input to the levators or to the frontalis muscle. The eye with the greater ptosis will require greater neurologic input. By Hering's law of equal innervation, the increased neural input will be transmitted to the less impaired levator on the other side. This excessive innervation results in a lid retraction in the less involved eye. When the more ptotic lid is covered or manually lowered, the contralateral lid retraction disappears. If the more ptotic lid is elevated manually, the previously retracted lid may become more ptotic. This fall of the apparently retracted upper lid has been termed "enhanced ptosis" by Gorelick et al.[25]

The definitive diagnosis of MG is made by a positive response to the intravenous injection of edrophonium chloride (Tensilon test).[23] Small amounts of injected Tensilon (Roche Laboratories, Nutley, NJ) result in diminution of the ptosis or diplopia. The results are often equivocal and can be judged more accurately if performed in conjunction with electromyography or a red lens diplopia test. False negatives are often noted in the early stages of MG, and the Tensilon test should be repeated if suspicion still persists.

CLINICAL PEARL

The definitive diagnosis of MG is made by a positive response to the intravenous injection of edrophonium chloride (Tensilon test).

There are several chairside procedures that may be useful in diagnosing MG. A patient with MG often presents with a minimal ptosis that becomes marked if he or she sustains upgaze or blinks forcibly for several minutes. Sethi, Rivner, and Swift[26] describe an elegant test to diagnose MG by using an ice pack. An ice pack is held against the ptotic lid for 2 minutes so that the skin temperature is lowered to 29°C. The cooling results in an increased release of ACh and a decreased release of the enzyme that degrades ACh, acetylcholinesterase. Myasthenic ptosis thus decreases. Cogan[27] has described the lid-twitch sign as being characteristic of MG ptosis. When a saccade is made from downgaze to the primary position, the eyelid that is ptotic from MG overshoots upward and then drifts to its previous ptotic position.

Several treatment options may be of benefit to the MG patient. Oral pyridostigmine bromide (Mestinon [Roche Laboratories, Nutley, NJ]) acts to prevent the degradation of ACh within the neuromuscular junction. Systemic corticosteroids may be used alone or in conjunction with Mestinon to mitigate the attack on the ACh receptors by the circulating antibody. In isolated, ocular MG, steroids are used alone and tend to relieve symptoms in as many as 80% of patients.[22] Chest x rays or computed tomography scans should be administered to detect enlargements or masses within the thymus gland. Oosterhuis[28] notes that 10% to 20% of MG patients demonstrate an enlarged thymus gland due to hyperplasia or thymoma. Moreover, removal of the thymus mass often results in a remission of the disease. A ptosis crutch and Fresnel press-on prisms may be palliative until the steroids take effect.

CLINICAL PEARL

In isolated, ocular MG, steroids are used alone and tend to relieve symptoms in as many as 80% of patients.

Finally, the MG patient should avoid certain antibacterial drugs. The aminoglycosides (gentamycin, tobramycin, neomycin, polymyxin) have a curare-like effect on the myoneural junction and may exacerbate the ptosis or diplopia. Other drugs that might induce symptoms in the myasthenic patient include beta-blockers, phenothiazines, alcohol, quinine derivatives, and penicillamine.[29-33]

If the diagnosis of MG is untenable in a patient who presents with ptosis, ocular motility disturbances, and normal pupils, other causes must be considered. Specifically, the ptosis may be due to a generalized myopathy of the muscles of the lid or a pupil-sparing CN III palsy. The latter pathology is discussed in Chapter 1.

Chronic progressive external ophthalmoplegia (CPEO) is a broad category of myopathies that have in common the development of a slowly progressive, generally symmetric, external ophthalmoplegia. Some authors believe the CPEO is a clinical sign and not a distinct nosologic entity.[24,34] Bilateral, slowly progressive ptosis is an early sign in the CPEO diseases and may precede the ophthalmoparesis by months or years.

Other myopathies, which are variants of CPEO, manifest the ptosis and external ophthalmoplegia but have additional signs and symptoms. Kearns-Sayre syndrome is characterized by progressive external ophthalmoplegia and ptosis along with atypical retinitis pigmentosa and heart block. Myotonic dystrophy has an associated muscle wasting throughout the body as well as in the face. Other stigmata include an inability to release a hand grip, defective swallowing, polychromatic cataracts, and pigmentary changes in the retina.[24]

Neurogenic ptosis

Neurogenic ptosis usually is caused by a CN III deficit to the levator or a sympathetic innervational deficit to the superior palpebral muscle of Müller. Usually the lower motor neurons are compromised, but a bilateral cerebral ptosis has been reported by Lepore.[35] The patients in his series had sustained acute hemispheric damage that resulted in a compromise to the supranuclear innervation to the levator nuclear complex.

CLINICAL PEARL

Neurogenic ptosis usually is caused by a CN III deficit to the levator or a sympathetic innervational deficit to the superior palpebral muscle of Müller.

In cases of newly acquired unilateral ptosis, the size and reactivity of the ipsilateral pupil usually establish whether the cause is CN III involvement or sympathetic deficit. Cranial nerve III palsies from trauma or compressive lesions such as aneurysms or neoplasms result in a complete ptosis with a mydriatic, nonresponsive pupil. Extraocular muscle palsies also are present, and the eye is postured in a down-and-out position (see Chapter 1). Ophthalmoplegic migraine is a rare disorder, occurring in children under age 10, that may produce a similar presentation (see Chapter 9). Ischemic CN III palsies from diabetes, hypertension, or atherosclerosis produce ptosis and ocular muscle abnormalities, but spare the pupil.

Sudden, acquired CN III ptosis mandates further study to establish cause. If the pupil is involved, aneurysm is suspect, and neuroimaging, cerebral spinal fluid studies, and cerebral angiography are indicated. If the patient is more than 40 years old, and the pupil is spared, the patient should be tested for diabetes and hypertension. Elderly patients should have an erythrocyte sedimentation rate to rule out giant cell arteritis.

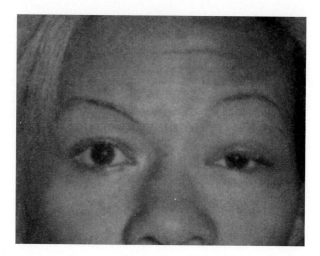

FIGURE 5-5 Traumatic ptosis caused by preseptal cellulitis.

Lesions involving the ocular sympathetics cause a partial ptosis, with retention of the lid fold, and pupillary miosis. Facial anhydrosis may be present if the lesion impacts the sympathetics proximal to the carotid bifurcation. This combination of signs defines the Horner's syndrome (see Chapter 3).

Traumatic ptosis

Traumatic ptosis results from damage to the levator or its tendon by trauma, inflammation, or tumor infiltration. As with mechanical ptosis, the lid is usually deformed as a result of the trauma (Figure 5-5).

One of the more common varieties of traumatic ptosis seen in the optometrist's office is that caused by an entrapped contact lens. The contact lens can migrate to the upper fornix and penetrate the conjunctiva. A granulomatous reaction may occur around the lens, resulting in a ptosis. Double eversion of the upper lid and careful inspection of the superior fornix usually will disclose the foreign body.

The optometrist also may encounter traumatic ptosis in patients who wear hard contact lenses. The removal of the hard contact lens usually is accomplished by the patient's tugging at the lateral canthus of the lids. This repeated, lateral, mechanical pull on the levator and pretarsal orbicularis at its juncture with the tarsal plate may disinsert and disrupt the flimsy attachments of the levator aponeurosis. Ptosis can result.

Traumatic ptosis may occur after blepharoplastic surgery or other common ophthalmic surgical procedures. The levator muscle–aponeurosis complex may become damaged from deep dissection into the upper eyelid, by the placement of a lid speculum, or by excessive manipulation of the superior rectus muscle with subsequent trauma to the levator.[36]

Pseudoptosis

Pseudoptosis includes those pathologic or anomalous lid affectations that mimic true ptosis but do not involve actual pathology to the lid elevators or contribute to excessive lid mass. The most common causes of pseudoptosis are blepharospasm, apraxia of lid opening, and illusory ptosis due to contralateral lid retraction.

CLINICAL PEARL

The most common causes of pseudoptosis are blepharospasm, apraxia of lid opening, and illusory ptosis due to contralateral lid retraction.

Blepharospasm

Blepharospasm is a voluntary or involuntary lowering of the upper lid brought about by forceful contraction of the orbicularis muscle. There is always an associated elevation of the lower lid and lowering of the brow (Figure 5-6).[37] The blepharospasm may be secondary to ocular irritation from keratitis, scleritis, uveitis, or other types of anterior segment inflammation or by meningeal inflammation (meningitis, subarachnoid hemorrhage). These patients can almost always open their eyes, however briefly, on command.

In the absence of ocular or meningeal inflammatory signs, the blepharospasm may be secondary to facial contracture after facial nerve palsy. The most common cause of facial nerve (CN VII)

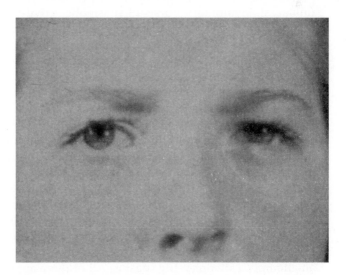

FIGURE 5-6 Blepharospasm of the left eye. Note the elevation of the lower lid and lowering of the brow.

disorders is Bell's palsy,[38] an acute peripheral facial palsy of unknown cause. In the recovery phase of the lower motor neuron facial palsy, the facial muscles on the involved side may become slightly contracted, resulting in a narrowing of the palpebral fissure. The contracture may be enhanced when the patient contracts the other facial muscles during pursing of the lips or smiling.

In cases of blepharospasm and facial weakness but no history of previous facial nerve palsy, the blepharospasm may be due to spastic-paretic facial contracture. The clinician should particularly look for superimposed vermiform (wormlike) movements of the orbicularis oculi and other facial muscles. These undulating movements are known as pathologic myokymia, and, when associated with ipsilateral tonic facial contracture and facial weakness, are pathognomic of spastic-paretic facial contracture.[39,40] The most common causes of spastic-paretic facial contracture are pontine neoplasms and compression of the medulla by tumor. It should be noted that myokymia and facial contracture may be complications of multiple sclerosis. The facial contracture and myokymia, however, are not accompanied by significant facial weakness. In addition, the facial contracture associated with multiple sclerosis usually remits in several months, whereas spastic-paretic facial contracture usually progresses.[40-44]

Pathologic facial myokymia should be differentiated from benign eyelid myokymia. Benign myokymia occurs in otherwise healthy patients and is characterized as a fine twitching of the upper and lower eyelids on one side. Episodes may last from hours to days and are usually secondary to fatigue, excessive coffee drinking, or anxiety.

Unilateral blepharospasm, in the absence of facial nerve palsy, may be due to hemifacial spasm. This condition is characterized by unilateral, involuntary bursts of spasmotic activity in the orbicularis oculi and other facial muscles. These spasms have no clear-cut precipitants, are usually brief, and may persist during sleep. The patients typically have no signs of facial weakness or pathologic myokymia and no evidence of epilepsy.[43]

Gardener and Sava[45] postulate that the CN VII is compressed by a stiff and tortuous cerebral vessel at its exit from the brain stem. Subsequently, an irritability and spontaneous firing occur. Neural impulses from damaged axons spread laterally and excite adjacent nerve fibers (ephaptic transmission). Thus impulses flowing in one direction set off similar neuronal firings in adjacent fibers, leading to spontaneous and simultaneous contraction of adjacent facial muscles. The treatment for hemifacial spasm ranges from suboccipital craniotomy and the placement of a sponge between the facial nerve and the offending artery to the use of oral carbamazepine (Tegretol [Geigy Pharmaceuticals, Ardsley, NY]) and injection of botulinum A toxin in an attempt to attenuate the spasms. All of these approaches have had some measure of success.[45]

Bilateral blepharospasm, in the absence of irritative external ocular disease or facial muscle weakness, may be associated with Parkinson's disease, myotonic dystrophy, Gilles de la Tourette's disease, Huntington's chorea, tardive dyskinesia, or Meiges' syndrome. All of these clinical entities have other neurologic signs and symptoms in addition to the bilateral blepharospasm. A large group of older patients remains who manifest bilateral blepharospasm or facial grimacing with no other associated neurologic stigmata. These patients are considered to have idiopathic (essential) blepharospasm. There appears to be a psychogenic substrate to this limited form of blepharospasm.[37]

Apraxia of Lid Opening

Apraxia of lid opening is the inability to voluntarily open the eyes despite normal functioning of the muscles and nerves that subserve lid opening. Lid opening may be accomplished by thrusting the head backward or by lifting the lid with the finger. This condition is not related to blepharospasm and displays no concomitant contraction of the orbicularis oculi muscle. Rather, these patients often have a supranuclear disorder such as Parkinson's disease, progressive supranuclear palsy, or frontal lobe disease.[9,46]

Illusory Ptosis Due to Contralateral Lid Retraction

Subtle lid retraction of one upper lid may create the illusion of ptosis of the other lid. The apparently normal lid is positioned above the superior limbus so that superior sclera is visible. This abnormal position is pathognomic of lid retraction and implies that the other lid is not truly ptotic.

CLINICAL PEARL

Subtle lid retraction of one upper lid may create the illusion of ptosis of the other lid.

Lid Retraction

The upper lid margin normally lies just below the superior limbus. Any sclera visible between the superior limbus and the upper lid is considered to be abnormal, and the abnormally elevated lid is said to be retracted (Figure 5-7). Lid retraction may occur in a variety of conditions (see the box on p. 144).

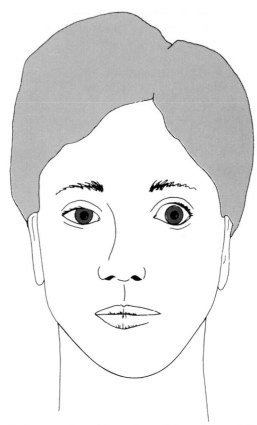

FIGURE 5-7 Lid retraction. Note the white sclera visible above the left limbus.

Etiologies of Lid Retraction

1. Pseudo-lid retraction
   A. May result from unilateral exophthalmos
      Unilateral orbital mass
      Congenital glaucoma (buphthalmos)
      Small orbit
   B. Parietal contralateral ptosis with Hering's and Sherrington's laws causing a lid retraction on the opposite side due to exerted efforts to raise the ptotic lid
2. True lid retraction
   A. Thyroid eye disease is the most common etiology (Dalrymple's sign)
   B. Other etiologies include: abnormal scarring, fibrosis, or innervational contracture of the lid elevators

Pseudo-lid retraction may result from an abnormally widened interpalpebral aperture due to excessive bulging of the globe. The excessive protrusion is usually due to an orbital mass but may reflect a unilateral, congenital glaucoma (buphthalmos) or an abnormally configured orbit. Another manifestation of pseudo-lid retraction is that which often accompanies partial ptosis. In cases of partial ptosis, the contralateral lid may be relatively retracted because of an increased effort to overcome the ptosis. According to Hering's law of equal and opposite innervation, the excessive innervation required to elevate the ptotic lid is transferred to the nonptotic lid. If the ptotic eye is occluded or the ptotic lid is mechanically raised, the contralateral retraction subsides.[23]

True lid retraction is most often caused by either abnormal cicatricial fibrosis or innervational contraction of the lid elevators. Thyroid eye disease is the most common cause.[47]

Thyroid Eye Disease

Thyroid eye disease (Graves' disease, Graves' ophthalmopathy, dysthyroid orbitopathy) is most commonly found in persons with a strong familial history of thyroid dysfunction. Women are generally affected more than men by a ratio of 2.3 to 1.[48] Invariably, the patients indicate a previous history of hyperthyroidism with clinical manifestations of thyrotoxicosis (diarrhea, tachycardia, anxiety, tremor, weight loss, and intolerance to heat). The eye signs, however, are independent of the level of thyroid activity, and the patient may be euthyroid or hypothyroid and still manifest significant thyroid eye disease. An autoimmune mechanism is the most likely explanation of the ophthalmopathy.[47]

The principal signs of Graves' ophthalmopathy are lid retraction (Dalrymple's sign), proptosis, edema of the lid and conjunctiva, and diplopia. Secondarily, corneal exposure leading to drying and compressive optic neuropathy may occur. Werner[49] has classified the clinical manifestations of thyroid eye disease (Tables 5-2 and 5-3). The optometrist can participate in the management of these patients in the early stages of their disease.

CLINICAL PEARL

The principal signs of Graves' ophthalmopathy are lid retraction (Dalrymple's sign), proptosis, edema of the lid and conjunctiva, and diplopia.

TABLE 5-2

Werner's Classification of Thyroid Eye Disease

Numerical class	Pneumonic letter	Definition
0	N	No signs, no symptoms
1	O	Only signs, no symptoms
2	S	Soft tissue involvement
3	P	Proptosis
4	E	Extraocular muscle involvement
5	C	Corneal involvement
6	S	Sight loss secondary to optic nerve involvement

TABLE 5-3

Thyroid Eye Disease Quick Reference

Class	Signs and symptoms	Treatment
0	No ocular signs. Patients may under go weight loss with increased appetite, nervousness, palpitation, tachycardia at rest, and systolic hypertension.	Referral to GP for blood work. Rule out systemic hypertension, diabetes. No ocular modalities.
1	Systemically, patients may suffer from increased anxiety. Ocularly, mild periorbital edema, startled or staring look. Mild corneal stippling inferiorly.	Copious artificial tear solutions and ointments. Monitor for progression.
2	Lid retraction (Darymple's sign), increased stare, possibly unilateral proptosis, lid lag (von Graefe's sign), dry eye with gritty sensation, more corneal compromise.	Copious artificial tear solutions and ointments. More ointment may now be necessary. Supportive patient education. Consult GP for possibility of initiating systemic therapy.
3	Proptosis, positive > 22 mm, increased lid retraction. Restrictive myopathy; positive forced duction test. Difficulty everting eyelid (Gifford's sign). Decreased blink posture (Stellwag's sign).	Copious artificial tear solutions and ointments. Depending on the severity of the blink posture, moisture chamber patches, blindfolds, or lid taping may be required.
4	Extraocular muscle involvement increases. More restriction leads to intermittent diplopia, which is slowly progressive. Positive forced duction testing. IOP rises by 4 mm or more upon upward gaze. Positive "30 degree" test on A-B-scan.	Referral to GP to initiate systemic corticosteroid therapy, 40 to 80 mg daily. Fresnel press-on prisms or occlusive therapy to eliminate diplopia. Consider partial surgical removal of thyroid.
5	Corneal epithelium is compromised and threatened by proptosis. Ulceration is possible. Severe dryness.	More corneal support. May require antibiotic ointments. If dryness threatens to provoke permanent visual disability, consider tarsorraphy. May try increased steroid dosage, 40 to 100 mg.
6	Compressive sight loss secondary to orbital congestion. Central, paracentral, and arcuate scotomata apparent.	Surgical innervation required. Supervoltage orbital irradiation, 1600 to 2000 rads directed toward the orbital apex. Orbital decompression as a last resort, Krönlean, Ogura, or two wall procedures (Leone et al[16]).

GP: general practitioner; IOP: intraocular pressure.

The cause of the lid retraction is not completely understood. It is thought that initially the retraction is due to excessive sympathetic innervation to Müller's muscle.[47] Subsequently, Müller's muscle as well as the levator become infiltrated with lymphocytes, macrophages, mast cells, and excessive mucopolysaccharides, leading to enlargement and fibrotic contracture. As a consequence of the lid retraction, the patient may manifest a "stare" appearance and give the illusion of proptosis even if none is present. In addition, the upper lid may lag in following the eye as it moves into downgaze (von Graefe's sign). Other eyelid signs that may accompany Graves' disease are tremor of the closed lid (Rosenbach's sign) and infrequent blinking (Stellwag's sign). Finally, the congestion and fibrosis in the lid makes eversion of the lid very difficult (Gifford's sign).

The diplopia that occurs in Graves' ophthalmopathy stems from the infiltration of the extraocular muscles, particularly the inferior rectus and medial rectus. The subsequent fibrosis and enlargement of the muscles, which can be visualized with computed tomography, magnetic imaging, or ultrasonography, create a tautness that results in a tethering of the globe. If the inferior rectus is involved, upward rotation of the globe is restricted. If the medial rectus is involved, an abduction deficit will result. The presence of a mechanical restriction affecting the extraocular muscles may be confirmed by the forced duction test (see Chapter 4 for a more complete discussion).

Lid retraction is an important component of the dorsal midbrain syndrome (Parinaud's syndrome, sylvian aqueduct syndrome).[50] The lid retraction is usually bilateral (Collier's sign) with no retraction in downgaze as in dysthyroid orbitopathy. Other pathognomic findings include mid-dilated pupils that are fixed to light but reactive to near-effort, supranuclear upgaze paresis with retraction-convergence nystagmus when upgaze is attempted, and convergence dysfunction. The most common cause is tumor of the pineal gland with subsequent compression of the structures contiguous to the cerebral aqueduct.

Workup and Management of Lid Dysfunction

The clinical evaluation of lid dysfunction requires deliberate, intuitive history-taking and exquisite observation with precise measurements of lid position, ocular motility, pupil function, and visual status.

The clinician must first decide whether the ptosis or lid retraction is real or apparent. As mentioned, the appearance of lid retraction on one side actually may represent an attempt by the patient to correct a ptosis on the other side. Similarly, the appearance of a ptosis on one side may be illusory because of a lid retraction contralaterally. Moreover, the clinician must carefully evaluate for the masqueraders of abnormal lid function (e.g., proptosis, blepharospasm, and apraxia of lid opening).

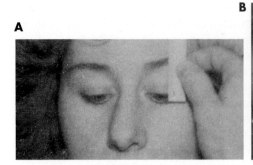
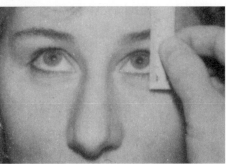

FIGURE 5-8 A, The patient is instructed to look down so that the ruler may be zeroed on the upper lid margin. **B**, The patient is instructed to look up. The amount of lid excursion of one eye is compared to that of the other eye.

A thorough history then must be elicited. The optometrist should inquire particularly about the time of onset and whether the abnormal lid position waxes and wanes. A review of old photographs may be helpful in this regard. Other important considerations are the current state of the patient's general and ocular health, a history of past ocular injury, past and present medications, the presence of lid dysfunction in family members, and a history of diplopia, transient visual loss, or other visual anomalies.

A careful examination must be performed to determine if an abnormal lid position is unilateral or bilateral. The absence or reduction of the lid fold with the eyes in primary gaze implies diminished integrity of the levator. A specific maneuver can be performed, however, to quantify the degree of levator function in each eye. The technique is as follows: A millimeter rule is placed in front of the eyes. Any accessory elevation being supplied to the lid is eliminated by applying downward pressure to the frontalis muscle. The patient is instructed to look down so that the ruler may be zeroed on the upper lid margin. The patient then is instructed to look up (Figure 5-8). The amount of lid excursion of one eye is compared with its fellow. The superior rectus contributes approximately 2 mm to this value and must be subtracted to obtain an accurate assessment of pure levator function. Normal levator function varies between 13 and 15 mm, but an excursion of 8 mm or more is considered to be satisfactory. Orbicularis oculi function can be estimated by having the patient forcibly close the eyes against the examiner's resistance. Diminished strength may indicate a previous CN VII palsy or MG.

CLINICAL PEARL

The absence or reduction of the lid fold with the eyes in primary gaze implies diminished integrity of the levator.

If MG is suspect, the clinician should attempt to induce fatigue by the previously described clinical procedures or refer for Tensilon testing. If Graves' ophthalmopathy is suspected, the optometrist should look for enlarged extraocular muscles with orbital scans. Additionally, the patient's metabolic status can be evaluated by laboratory testing of triiodothyronine and thyroxine levels along with thyroid-stimulating hormone profiles.

The management of eyelid dysfunction is directed at eliminating the underlying cause and applying supportive, palliative treatment. The management of MG and thyroid eye disease has been discussed in previous sections. In the case of congenital ptosis, surgical treatment is usually delayed until the patient is 3 years old. If the ptosis is complete and threatens to cause occlusion amblyopia, however, surgery may be performed as early as 6 months of age. The surgical procedure chosen for the correction of any ptosis depends on the degree of levator function. Ptosis with moderate levator function is usually corrected by levator resection. If levator function is severely limited, frontalis suspension is the procedure of choice. Ptosis crutches may be considered when surgery is contraindicated or refused.

References

1. Goldberg, RA, Lufkin R, Farahani K, Wu JC, et al: Physiology of the lower eyelid retractors: tight linkage of the anterior capsulopalpebral fascia demonstrated using dynamic ultrafine surface coil MRI, *Ophthal Plast Reconstr Surg* 10(2):87-91, 1994.
2. Rathbun JE: *Eyelid surgery*, Boston, 1991, Little, Brown, 1-10.
3. Clemente CD: In Clemente CD, ed: *Gray's anatomy of the human body*, 1985, Philadelphia, 1985, Lea & Febiger, 1305-1312.
4. Aramideh M, Ongerboer-de-Visser BW, Koelman JH, Bour LJ, et al: Clinical and electromyographic features of levator palpebrae superioris muscle dysfunction in involuntary eyelid closure, *Mov Disord* 9(4):395-402, 1994.
5. Bosniak SL, ed: *Cosmetic blepharoplasty*, New York, 1990, Raven Press, 1-23.
6. Duane T, ed: Neuro-opthalmology and the orbit. In *Clinical ophthalmology*, Philadelphia, 1990, Harper & Row, 6-7.
7. Spalton DJ, Hitchings RA, Hunter PA, eds: *Atlas of clinical ophthalmology*, Philadelphia, 1984, JB Lippincott, 2·2-2·16.
8. Shorr N, Cohen M: Cosmetic blepharoplasty, *Ophthalmol Clin North Am* 4(1):17-33, 1991.
9. Roy FH, ed: *Ocular diagnosis*, ed 4, Philadelphia, 1989, Lea & Febiger, 4-113.
10. Nunery WR, Cepela M: Levator function in the evaluation and management of blepharoptosis, *Ophthalmol Clinics North Am* 4(1):1-15, 1991.
11. McCord CD: The evaluation and management of patients with ptosis, *Clin Plastic Surg* 15:169-184, 1988.
12. Berke RN: Congenital ptosis: a classification of two hundred cases, *Arch Ophthalmol* 41:188-197, 1949.
13. Drachman DB: Myasthenia gravis, *N Engl J Med* 298:136-140, 1978.
14. Eve RF: Pterygoid-levator synkinesis: the Marcus Gunn jaw winking phenomenon, *J Clin Neuro Ophthalmol* 7:61-62, 1987.
15. Beard C, ed: *Ptosis*, ed 2, St Louis, 1976, Mosby, 42-77.
16. Leone CR, Piest KL, Newman RJ: Medial and lateral wall decompression for thyroid ophthalmopathy, *Am J Ophthalmol* 108:160-166, 1989.

150 Ocular Manifestations of Neurologic Disease

17. Haskes LP, Oshinskie LJ: Transient acquired ptosis, *J Am Optom Assoc* 60:668-675, 1989.
18. Barresi BJ: Ocular assessment. In Barresi BJ, ed: *The manual of diagnosis for office practice*, Boston, 1984, Butterworth, 282-283.
19. Pavan-Langston D, ed: *Manual of ocular diagnosis and therapy*, Boston, 1991, Little, Brown, 339-340.
20. Yanoff M, Fine B, eds: *Ocular pathology*, ed 2, Philadelphia, 1982, Harper & Row, 33-34.
21. Pearl RM: Acquired ptosis: a re-examination of etiology and treatment, *Plast Reconstr Surg* 76:54-66, 1985.
22. Rodgin SE: Ocular and systemic myasthenia gravis, *J Am Optom Assoc* 61:384-389, 1990.
23. Kansu T, Subutay N: Lid retraction in myasthenia gravis, *J Clin Neuro Ophthalmol* 7(3):145-148, 1987.
24. Francis IC, Nicholson GA, Kappagoda MB: An evaluation of signs in ocular myasthenia gravis and correlation with acetylcholine receptor antibodies, *Aust N Z J Ophthalmol* 13:395-399, 1985.
25. Gorelick PB, Rosenberg M, Pagano RJ: Enhance ptosis in myasthenia gravis, *Arch Neurol* 38:531-534, 1981.
26. Sethi KD, Rivner MH, Swift TR: Ice pack test for myasthenia gravis, *Neurology* 37:1383-1384, 1987.
27. Cogan DG: Myasthenia gravis: a review of the disease and description of lid twitch as a characteristic sign, *Arch Ophthalmol* 74:217-221, 1965.
28. Oosterhuis HJ: The ocular signs and symptoms of myasthenia gravis, *Doc Ophthalmol* 52:363-378, 1982.
29. Martens EL, Ansink BJ: A myasthenia-like syndrome and polyneuropathy complications of gentamycin therapy, *Clin Neurol Neurosurg* 81:241-246, 1979.
30. Shaivitz SA: Timolol and myasthenia gravis, *JAMA* 242:1611-1612, 1979.
31. Acers TE: Ocular myasthenia gravis mimicking pseudo-internuclear ophthalmoplegia and variable esotropia, *Am J Ophthalmol* 88:319-321, 1979.
32. Shy ME, Lange DJ, Howard JW, et al: Quinidine exacerbating myasthenia gravis: a case report and intracellular readings, *Ann Neurol (Abstract)* 1:120, 1985.
33. Katz JL, Lesser RL, Merikangas JR, Silverman JP: Ocular myasthenia gravis after d-penicillamine administration, *Br J Ophthalmol* 73:1015-1018, 1989.
34. Rowland LP: Progressive external ophthalmoplegia. In Vinken PJ, Bruyn GW, Delong JMBV, eds: *Systems disorders and atrophies: handbook of clinical neurology*, New York, 1975, American Elsevier, 177-202.
35. Lepore FE: Bilateral cerebral ptosis, *Neurology* 37:1043, 1987.
36. Linberg JV, McDonald MB, Safir A, et al: Ptosis following radial keratotomy performed using a rigid eyelid speculum, *Ophthalmology* 93:1509-1512, 1986.
37. Aramideh M, Bour LJ, Koelman JH, Speelman JD, et al: Abnormal eye movements in blepharospasm and involuntary levator palpebrae inhibition. Clinical and pathophysiological considerations, *Brain* 117:1457-1474, 1994.
38. Wesley RE, Jackson CG, Tiepeken P, Glassock M: Reconstruction of the eyelid after facial nerve paralysis, *Ophthalmol Clin North Am* 4(1):47-71, 1911.
39. Gausas RE, Lemke BN, Sherman DD, Dortzbach RK: Oculinum injection–resistant blepharospasm in young patients, *Ophthal Plast Reconstr Surg* 10(3):193-194, 1994.
40. Waybright EA, Gutmann C, Chou SM: Facial myokymia: pathologic features, *Arch Neurol* 36:244-245, 1979.
41. Tenser RB: Myokymia and facial contraction in multiple sclerosis, *Arch Intern Med* 136:81-83, 1976.
42. deSilva KL, Pierce J: Facial myokymia: a clue to the diagnosis of multiple sclerosis, *Postgrad Med J* 48:657-661, 1972.
43. Andermann F: Facial myokymia in multiple sclerosis, *Brain* 85:31-44, 1961.
44. Auger RG: Hemifacial spasm: clinical and electrophysiological observations, *Neurology* 29:1261-1272, 1979.

45. Gardener WJ, Sava GA: Hemifacial spasm: a reversible pathophysiological state, *J Neurosurg* 10:240-245, 1962.
46. Krack P, Marion MH: "Apraxia of lid opening," a focal eyelid distonia: clinical study of 32 patients, *Mov Disord* 9(6):610-615, 1994.
47. Barker AB, Joynt RJ: *Clinical neurology: disorders of the brainstem and its cranial nerves*, New York, 1988, Harper & Row, 3:28-40.
48. McGarvey EJ: Thyroid disease: review and case reports, *J Am Optom Assoc* 61(9):689-698, 1990.
49. Werner SC: Classification of the eye changes in Graves' disease, *J Clin Endocrinol Metab* 29:982-984, 1969.
50. Poppen JL, Marino R: Pinealoma and tumors of the posterior portion of the third ventricle, *J Neurosurg* 28:357-364, 1968.

6

Optic Disc Edema

Anthony B. Litwak

Key Terms

anterior ischemic optic neuropathy	papilledema pseudotumor cerebri	toxic optic neuropathies
giant cell arteritis nonarteritic AION optic neuritis demyelinating disease	pseudopapilledema optic disc drusen infiltrative optic neuropathies	Leber's optic neuropathy

Establishing the specific cause in a patient who presents with optic disc edema is arduous. The disc swelling may be the result of infarction, inflammation, infiltration, increased intracranial pressure, toxicity, or hereditary factors. Most often the cause of the nerve head swelling is determined by integrating the clinical appearance of the disc, patient symptoms, other clinical findings, laboratory test results, and neuroimaging studies.

This chapter discusses the more common causes of optic disc edema: anterior ischemic optic neuropathy, optic neuritis, papilledema,

For color illustrations, see color plates following p. 172.

pseudopapilledema, pseudotumor cerebri, and compressive, infiltrative, toxic, and hereditary optic neuropathies. The natural history, clinical findings, auxiliary testing, differential diagnosis, and management are stressed.

Anterior Ischemic Optic Neuropathy

Anterior ischemic optic neuropathy (AION) is characterized by a sudden, painless, unilateral loss of vision or visual field secondary to infarction of the optic nerve at the level of the lamina cribrosa. It is the most common cause of optic disc swelling in the elderly.[1] The visual acuity can range from 20/20 to no light perception. There is reduced color vision in proportion to the visual acuity loss. An afferent pupillary defect is present. The most common type of visual field loss is an altitudinal defect; however, a central scotoma can occur in 20% to 30% of the patients.[2] The fundus will show a pale swollen optic nerve head (Plate 1, A), often with peripapillary hemorrhages in a sectoral pattern. The disc swelling is usually confined to within one disc diameter of the optic nerve head and occurs in the superior pole, compared with the inferior pole, by a ratio of $3:1$.[3] The retinal arterioles are attenuated in half of the cases.[4] Fluorescein angiography will show delayed filling of the peripapillary choroidal vasculature, which suggests an occlusion of the short posterior ciliary arteries as the cause of AION (Figure 6-1). There is normal filling of the retinal vasculature. In the late phase of the fluorescein angiogram, there is diffuse leakage from the disc capillaries.

CLINICAL PEARL

Anterior ischemic optic neuropathy (AION) is characterized by a sudden, painless, unilateral loss of vision or visual field secondary to infarction of the optic nerve at the level of the lamina cribrosa. It is the most common cause of optic disc swelling in the elderly.

After 2 to 8 weeks, the disc swelling and hemorrhages resolve; however, atrophy of the disc in the form of pallor and nerve fiber layer loss are apparent (Plate 1, B). There is usually very little or no improvement in visual function after the event, and recurrences to the same eye are rare.[5] The visual field defects in AION may mimic glaucoma; however, the history of sudden visual loss accompanied by pallor of the remaining neural-retinal rim tissue of the disc help to differentiate AION from glaucomatous optic neuropathy.

Anterior ischemic optic neuropathy can be associated with a variety of systemic diseases (see the box on pp. 155-156), but none more

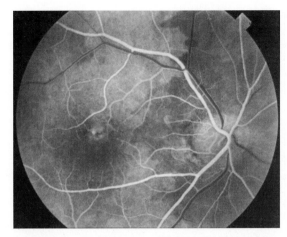

FIGURE 6-1 Fluorescein angiography of acute AION. Note the nonfilling of the choroidal vasculature around the optic nerve head. Mild disc leakage is seen in the later stages of the fluorescein angiogram. (From Litwak AB: Ischemic optic neuropathy. In Onofrey BE, ed: *Optometric pharmacology and therapeutics,* Philadelphia, 1991, JB Lippincott, 51:1-18. Reprinted by permission of JB Lippincott, 1991.)

important than giant cell arteritis (termed arteritic AION) (Plate 2); however, it is associated with AION in only 6% to 18% of cases.[2] Anterior ischemic optic neuropathy not associated with giant cell arteritis (nonarteritic AION) is more commonly associated with systemic vasculopathies such as hypertension (41%), diabetes mellitus (17%), and arteriosclerosis (14%).[6] Approximately one fourth of patients with nonarteritic AION have no systemic illness and are classified as idiopathic.

Systemic Associations of AION

Arteritic AION
  Giant cell arteritis
  Systemic lupus erythematosus
  Polyarteritis nodosa
  Allergic vasculitis
  Rheumatoid arthritis
  Pulseless disease
  Buerger's disease
  Crohn's disease
  Herpes zoster
  Behçet's disease
  Syphilis

Systemic Associations of AION— cont'd

Nonarteritic AION
  Hypertension
  Atherosclerosis
  Diabetes mellitus
  Migraine
  Waldenstrom's macroglobulinemia
  Sickle cell disease
  Polycythemia
  Preeclampsia
  Carotid artery occlusive disease
  Acute blood loss
  Chronic papilledema
  S/P cataract surgery
  Idiopathic

S/P, status post.

Arteritic AION

Giant cell arteritis is an inflammatory vasculitis that affects medium-and large-sized arteries throughout the body, leading to vessel narrowing and occlusion. It is believed to be caused by an auto-immune or allergic response to elastic tissue in the artery.[7] Patients with giant cell arteritis tend to be older than 60 years old, with a female to male ratio of 3:1.[8] The disease is more common in caucasians and is unusual in blacks and Asians.[9]

It is extremely important to differentiate those patients with giant cell arteritis from those with nonarteritic disease (Table 6-1) because the former are at imminent risk of developing AION in their unaffected eye, resulting in permanent bilateral blindness.[10] Giant cell arteritis is a true ocular and medical emergency that requires prompt treatment with systemic corticosteroids.

CLINICAL PEARL

It is extremely important to differentiate patients with giant cell arteritis from those with nonarteritic disease because the former are at imminent risk of developing AION in their unaffected eye, resulting in permanent bilateral blindness.

All patients with AION should be questioned for symptoms of giant cell arteritis, such as headaches, scalp tenderness, jaw claudication, and muscle stiffness in the neck and shoulders (see the box on pp. 157-158).

TABLE 6-1
Differential of Arteritic and Nonarteritic AION

	Arteritic AION	Nonarteritic AION
History	See symptoms GCA	Lacking symptoms
Age (years)	Over 70	40–65
Sex	F > M	Equal
Race	More common in caucasians; unusual in blacks and Asians	No preference
Ocular associations	Amaurosis fugax, diplopia, central retinal artery occlusion	Small optic disc or cup
Systemic associations	Giant cell arteritis	Hypertension, diabetes, arteriosclerosis, migraine
Visual acuity	18% 20/40 or better	45% 20/40 or better
	24% 20/40–20/200	13% 20/40–20/200
	58% 20/200 or worse	42% 20/200 or worse
Visual fields	Inferior altitudinal, 30% central scotoma	Inferior altitudinal, 20% central scotoma
Fundus findings	Chalky pale disc	Pale or hyperemic disc
Bilaterality	65% within days if untreated	25% to 40% over months to years
Laboratory testing	ESR over 40 mm/hr; anemia	ESR under 35 mm/hr
TA biopsy	Positive for GCA	Normal
Risk CVA, MI	No higher risk	Risk suggested
Response to steroids	Dramatic relief of symptoms; little improvement of VA; prevents visual loss in the fellow eye	No proven efficacy

GCA, giant cell arteritis; ESR, erythrocyte sedimentation rate; CVA, cerebral vascular accident; MI, myocardial infarction; VA, visual acuity; TA, temporal artery.
From Litwak AB: Ischemic optic neuropathy. In Onofrey BE, ed: *Optometric pharmacology and therapeutics,* Philadelphia, 1991, JB Lippincott, 51:1-18. Reprinted by permission of JB Lippincott, 1991.

Patients with giant cell arteritis may experience episodes of amaurosis fugax, days or months before AION occurs.[4] Other ocular signs of giant cell arteritis include ophthalmoparesis[10] and central retinal artery occlusion.[11] Giant cell arteritis should always be included in the differential diagnosis of any elderly patient who presents with diplopia, amaurosis fugax, or sudden visual loss.

Clinical Symptoms of Giant Cell Arteritis

Headaches (often temporal)
Scalp tenderness
Swollen, tender temporal arteries
Jaw claudication
Jaw pain (toothache)
Ear pain

Clinical Symptoms of Giant Cell Arteritis — cont'd

Deafness
Malaise
Weight loss
Intermittent fevers
Arthralgias
Myalgias
Muscle stiffness in the neck
Anorexia
Depression
Dementia

Anterior ischemic optic neuropathy patients older than 60 years of age or patients with symptoms of giant cell arteritis should have an immediate erythrocyte sedimentation rate (ESR) measured (Figure 6-2). The ESR is elevated in more than 80% of the patients with giant cell arteritis.[12] The Westergren method is preferred, with normal values below 35 to 40 mm/hour. The diagnosis of giant cell arteritis is confirmed by biopsy of the temporal artery, which shows a granulomatous inflammation of the arterial wall with infiltration of epithelioid cells, lymphocytes, and giant cells.[12] A suspected giant cell arteritis patient with an elevated ESR and normal temporal artery biopsies on both sides should be evaluated for a collagen vascular disease or an occult malignancy.[13]

The treatment for arteritic AION is immediate high-dose systemic corticosteroids. Treatment is initiated based on patient symptomatology and an elevated ESR. The initiation of systemic corticosteroids should never be delayed while waiting for temporal artery biopsy confirmation. The biopsy remains positive for several weeks after the initiation of corticosteroids.[14] The goal of therapy is to prevent AION in the contralateral eye, which may occur within hours or days without sufficient treatment. Corticosteroids will not improve vision in the affected eye.

CLINICAL PEARL

The treatment for arteritic AION is immediate high-dose systemic corticosteroids.

Management of steroid therapy is best directed by a rheumatologist familiar with the complications of corticosteroids in the elderly

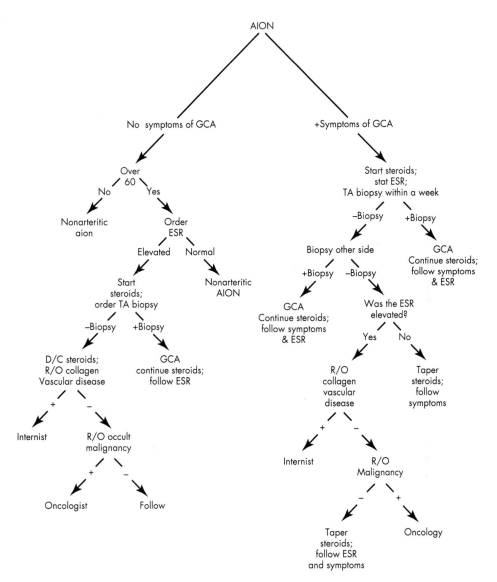

FIGURE 6-2 Flowchart of the management of AION. (From Litwak AB: Ischemic optic neuropathy. In Onofrey BE, ed: *Optometric pharmacology and therapeutics,* Philadelphia, 1991, JB Lippincott, 1-18. Reprinted by permission of JB Lippincott, 1991.)

population. The corticosteroids are gradually tapered over a period of weeks to months, depending on the patient's symptomatology and ESR. Exacerbations are common if the steroids are reduced too quickly. Many patients require long-term corticosteroid therapy and must be monitored closely for possible steroid-induced complications.

Nonarteritic AION

Patients with nonarteritic AION tend to be younger (between 40 and 65) than patients with giant cell arteritis. Both sexes are equally affected and there is no racial preference. Nonarteritic patients in general have less severe visual acuity and field loss than do arteritic patients; however, acuity and field loss should not be used as parameters to separate the two groups (see Table 6-1). Nonarteritic patients lack clinical symptoms of giant cell arteritis and have normal sedimentation rates.

CLINICAL PEARL

Patients with nonarteritic AION tend to be younger (between 40 and 65) than patients with giant cell arteritis. Both sexes are equally affected and there is no racial preference.

Another important finding in the differentiation between the two groups is the appearance of the disc and cup size in the contralateral eye. Nonarteritic AION occurs in patients with small discs with little or no optic cupping[15] (see Plate 1, C). It has been proposed that a small, compact optic disc in conjunction with a small vessel disease (i.e., hypertension, diabetes) may predispose the optic nerve to infarction.[16,17] Disc and cup size does not play a role in the pathogenesis of arteritic AION.

CLINICAL PEARL

Nonarteritic AION occurs in patients with small discs with little or no optic cupping.

The treatment of nonarteritic AION is controversial. Hayreh[18] recommends high-dose systemic corticosteroids in the initial phase of disc swelling; however, other studies have shown no benefit from the use of systemic corticosteroids in the treatment of nonarteritic AION.[4] A randomized, prospective clinical trial is necessary to determine the effectiveness of corticosteroids in the treatment of nonarteritic AION. At this time, there is insufficient evidence to advocate corticosteroid treatment in nonarteritic AION.[2] Patients with nonarteritic AION should have a general medical examination to uncover undiagnosed hypertension or diabetes. Guyer and co-workers[6] found a three times greater incidence of cerebral vascular accidents or myocardial infarction in nonarteritic patients with hypertension.[6] Nonarteritic patients also have a 25% to 40% chance of developing AION in their fellow eye in the next 3 to 5 years.[2] There is no known prevention. Bilateral, nonsimultaneous AION should not be confused with the Foster-Kennedy syndrome.[19] Foster-Kennedy syndrome is caused by a large subfrontal mass in the brain that compresses one optic nerve, leading to optic atrophy and increased intracranial pressure, resulting in papilledema (without visual loss) in the contralateral eye.

The ischemic optic neuropathy decompression trial for nonarteritic anterior ischemic optic neuropathy (NAION) has demonstrated that nerve sheath decompression does not provide a benefit over observation for the improvement of visual acuity or visual fields.[20] In fact, patients operated on had a significantly greater risk of losing vision (defined as losing three or more lines of Snellen acuity). Therefore, optic nerve sheath decompression plays no role in the treatment of NAION and may be harmful. The study has also established that approximately 42% of the patients with nonarteritic AION experience a spontaneous improvement of visual acuity of three lines or more.[20] This is in contrast to the previous impression that most patients do not show any visual improvement following an episode of NAION.

Optic Neuritis

Optic neuritis is an inflammation of the optic nerve usually seen in female patients between the ages of 20 and 50 years. Visual acuity loss is usually abrupt, but may progress over a period of several days to weeks. Visual acuity dysfunction can vary from 20/20 to no light perception. Color vision can be severely reduced in proportion to the visual acuity loss, with a notable desaturation to red test objects. A central scotoma is the most common visual field defect; however, any type of visual field loss, including altitudinal, arcuate, hemianoptic, and peripheral depression, may occur. An afferent pupillary defect is present in all unilateral cases. Ocular or orbital pain on extraocular eye movements is seen in 80% of the patients with optic neuritis, either before or at the time of visual loss. The ocular pain may be caused by the tugging on the inflamed nerve sheaths at the attachment sites of the extraocular muscles at the apex of the orbit.

About 40% of patients with optic neuritis present with optic nerve swelling (termed papillitis) (Plate 3, *A*). The degree of optic nerve swelling as well as the presence of disc hemorrhages and exudates is variable. The amount of disc swelling or hemorrhage does not correlate with the degree of visual loss or the overall prognosis for recovery.[21] About 50% of the patients with optic neuritis present without optic nerve swelling (termed retrobulbar optic neuritis). The only initial objective clinical finding is the presence of an afferent pupillary defect. Finally, about 10% of patients present with a sudden visual deficit and a pale, nonswollen optic nerve head, indicating that they have had episodes of optic neuritis in the past (termed recurrent).

There is almost always some improvement of visual function in patients with optic neuritis over a period of 1 to 8 weeks and sometimes up until 6 months. In the Perkin and Rose study,[22] visual acuity improved to 20/40 or better in 87% of the patients and was worse than 20/200 in 8%.[22] In some cases, the vision improves to 20/20; however, there is often a residual color deficit. The patients also indicate that their vision is not the same 20/20 as before the incident. The afferent pupillary defect may or may not resolve with the acuity improvement. The optic nerve usually develops some degree of pallor with nerve fiber layer dropout, indicating optic atrophy (Plate 3, B). Recurrent optic neuritis occurs in 11% to 24% of the patients and usually is associated with lesser degrees of visual recovery.[21]

Optic neuritis is often associated with demyelinating disease (multiple sclerosis [MS]). Studies show between a 12% and 85% incidence of developing MS after an episode of optic neuritis.[23] Many cases of optic neuritis have no underlying cause, except for a preceding viral illness. There are cases of optic neuritis that occur in patients with systemic lupus erythematosus, sarcoidosis, and syphilis. It is important to examine the vitreous for cells overlying the optic nerve swelling. A large number of vitreous cells, bilateral involvement, or extensive sheathing of the retinal vessels suggests an underlying systemic inflammatory disease as the cause of the optic neuritis. These patients with optic neuritis should have a complete blood count, ESR, antinuclear antibody (ANA) test, angiotensin converting enzyme (ACE) test, chest x ray, fluorescent treponemal antibody absorption test, and venereal disease research laboratory (VDRL) test. Patients with underlying collagen vascular disease improve with moderate doses of systemic corticosteroids. Patients with syphilitic optic neuritis improve with appropriate antibiotic therapy. Bilateral disc swelling associated with a systemic viral illness is a common presentation of optic neuritis in children.[24]

Patients with suspected retrobulbar optic neuritis who are atypical in their presentation or do not show visual improvement over time require neuroimaging to rule out the possibility of a compressive mass lesion. Visual field testing may disclose a field cut in the superior temporal quadrant in the contralateral eye from a compressive anterior chiasmal lesion. Magnetic resonance imaging testing also may disclose white matter lesions in the brain suggestive of multiple sclerosis.

CLINICAL PEARL

Patients with suspected retrobulbar optic neuritis who are atypical in their presentation or do not show visual improvement over time require neuroimaging to rule out the possibility of a compressive mass lesion.

The treatment of idiopathic optic neuritis with systemic corticosteroids is controversial. The optic neuritis treatment trial (ONTT) conducted a clinical trial to determine the efficiency of systemic corticosteroids in the treatment of idiopathic optic neuritis. Patients with first episodes of acute optic neuritis were randomized into three treatment categories; one group received intravenous steroids followed by oral prednisone, one group received oral prednisone, and the final group received oral placebo.

The results of the optic neuritis treatment trial showed that the use of oral prednisone alone has no benefit on the visual outcome of patients with optic neuritis.[25-27] Furthermore, patients treated with oral prednisone alone had a 27% recurrence of optic neuritis compared to 15% in the placebo group and 13% in the combination IV/oral steroid group. Therefore, oral prednisone alone is contraindicated in the treatment of optic neuritis. Treatment with IV methylprednisolone followed by oral prednisone resulted in faster visual recovery but had no significant advantage in long-term visual acuity compared to oral placebo. If the visual acuity is better than 20/40, there is no faster recovery with combination steroids compared to oral placebo.

Patients treated with IV and oral steroids experienced a delay in the development of multiple sclerosis, especially if the patient initially presented with demyelinating lesions on MRI.[28-30] Further studies may reveal whether patients with optic neuritis should be treated with a combination of IV and oral steroids or simply monitored without therapy.

Papilledema

Papilledema is optic disc swelling caused by increased intracranial pressure. It is almost always bilateral; however, it may be asymmetric in presentation. There is usually excellent visual acuity and no visual field defects except for an enlarged blind spot, unless there is an intracranial mass compressing the afferent visual pathway. An afferent pupillary defect is absent. The patient may be totally asymptomatic or may experience headaches, nausea, vomiting, focal neurologic symptoms, or transient obscurations of vision. These are momentary blackouts of vision that last 3 to 5 seconds and are often postural. Some patients may develop bilateral VI nerve palsies from compression of the abducens nerve as it transverses above the clivus at the base of the skull.

The disc swelling begins as blurring of the peripapillary nerve fiber layer with disc hyperemia from capillary dilation (Plate 4). There is loss of a superficial venous pulse (SVP) at the optic nerve head. The presence of an SVP indicates that the intracranial pressure is below 200 mm H$_2$O. Twenty percent of the normal population, however, will not have an SVP.[21] Therefore its presence is helpful to rule against increased intracranial pressure, but its absence is of limited use. With advanced disc swelling, the disc margins are blurred with splinter peripapillary hemorrhages, hard exudates, and cotton wool spots. Severe disc edema can extend into the macular area and result in reduction of visual acuity from serous macular detachment (Plate 5). Reduced venous return may lead to breakthrough hemorrhage into the subhyaloid space or vitreous. Chronic papilledema may show gliosis of the optic disc, optociliary shunt vessels, and pseudo-drusen bodies of the optic nerve head. Fluorescein angiography shows early disc hyperfluorescence with late leakage from the dilated disc capillaries.

Although visual field loss may initially be limited to an enlarged blind spot, severe or chronic papilledema can result in permanent optic nerve damage and atrophy. Visual field defects are similar to those that develop in glaucoma and include paracentral and arcuate scotomas and concentric constriction of the peripheral visual field.

All patients with bilateral disc swelling or suspected papilledema require immediate neurologic evaluation. Neuroimaging must be performed to rule out an intracranial mass. If the imaging study is normal and the ventricles are not dilated, a lumbar puncture with examination of the cerebrospinal fluid is necessary to rule out a meningitis, subarachnoid hemorrhage, or a diffuse tumor infiltration. The opening pressure of the lumbar puncture is often elevated (over 180 mm H$_2$O); however, the intracranial pressure can fluctuate, so a normal reading does not necessarily rule out papilledema.[21]

CLINICAL PEARL

All patients with bilateral disc swelling or suspected papilledema require immediate neurologic evaluation. Neuroimaging must be performed to rule out an intracranial mass.

Pseudotumor Cerebri

Pseudotumor cerebri is a diagnosis of exclusion. It usually occurs in young, obese women, but also can be seen in nonobese and male

Right eye   **Left eye**

A

Right eye   **Left eye**

B

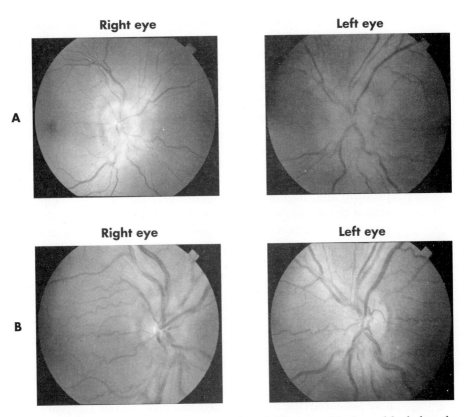

FIGURE 6-3 Pseudotumor cerebri. A 30-year-old obese, black female with complaint of headache and transient obscurations of vision. **A,** Note bilateral disc swelling. CT scan revealed no mass lesions. Light perception showed an increased opening pressure with normal CSF composition. The patient was encouraged to lose weight and was placed on oral acetazolamide. **B,** Six months later, after weight loss and treatment, the disc swelling has improved.

patients. The cause is usually unknown, but may be a blocked venous sinus, exogenous agents, endocrine abnormalities, or increased arachnoid resistance to cerebrospinal fluid drainage.[24] The patient usually presents with symptoms of headache that are worse in the morning and exacerbated by coughing or a Valsalva maneuver. The patient also may experience nausea, vomiting, diplopia, tinnitus, and transient obscurations of vision. Some patients are totally asymptomatic. The visual acuity and field are normal except for an enlarged blind spot. The patient has bilateral optic disc swelling (Figure 6-3, *A*), but no intracranial mass lesions on neuroimaging studies. The lumbar puncture shows an increased opening pressure with normal cerebrospinal fluid composition. Approximately 25% of the patients develop visual acuity or field loss over the course of their disease.[21] It is extremely important to monitor these patients closely with visual acuity, color vision, serial visual fields, and disc photography.

The treatment of pseudotumor cerebri is to first rule out an exogenous agent such as excessive vitamin A, certain acne medications such as isotretinoin (Accutane [Roche Laboratories, Nutley, NJ]), oral contraceptives, tetracycline, lithium, or corticosteroids as the cause. Increased intracranial pressure may be reduced with weight loss, oral Diamox (Lederle Laboratories, Pearl River, NY), or Lasix (Hoechst, Somerville, NJ) (Figure 6-3, B). If there is progressive visual damage or severe, unrelenting headaches, various surgical procedures such as a lumboperitoneal shunt can be performed to reduce the intracranial pressure and, it is hoped, to preserve vision function.[21] Optic nerve sheath decompression has recently been advocated in patients with pseudotumor cerebri and optic nerve compromise.[31] This procedure is recommended at the first sign of progressive visual dysfunction and is less beneficial in patients with chronic atrophic papilledema.

Pseudopapilledema of the Optic Nerve Head

The development of optic nerve head drusen is the most frequent cause of pseudodisc swelling, occurring in 75% of the cases.[21] Optic disc drusen are hyalin bodies deposited either on the surface of the disc (Plate 6) or buried within the optic nerve head (Plate 7). They may cause the disc to be elevated and give a choked appearance. The disc margins may appear blurred with a deep yellow smudging; however, unlike true papilledema, the overlying retinal vessels are distinctly visible and the disc is not hyperemic. Optic nerve head drusen are often associated with anomalous branching of disc vessels and a small optic nerve head with little or no cup. The condition is often bilateral and familial. When drusen bodies are located beneath the surface of the optic nerve head, ultrasonography and computed tomography may be helpful in making the diagnosis. Disc drusen give highly reflective echoes because of their calcification (Figure 6-4). Visual acuity loss and visual field and nerve fiber layer defects may be present and are sometimes progressive. These patients should be monitored with visual acuity, color vision, visual fields, and disc photography. Progressive visual dysfunction warrants a neuroimaging study to rule out the possibility of a concurrent intraorbital or intracranial tumor.

CLINICAL PEARL

Optic nerve head drusen are the most frequent cause of pseudodisc swelling, occurring in 75% of the cases.

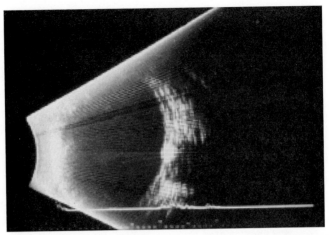

FIGURE 6-4 Ultrasonography shows highly reflective echo of calcified optic nerve head drusen.

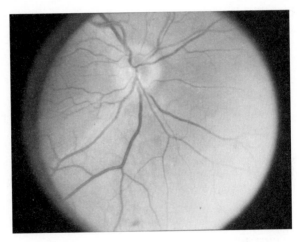

FIGURE 6-5 Optic nerve hypoplasia. Note small size of optic nerve in relation to normal-sized disc vessels.

Other causes of pseudopapilledema include high hyperopia with disc hypoplasia (Figure 6-5), tilted discs (Figure 6-6), myelinated nerve fibers (Figure 6-7), and peripapillary choroidal neovascular membranes (Plate 8).

Compressive Optic Neuropathy

An intraorbital expanding mass lesion may compress the optic nerve, resulting in progressive visual loss with or without concurrent disc swelling. An expanding mass in the orbit may also lead to

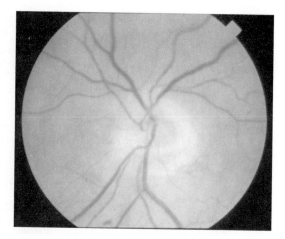

FIGURE 6-6 Tilted disc. Note oblique insertion of the optic nerve with inferior peripapillary crescent.

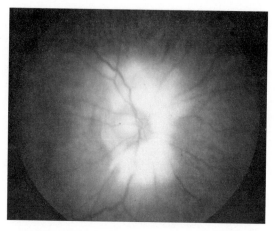

FIGURE 6-7 Myelinated nerve fiber layers. Note white feathery edges of medullated retinal nerve fibers without visibility of underlying retinal vessel.

proptosis, extraocular movement restriction, episcleral congestion, lid abnormalities, optociliary disc vessels, and choroidal folds. Eventually, the disc swelling resolves as axons atrophy and the optic nerve becomes pale. The differential diagnosis includes optic nerve glioma in a child, optic nerve sheath meningioma in a middle-aged adult, dysthyroid optic neuropathy, orbital pseudotumor, and other space-occupying intraorbital tumors. A computed tomography scan or magnetic resonance imaging with surface coils of the orbits are indicated in any patient with progressive, unexplained visual acuity loss. Treatment will depend on the underlying cause.

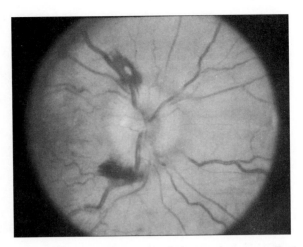

FIGURE 6-8 Leukemic infiltration of the optic nerve. Patient noted acute vision loss with 360° of disc swelling with peripapillary hemorrhages. Diagnosis of leukemia was already established.

Infiltrative Optic Neuropathy

Infiltrative optic neuropathies can present with or without disc swelling and can be unilateral or bilateral. There is usually painless, progressive, severe visual acuity loss. Vitreous or tumor cells are often seen overlying the swollen optic nerve head. The disc swelling results from tumor infiltration of the optic nerve (Plate 9 and Figure 6-8) or from increased intracranial pressure. These patients are usually already diagnosed with a systemic illness such as leukemia, lymphoma, or metastatic disease. Patients with infiltrative optic neuropathy may respond to chemotherapy or low doses of irradiation to the orbit. If the patient is not diagnosed with a systemic illness, the patient should be worked up for a granulomatous disease such as sarcoidosis or syphilis.

Toxic Optic Neuropathy

Toxic optic neuropathies from methanol, streptomycin, chloramphenicol, ethylene glycol (antifreeze), ethambutol, and lead ingestion can present with bilateral disc swelling in the acute phase. The visual acuity loss is progressive. The disc swelling eventually resolves to optic atrophy. Treatment is to discontinue or prevent the ingestion of the offending agent. Prognosis is related to the toxicity of the agent and the amount and duration of exposure.

Chronic alcohol abuse can lead to a slow progressive retrobulbar optic neuropathy that does not usually present with optic nerve head swelling. A nutritional component may be equally responsible for the

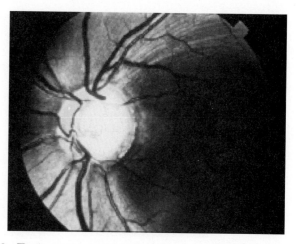

FIGURE 6-9 Toxic optic neuropathy. 50-year-old black male with a 30-year history of alcohol abuse and poor nutrition. The patient reported bilateral, progressive visual acuity loss with 20/80 vision, poor color vision, and a cecocentral scotoma. Red-free photograph showing nerve fiber layer dropout in the papillomacular bundle in the left eye.

optic neuropathy in alcohol-nutritional amblyopia, which is more commonly seen in men of middle to older age. The visual acuity loss is progressive over many years. Color vision loss and desaturation to red often precede the visual acuity loss. The visual field defect is often a central or cecocentral scotoma. Because this is a bilateral disease, an afferent pupillary defect is not seen. There is eventual disc pallor, usually of the temporal rim with nerve fiber layer dropout in the papillomacular bundle (Plate 10 and Figure 6-9). The history of alcohol abuse is often not given by the patient, but can be obtained from a family member. Laboratory work-up includes a red blood cell folate and serum B_{12} levels. The patient should be directed to an Alcoholics Anonymous counseling group and a nutritionist. Folate and B vitamin supplements may be given; however, the prognosis for visual improvement once atrophy has occurred is guarded. A computed tomography or magnetic resonance imaging scan may be required to rule out the possibility of a compressive lesion.

Leber's Hereditary Optic Neuropathy

Leber's optic neuropathy affects young men between the ages of 15 and 30. The disease is not inherited as a sex-linked transmission, although males are affected by a 9 : 1 ratio. It is believed to be caused by a genetically transmitted mitochondrial DNA mutation.[32-34] There is severe, rapid, unilateral visual acuity loss with most patients 20/200 or worse and sometimes with no light perception. The visual field loss is a central or cecocentral scotoma. The contralateral eye has a similar episode of acute visual loss within days or weeks of the first eye's episode.

CLINICAL PEARL

Leber's optic neuropathy affects young men between the ages of 15 and 30.

The optic disc appears mildly elevated (pseudoedema) with peri-papillary vessel telangiectasia (Plate 11) that do not leak on fluorescein angiography. Within a couple of weeks, the disc swelling and telangiectasia resolve and optic pallor and nerve fiber layer loss become apparent. The visual recovery is variable, but the overall visual prognosis is poor. There are cases of improved visual acuity after years of poor vision.[35] Repeat episodes of visual loss to the same eye once vision has improved are uncommon.[21] The appropriate diagnosis is made by history, fluorescein angiography, examination of other family members, and genetic analysis of mitochondrial DNA mutation.[35] Female carriers may show abnormal disc vasculature or telangiectatic microangiopathy. Early and correct diagnosis can save the patient unnecessary neurologic work-up. Patients with Leber's optic neuropathy should consult a cardiologist because of the association with electrocardiographic abnormalities.[36,37]

Other Causes of Optic Disc Swelling

Other causes of optic nerve head swelling include diabetic papillopathy, central retinal vein occlusions, hypertensive papillopathy, posterior uveitis, and hypotony. These entities are differentiated by the patient's systemic medical history, symptomatology, and related clinical findings.

Summary

When a patient presents with swelling of the optic disc, the practitioner must take a careful history, gather the pertinent clinical findings, and order the necessary laboratory or neuroimaging tests to make the correct diagnosis (Table 6-2). Once the proper diagnosis is made, the appropriate management or referral plan should be initiated to prevent further ocular or systemic complications.

TABLE 6-2
Differential of Optic Disc Swelling

	Nonarteritic AION	Optic neuritis	Pseudotumor cerebri	Infiltrative neuropathy
Age	Over 40	Under 45	2nd–4th decade	Any age
Ocular pain	No	Yes	Headaches	Rare
Clinical symptoms	None	Symptoms of MS	Nausea, vomiting	Systemically ill
Related ocular findings	Small optic disc with no cupping	Ocular pain on eye movements	Diplopia, TOV	Cells in vitreous
APD	Yes	Yes	No	Common
Visual acuity	Usually reduced	Reduced	Normal	Progressive loss
Visual field	Altitudinal defect	Central scotoma	Enlarged blind spot	Central scotoma
Color vision	Reduced pallid	Reduced	Normal	Reduced
Disc swelling		50% present, 50% retrobulbar	Bilateral hyperemic	Common, can be retrobulbar
Recurrences	Rare	Common in MS	Persistent without treatment	Persistent without treatment
Bilaterality	25% to 40% over months to years	Rare except in MS	Yes	Common
Systemic associations	HTN, DM, migraine, arteriosclerosis	MS, CVD, viral illness	Obesity, small cerebral ventricles	Leukemia, lymphoma, metastatic disease
Recovery	Rare	Yes 2–8 weeks	75% maintain good vision	Gets worse with time
Treatment	Steroids?	Steroids?	Weight loss, Diamox, shunt procedures	Good response to radiation treatment

TOV, transient obscurations of vision; CVD, collagen vascular disease; DM, diabetes mellitus; HTN, hypertension; APD, afferent pupillary defect; MS, multiple sclerosis.

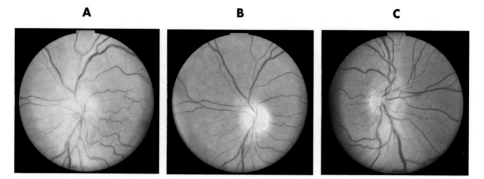

PLATE 1 Nonarteritic AION. A 60-year-old white male with sudden visual loss in the left eye with normal ESR and no clinical symptoms of GCA. **A,** Note 360° of pale optic disc swelling with greater swelling in the superior pole. **B,** Six weeks later, the disc swelling resolved with the development of optic atrophy and diffuse nerve fiber layer dropout. The VA did not improve. **C,** Fellow eye of patient in *A* and *B*. Patients with nonarteritic AION typically have a small disc with very little or no optic cupping. This anatomic crowding of nerve fiber axons in the presence of arteriosclerosis may predispose patients to disc infarction.

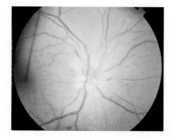

PLATE 2 Arteritic AION. A 70-year-old white male with sudden visual loss in the right eye. Patient had headaches, scalp tenderness, and jaw claudication with an elevated sedimentation rate and a positive temporal artery biopsy for giant cell arteritis. Note superior, pale disc swelling with peripapillary splinter hemorrhages and an associated inferior altitudinal visual field defect.

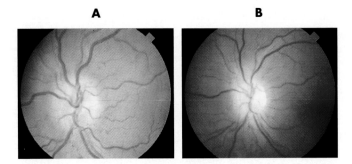

A   **B**

PLATE 3 Optic neuritis. A 32-year-old white male with a 3-day history of left ocular pain especially on eye movements. **A,** Patient developed abrupt visual loss in the left eye with 20/80 VA, poor color vision, and an afferent pupillary defect. Note mild disc swelling without hyperemia. After 2 weeks the VA improved to 20/20 but patient still had a color deficit and noticed asymmetry in the vision. **B,** Three weeks later, the disc swelling had begun to resolve with the appearance of optic pallor.

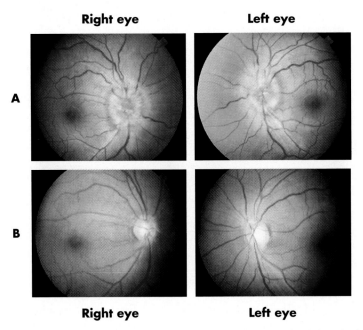

Right eye   **Left eye**

A

B

Right eye   **Left eye**

PLATE 4 Papilledema. A 38-year-old black male who had headaches but normal VA, color vision, and visual fields (except for enlarged blind spot). **A,** Note bilateral, hyperemic optic nerve swelling. A CT scan showed a large posterior fossa tumor, which was treated with irradiation and corticosteroids to reduce cerebral edema. **B,** Eight weeks later, the symptoms and disc swelling improved. (From Litwak AB: Ischemic optic neuropathy. In Onofrey BE, ed: *Optometric pharmacology and therapeutics,* Philadelphia, 1991, JB Lippincott, 51:1-18. Reprinted by permission of JB Lippincott, 1991.)

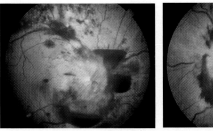 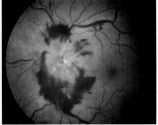

Right eye **Left eye**

PLATE 5 Papilledema. A 34-year-old black male with AIDS and *Cryptococcus meningitis* causing increased intracranial pressure. Note extensive bilateral disc swelling with intraretinal and preretinal hemorrhage from poor venous return. Edema extended into the macular area in the right eye, causing reduced central acuity. Patient had concurrent CMV retinitis in the superior arcades in the right eye.

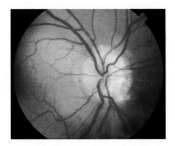

PLATE 6 Pseudodisc swelling. Optic nerve head drusen. Note highly visible drusen bodies on the surface of the optic disc, with no cupping, and extensive disc vessel branching.

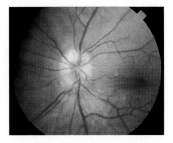

PLATE 7 Buried optic nerve head drusen. Note deep yellow smudging of the disc margins without blurring of the overlying retinal vessels and without disc hyperemia.

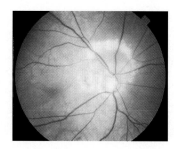

PLATE 8 Peripapillary choroidal neovascular membrane. Note superior leakage of subretinal fluid and exudate. Fluorescein angiography helps diagnose and identify the location of the leaking membrane.

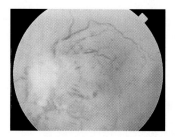

PLATE 9 Infiltrative optic neuropathy. A 66-year-old white male with acute visual loss in the left eye and systemic diagnosis of metastatic carcinoma. Note visibility of tumor infiltration on the surface of the optic disc with peripapillary hemorrhages and overlying vitreous and tumor cells. (From Litwak AB: Ischemic optic neuropathy. In Onofrey BE, ed: *Optometric pharmacology and therapeutics*, Philadelphia, 1991, JB Lippincott, 51:1-18. Reprinted by permission of JB Lippincott, 1991.)

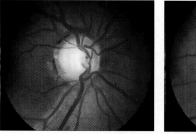 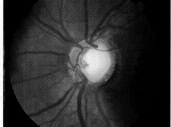

Right eye   **Left eye**

PLATE 10 Toxic optic neuropathy. A 50-year-old black male with a 30-year history of alcohol abuse and poor nutrition. Patient reported bilateral, progressive visual acuity loss with 20/80 vision, poor color vision, and a cecocentral scotoma. Note temporal optic nerve rim pallor.

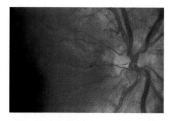

PLATE 11 Leber's hereditary optic neuropathy. A 15-year-old white male who experienced sudden visual decrease in his left eye with the best corrected vision being count fingers. Several weeks later he experienced visual decrease in his right eye with best corrected vision being 20/400. Additionally, he manifested a central scotoma in that eye. Note thickish white opacity in the circumpapillary nerve fiber layer (pseudoedema) with tortuous peripapillary vessels. The disc vessels showed no leakage on fluorescein angiography. The pseudo-disc edema and telangiectasia resolved over several weeks with the development of optic nerve pallor. (Photo courtesy Cindy Guenzel, OD.)

References

1. Miller NR: Anterior ischemic optic neuropathy: diagnosis and management, *Bull NY Acad Med* 56:643-654, 1980.
2. Litwak AB: Ischemic optic neuropathy. In Onofrey BE, ed: *Optometric pharmacology and therapeutics*, Philadelphia, 1991, JB Lippincott, 51:1-18.
3. Repka MX, Savino PJ, Schatz NJ, Sergott RC: Clinical profile and long-term implications of anterior ischemic optic neuropathy, *Am J Ophthalmol* 96:478-483, 1983.
4. Boghen DR, Glaser JS: Ischemic optic neuropathy. The clinical profile and history. *Brain* 98:689-708, 1975.
5. Burde RM: Ischemic optic neuropathy. In Smith JL, ed: *Neuro-ophthalmology*, St Louis, 1973, Mosby.
6. Guyer DR, Miller NR, Auer CL, Fine SL: The risk of cerebrovascular and cardiovascular disease in patients with anterior ischemic optic neuropathy, *Arch Ophthalmol* 103:1136-1142, 1985.
7. Healey LA, Wilske KR: *The systemic manifestations of temporal arteritis*, New York, 1978, Grune & Stratton.
8. Hunder GG: Giant cell (temporal) arteritis, *Rheum Dis Clin North Am* 16:399-409, 1990.
9. Liang GC, Simkin PA, Hunder GG, et al: Familiar aggregation of polymyalgia rheumatica and giant cell arteritis, *Arthritis Rheum* 17:19, 1974.
10. Keltner JL: Giant-cell arteritis. Signs and symptoms, *Ophthalmology* 89:1101-1110, 1982.
11. Cullen JF: Occult temporal arteritis. A common cause of blindness in old age, *Br J Ophthalmol* 51:513-525, 1967.
12. Tang RA: Giant cell arteritis: diagnosis and management, *Semin Ophthalmol* 3:244-248, 1988.
13. Hedges TR, Gieger GL, Albert DM: The clinical value of negative temporal artery biopsy specimens, *Arch Ophthalmol* 101:1251-1254, 1983.
14. McDonnell PJ, Moore GW, Miller NR, et al: Temporal arteritis. A clinicopathologic study, *Ophthalmology* 93:518-530, 1986.
15. Jonas JB, Gusek GC, Naumann OH: Anterior ischemic optic neuropathy: nonarteritic form in small and giant cell arteritis in normal sized optic discs, *Int Ophthalmol* 12:119-125, 1988.
16. Mansour AM, Shoch D, Logani S: Optic disk size in ischemic optic neuropathy, *Am J Ophthalmol* 106:587-589, 1988.
17. Feit RH, Tomsak RL, Ellenberger C Jr: Structural factors in the pathogenesis of ischemic optic neuropathy, *Am J Ophthalmol* 98:105-108, 1984.
18. Hayreh SS: Anterior ischaemic optic neuropathy. III. Treatment, prophylaxis, and differential diagnosis, *Br J Ophthalmol* 58:981-989, 1974.
19. Miller NR, Keltner JL, Gittinger JW, Burde RM: Giant cell (temporal) arteritis: the differential diagnosis, *Surv Ophthalmol* 23:259-263, 1979.
20. The Ischemic Optic Neuropathy Decompression Trial Research Group: Optic nerve decompression surgery for nonarteritic anterior ischemic optic neuropathy (NAION) is not effective and may be harmful: results of the Ischemic Optic Neuropathy Decompression Trial (IONDT), *JAMA* 273:625-632, 1995.
21. Miller NR: *Walsh and Hoyt's clinical neuro-ophthalmology*, ed 4, vol 1, Baltimore, 1982, Williams & Wilkins.
22. Perkin GD, Rose FC: *Optic neuritis and its differential diagnosis*, Oxford, 1979, Oxford Medical Publications.
23. Cohen MM, Lessell S, Wolf PA: A prospective study of the risk of developing multiple sclerosis in uncomplicated optic neuritis, *Neurology* 29:208, 1979.
24. Burde RM, Savino PJ, Trobe JD: *Clinical decisions in neuro-ophthalmology*, St Louis, 1985, Mosby.

25. Beck RW: Optic Neuritis Study Group. A randomized controlled trial of corticosteroids in the treatment of acute optic neuritis, *N Engl J Med* 326:581-588, 1992.
26. Beck RW: Optic Neuritis Study Group. Optic neuritis treatment trial—one year follow-up results, *Arch Ophthalmol* 111:773-775, 1993.
27. Harkins T: A summary of the optic neuritis treatment trial, *Clin Eye Vis Care* 6(1):33-40, 1994.
28. Beck RW, Cleary PA, Trobe JD, et al: The effect of corticosteroids for acute optic neuritis on the subsequent development of multiple sclerosis, *N Engl J Med* 329:1764-1769, 1993.
29. Trobe JD: High-dose corticosteroid regimen retards development of MS in optic neuritis treatment trial, *Arch Ophthalmol* 112:35-36, 1993.
30. Harkins T: Treating multiple sclerosis, *Clin Eye Vis Care* 6(3):133-136, 1994.
31. Spoor TC, Ramocki JM, Madion MP, et al: Treatment of pseudotumor cerebri by primary and secondary optic nerve sheath decompression, *Am J Ophthalmol* 112:177-185, 1991.
32. Singh G, Lott MT, Wallace DC: A mitochondrial mutation as a cause of Leber's hereditary optic neuropathy, *N Engl J Med* 320(20):1300-1305, 1989.
33. Parker WD, Oley CA, Parks JK, A defect in mitochondrial electron-transport activity (NADH-coenzyme Q oxidoreductase) in Leber's hereditary optic neuropathy, *N Engl J Med* 320(20):1331-1333, 1989.
34. Yoneda M, Tsuji S, Yamauchi T, et al: Mitochondrial DNA mutation in family with Leber's hereditary optic neuropathy, *Lancet* 1(8646):1076-1077, 1989.
35. Newman NJ, Loft MT, Wallace DC: The clinical characteristics of pedigrees of Leber's hereditary optic neuropathy with the 11778 mutation, *Am J Ophthalmol* 111:750-762, 1991.
36. Nikoskelainen E, Wanne O, Dahl M: Pre-excitation syndrome and Leber's hereditary optic neuroretinopathy, *Lancet* 1:969, 1985.
37. Rose FC, Bowden AN, Bowden PM: The heart in Leber's optic atrophy, *Br J Ophthalmol* 54:388, 1970.

7

Transient Visual Loss

Barbara J. Jennings

Key Terms

transient ischemic attack	thrombosis	angiography
	embolization	magnetic resonance
transient visual loss	auscultation	angiography
atherosclerosis	bruit	carotid
carotid artery disease	duplex ultrasonography	endarterectomy
vertebrobasilar insufficiency	periorbital Doppler	

If the blood supply to the brain is diminished for any length of time, patients will experience either transient or permanent symptoms and signs that indicate the part of the brain that experienced the ischemia. The concepts of cerebrovascular disease and the premonitory symptoms associated with it are not new, but were described by Gowers,[1,2] in the late 19th century.

If the ischemic event results in permanent dysfunction, the patient is said to have suffered a stroke. When the ischemia results in only temporary dysfunction, the patient has experienced a transient ischemic attack (TIA). Both stroke and TIA can have visual and ocular signs and symptoms, and it is therefore essential for the optometrist to understand the presenting complaints for these patients, as well as the appropriate treatment and referrals to make when necessary. Because stroke is the third leading cause of death in the United States,[3] after heart disease and cancer, and the leading cause of major disability,[4-6] it is expected that optometrists will not only diagnose stroke and potential stroke victims, but will work closely with neurologists toward the rehabilitation of stroke victims.

Epidemiology and Risk Factors for Transient Visual Loss and Stroke

Transient visual loss (TVL), or amaurosis fugax, is a sudden, transient monocular blindness (TMB) due to an abrupt reduction of perfusion to one eye. This is a common complaint in clinical practice.[7] Patients experience increasing numbers of episodes of TVL in the 60- to 70-year age group.[8] Between 40 and 80 years of age, men experience more episodes of TVL than women by a 2.3/1.0 margin. Just as with stroke victims, there is a high incidence of cigarette smoking in patients who experience TVL (55%), and elevated blood pressure and ischemic heart disease each are seen in about 20% of cases. The natural history of untreated patients with TVL remains somewhat unclear. Different studies report an incidence of eventual stroke in patients with episodes of TVL as 12.5%,[9] 34%,[10] and 40%.[11] In an additional study,[12] 110 medically treated TVL patients were followed for an average of 8 years. Survival curves were generated, and an increased mortality rate in TVL patients compared with a control population in the United Kingdom was noted.[12] Furthermore, survival of patients free of ischemic heart disease was significantly less frequently noted in the TVL patients. When patients demonstrate embolic cholesterol plaques in retinal arteries with associated visual loss, the life expectancy also is significantly shorter than in control subjects.[13] Thus TVL should not be ignored, because it may indicate vascular disease in the coronary or cerebral circulations.[8]

CLINICAL PEARL

Transient visual loss (TVL), or amaurosis fugax, is a sudden, transient monocular blindness (TMB) due to an abrupt reduction of perfusion to one eye.

CLINICAL PEARL

When patients demonstrate embolic cholesterol plaques in retinal arteries with associated visual loss, the life expectancy is significantly shorter than in control subjects.

Although there are several causes of strokes, only those resulting from occlusion of a blood vessel with subsequent ischemia to the brain will be considered here. This type of stroke, caused by thrombosis or embolism, accounts for approximately 80% of all strokes,[14-17] half of which have premonitory symptoms.[18]

No matter what the cause of infarction of brain tissue, mortality associated with stroke remains quite high, and there has been little change in the rate of death among these patients in the past 20 years.[19] Between 30% and 52% of patients suffering an ischemic stroke will die within 1 year of the event.[14,20,21]

Risk factors for stroke include hypertension, cardiac disease, TIAs, elevated hematocrit values, diabetes mellitus, previous stroke, and others (see the box below).[22] Black patients are at substantially greater risk for stroke.[23-25] The most important risk factor for stroke has been considered to be hypertension; moreover, the higher the blood pressure, the more the risk increases.[26] When hypertension is adequately treated, both the incidence of stroke and mortality associated with it are reduced.[27-30] However, more recent studies show that the presence of other cardiovascular diseases may in fact be greater risk factors for stroke. Although hypertensive patients were shown to suffer strokes more than three times more frequently than nonhypertensive patients in the Framingham cohort, patients with cardiac failure demonstrated a fourfold excess of stroke development;[31] furthermore, atrial fibrillation appeared to be the most important risk factor for stroke, particularly with increasing age.[31-33]

Risk Factors for Stroke

I. Single risk factor
   A. Well documented
      1. Treatment effective
         a. Hypertension
         b. Cardiac disease
         c. Transient ischemic attacks
         d. Increasing hematocrit
      2. Value of treatment not established
         a. Diabetes mellitus
         b. Previous stroke
         c. Increasing blood fibrinogen
         d. Sickle cell disease
         e. Asymptomatic carotid bruits
      3. Treatment not feasible
         a. Age
         b. Gender

Risk Factors for Stroke — cont'd

        c. Heredofamilial
        d. Race
   B. Less well documented
     1. Treatable
        a. Elevated blood cholesterol and lipids
        b. Cigarette smoking
        c. Alcohol consumption
        d. Oral contraceptives
        e. Sedentary physical activity
        f. Obesity
     2. Treatment not feasible
        a. Geographic location
        b. Season and climate
        c. Socioeconomic factors
II. Multiple risk factors
   A. Framingham profile
     1. Systolic blood pressure
     2. Serum cholesterol
     3. Glucose intolerance
     4. Cigarette smoking
     5. Abnormal ECG (left ventricular hypertrophy)
   B. Paffenbarger and Williams study
     1. Cigarette smoking, systolic blood pressure, and low ponderal index
     2. Body height, a parent dead, and not a varsity athlete
   C. Women of childbearing age
     1. Oral contraceptives
     2. Cigarette smoking
     3. Older than 35 years

From Dyken ML: Risk factors predisposing to stroke. In Moore WS, ed: *Surgery for cerebrovascular disease,* New York, 1987, Churchill Livingstone, p. 80. Reprinted by permission of Churchill Livingstone, 1987. Also modified from Dyken ML, et al: *Stroke* 15 1105, 1984. Courtesy the American Heart Association.

Because of the many potential risk factors for stroke, the best method of determining which patients are at greatest risk for developing stroke is to take a multifactorial approach to the analysis. Studying patients in the 55- to 84-year range, a recent analysis of the Framingham cohort developed a risk profile for stroke.[34] The authors were able to develop a point system for male and female patients to determine the probability that a patient would suffer a stroke given certain existent risk factors. Using this multifactorial point system, it is possible to predict which patients have the greatest likelihood for suffering a stroke, so that those risk factors can be addressed.

Anatomic Correlates

The blood supply to the brain transports oxygen and nutrients to it. Additionally, metabolic byproducts are transported from the brain through the blood supply. The brain does not store large amounts of glucose or oxygen, so that the glucose supply used for energy by the brain must be delivered to it through the continuous flow of blood. When the blood supply to the brain is cut off, loss of consciousness occurs in less than 1 minute. Irreparable damage to the brain tissue occurs within 5 minutes after the blood supply to the brain has been stopped.

The brain receives its blood supply from two pairs of arterial trunks, resulting in separate anterior and posterior circulatory systems that join each other at the circle of Willis (Figure 7-1). The major arteries extending off the circle of Willis (Figure 7-2) each supply a specific territory of the brain. These territories are separated from each other by "watershed areas." Because of the distribution of individual arteries to specific territories in the brain, localization of vascular

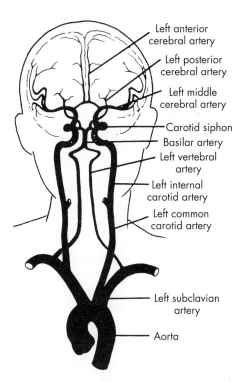

FIGURE 7-1 Cerebral arteries. (From de Groot J: *Correlative neuroanatomy,* ed 21, Norwalk, Conn, Appleton & Lange, 129. Reprinted by permission of Appleton & Lange, 1991.)

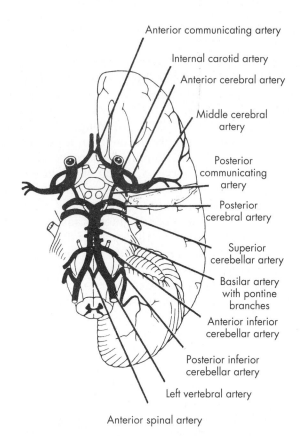

Anterior communicating artery

Internal carotid artery

Anterior cerebral artery

Middle cerebral artery

Posterior communicating artery

Posterior cerebral artery

Superior cerebellar artery

Basilar artery with pontine branches

Anterior inferior cerebellar artery

Posterior inferior cerebellar artery

Left vertebral artery

Anterior spinal artery

FIGURE 7-2 Circle of Willis and principal arteries of the brain stem. (From de Groot J: *Correlative neuroanatomy,* ed 21, Norwalk, Conn, 1991, Appleton & Lange, 130. Reprinted by permission of Appleton & Lange, 1991.)

occlusions are rather straightforward because the signs and symptoms present in the patient will correlate with the area of the brain suffering decreased perfusion.

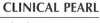

CLINICAL PEARL

The brain receives its blood supply from two pairs of arterial trunks, resulting in separate anterior and posterior circulatory systems that join each other at the circle of Willis.

The anterior circulation to the brain begins as the extracranial carotid arterial system. The left common carotid artery arises directly from the aortic arch. The left subclavian artery also arises directly from the aortic arch. On the right side, the brachiocephalic trunk arises from the aortic arch to form the innominate artery, and then bifurcates into the right common carotid and subclavian arteries. On both sides, the common carotid artery travels in the anterior triangle of the neck, medial to the sternocleidomastoid muscle. At the upper level of the thyroid cartilage, the common carotid artery bifurcates into the internal and external carotid vessels. The branches of the external carotid artery are the following:

Superior thyroid artery
Ascending pharyngeal artery
Lingual artery
Facial artery
Occipital artery
Posterior auricular artery
Superficial temporal artery
Maxillary artery

These branches supply the face and scalp and not the brain.

The internal carotid artery continues through the carotid canal in the petrous bone to eventually supply the brain. The two terminal branches of the internal carotid artery are the middle cerebral artery and the anterior cerebral artery (Figures 7-3 and 7-4). In general, the middle cerebral artery supplies the lateral surfaces of the frontal,

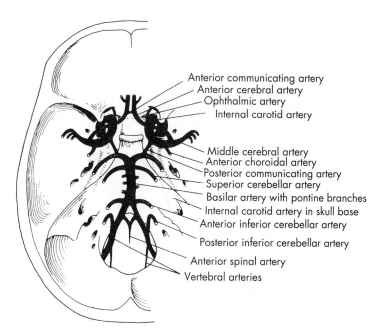

Anterior communicating artery
Anterior cerebral artery
Ophthalmic artery
Internal carotid artery

Middle cerebral artery
Anterior choroidal artery
Posterior communicating artery
Superior cerebellar artery
Basilar artery with pontine branches
Internal carotid artery in skull base
Anterior inferior cerebellar artery

Posterior inferior cerebellar artery

Anterior spinal artery
Vertebral arteries

FIGURE 7-3 Principal arteries on the floor of the cranial cavity (brain removed). (From de Groot J: *Correlative neuroanatomy*, ed 21, Norwalk, Conn, 1991, Appleton & Lange, 131. Reprinted by permission of Appleton & Lange, 1991.)

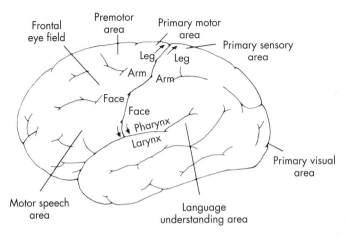

FIGURE 7-4 Lateral view of the left hemisphere, showing the functions of the cortical areas. (From de Groot J: *Correlative neuroanatomy,* ed 21, Norwalk, Conn, 1991, Appleton & Lange, 108. Reprinted by permission of Appleton & Lange, 1991.)

parietal, and temporal lobes. The anterior cerebral artery serves the anterior frontal lobe and the medial surfaces of the hemisphere, including the medial surface of the frontal and parietal lobes. Each internal carotid artery gives rise to one set of vessels on each side, and therefore each carotid artery serves the ipsilateral cerebral hemisphere. When one considers the functions served by the various cortical areas supplied by the branches of the internal carotid artery, a loss of blood supply to a specific area of the brain will result in a dysfunction of that part of the body innervated by that portion of the brain (Figure 7-4).

The posterior circulation to the brain begins as the vertebral arteries, which originate as the first branches of the subclavian arteries on each side. At the sixth cervical vertebra, the vertebral arteries enter the foramina transversaria and move caudally through each successively higher vertebra. The vertebral arteries enter the posterior fossa through the foramen magnum. The vertebral arteries give off the anterior and posterior spinal arteries, which descend ventrally and dorsally, respectively, to supply the spinal cord. At the pontomedullary junction, the vertebral arteries join to form one vessel, the basilar artery. The terminal branches of the basilar artery are the posterior cerebral arteries, which are formed from the bifurcation of the basilar artery at the midbrain level. The vertebral and basilar arteries are the only source of blood supply for the cervical spinal cord, medulla, pons, midbrain, and cerebellum. The posterior cerebral arteries supply the primary visual cortex (Brodmann's area 17) in the occipital lobe.

Joining the anterior and posterior territory circulation is the circle of Willis (Figure 7-2). The complete circle is formed from the posterior and anterior cerebral arteries, joined by the posterior communicating arteries. The anterior communicating artery joins the two anterior cerebral arteries, completing the circle. Under normal conditions, there is little exchange of blood between the right and left cerebral hemispheres.[35,164] Although it is possible for the circle of Willis to equalize blood flow to both sides of the brain, the communicating arteries apparently do not form adequate anastomoses, which is why serious alterations in blood flow to the brain can occur when occlusion of a carotid artery occurs.

Because the patterns of blood supply to the brain are well established, it should be quite easy to determine which vessel is affected when a stroke patient presents with specific complaints. For example, if a patient presents with a monocular visual disturbance associated with a vascular occlusion, the patient must have ipsilateral carotid artery disease, because the ophthalmic artery on that side branches off the ipsilateral carotid artery. If the patient complains of weakness, numbness, or tingling of the arm and leg on the right side, the left side of the brain is affected, because the nerves involved cross to the right arm and leg from the left cerebral hemisphere. Table 7-1[36] summarizes the findings associated with occlusion of blood flow to each of the major arteries to the brain. Although the general concepts summarized in the table hold true, recent literature[37,38] demonstrates that there may be more variability between patients than previously believed, and that there remains some controversy as to the exact areas of the brain supplied by each vessel.

CLINICAL PEARL

If a patient presents with a monocular visual disturbance associated with a vascular occlusion, the patient must have ipsilateral carotid artery disease, because the ophthalmic artery on that side branches off the ipsilateral carotid artery.

Atherosclerosis

Approximately three fourths of all strokes are a result of cerebral infarction associated with blood vessels arising from the carotid and vertebral arteries.[39] The data from the Framingham study showed that 78% of strokes have a thromboembolic origin; however, only 2% of strokes resulted from cardiac emboli.[40] Of lesser importance in the cause of stroke are both subarachnoid hemorrhage, accounting for 8% to 12% of strokes, and primary intracerebral hemorrhage, accounting for 5% to 10% of all strokes.

TABLE 7-1
Occlusion of Major Arteries to the Brain

Artery and Findings	Area Involved in Lesion
I. Anterior cerebral artery	
A. Contralateral monoplegia (leg)	Paracentral lobule
B. Contralateral sensory loss	Thalamocortical radiations
C. If on dominant side	
1. Mental confusion	Frontal lobe
2. Apraxia, aphasia	Corpus callosum, cortical speech area
II. Anterior choroidal artery	
A. Homonymous hemianopsia	Geniculocalcarine tract (optic radiation)
B. Contralateral	
1. Hemiplegia	Corticospinal fibers of internal capsule
2. Hemianesthesia	Posterior limb of internal capsule
III. Middle cerebral artery	
A. Homonymous hemianopsia	Optic tract
B. Contralateral	
1. Hemiplegia and hemianesthesia	Anterior and posterior limbs of internal capsule
C. If on dominant side	
1. Global aphasia	Motor and sensory speech areas
IV. Posterior cerebral artery	
A. Homonymous hemianopsia	Optic radiations
B. Contralateral	
1. Hemiplegia, ataxia	Internal capsule, spinocerebellar tract
2. Impaired sensation	Posterolateral ventral nucleus of thalamus
3. Burning pain	Dorsal nucleus of thalamus
4. Choreoathetoid movements	Red nucleus
V. Superior cerebellar artery	
A. Homolateral	
1. Cerebellar ataxia	Spinocerebellar tract
2. Choreiform movements	Red nucleus
3. Horner's syndrome	Reticular formation
B. Contralateral	
1. Loss of pain and temperature (face and body)	Spinal nucleus of V and lemniscus system
2. Central facial weakness	Corticobulbar fibers to nucleus of VII
3. Partial deafness	Lateral lemniscus
VI. Anterior inferior cerebellar artery	
A. Homolateral	
1. Cerebellar ataxia, deafness	Spinocerebellar tract, cochlear nuclei
2. Loss of sensation (face)	Spinal tract and nucleus of V
B. Contralateral	
1. Loss of pain and temperature (body)	Lemniscus system (spinothalamics)
VII. Posterior inferior cerebellar artery	
A. Homolateral	
1. Cerebellar ataxia, nystagmus	Spinocerebellar tract
2. Horner's syndrome	Reticular formation
3. Loss of sensation (face)	Spinal tract and nucleus of V
4. Dysphagia and dysphonia	Nucleus ambiguus, to IX and to X
B. Contralateral	
1. Loss of pain and temperature (body)	Lateral spinothalamic tract

From Pansky B, House EL: *Review of gross anatomy,* ed 3, New York, 1975, MacMillan pp. 92. Reprinted by permission of McGraw-Hill, 1975.

CLINICAL PEARL

Approximately three fourths of all strokes are a result of cerebral infarction associated with blood vessels arising from the carotid and vertebral arteries.

The most common disorder producing brain ischemia is atherosclerosis of the cerebral vessels.[41,42] Atherosclerosis is a type of arteriolosclerosis that results in changes in small portions of vessels, rather than diffuse changes. The earliest lesion noted is the fatty streak, in which lipid-laden smooth muscle cells and macrophages, foam cells, and fibrous tissues accumulate in focal areas of the intima. Fatty streaks are common findings in children, and may be present in as much as 30% to 50% of the aortic surface by the age of 25 years.[43] Fatty streaks do not cause stenosis of the vessel.

When the lesion becomes more advanced and involves the inner layers of the vessel wall protruding into the lumen, a fibrous plaque has evolved. These plaques contain a central core of extracellular lipids and cholesterol esters,[44,45] necrotic cell debris, and occasionally calcium salts precipitated in the tissue, resulting in calcification of the lesion.[46] Fibrous plaques are termed complicated lesions when they demonstrate such calcification, or when necrosis, thrombosis, or ulcerations of the surface are present. The pathologic findings include either well-defined hemorrhaging covered with fibrous and calcified tissue or highly vascular atheromas. Embolization of plaque material may occur when fragments of the lesion break off and circulate to smaller vessels, thus occluding them.[47] Stroke also may result from hemorrhaging into the vascularized plaque. Carotid plaques tend to demonstrate more hemorrhaging and vascularization than do those of the vertebral arteries.

Atherosclerosis of the vertebral arteries tends to present with less hemorrhaging, but more fibrosis and calcification.[42] Plaques in the vertebral arteries tend to be located at the origin of the vessels.[48]

The atherosclerotic process is a diffuse, generalized one throughout all vessels. The most pronounced lesions, however, tend to be located at large arterial bifurcations and branches of arteries.[39] Consequently, the bifurcation of the common carotid artery into the internal and external vessels accounts for as many as 90% of ischemic stroke syndromes.[49]

The currently accepted theory on the cause of cerebral ischemia involves the embolization of particles from the atherosclerotic plaque in the extracranial vessels to distal vessels in the brain. Because TIAs occur with a sudden onset and only intermittently, the embolic theory is a likely explanation of their cause.

The plaque that forms at the carotid bifurcation is an important source of emboli. When the intimal layer of the artery becomes ulcerated, various materials can attach to the surface of the ulcer; furthermore, particles of the plaque itself can break off, with resultant embolization to smaller vessels distally. The emboli may be made up of aggregates of platelets, thrombotic material, cholesterol crystals, metabolic byproducts of intraplaque hemorrhage, or other portions of the atheromatous plaque itself.[42] Because of the numerous vessels that branch off the internal carotid artery distally, many symptoms may be experienced by the patient. Ulceration of the surface of the lesion is a common finding in patients with TIAs, whereas hemodynamically significant stenosis is found in less than 50% of these patients.[50-53]

The symptoms resulting from ischemia of the brain may be relieved when the emboli dissolve, become more fragmented, and travel to smaller, more distal branches of the vessel without obstructing blood flow, or when collateral channels open rapidly.

Although atherosclerosis is responsible for most cerebral ischemic attacks, there are other causes of ischemic strokes, such as fibromuscular dysplasia. Other causes of cerebral ischemia are noted in the box below.

Causes of Cerebral Ischemia

Atherosclerosis
Cardiogenic emboli to brain
Subarachnoid hemorrhage
Venous or dural sinus thrombosis
Takayasu's arteritis
Giant cell arteritis
Fibromuscular dysplasia[54]
Aneurysm
Spontaneous carotid dissection
Severe anemia[55]
Infectious arteritis
Cocaine use[56]
Amphetamine use
Fibrinoid necrosis and lipohyalinosis
Binswanger's disease (subacute arteriosclerotic
   encephalopathy)[57-59]
Idiopathic regressing arteriopathy
Amyloid angiopathy
Systemic cholesterol microembolization
   syndrome[60]
Polyarteritis nodosa and other connective tissue
   diseases
Wegener's granulomatosis
Moyamoya disease

Symptoms of Transient Visual Loss

Regardless of the mechanism for cerebral ischemia, the symptoms described by patients experiencing transient occlusion of cerebral arteries are classic. The duration of symptoms is extremely important. A TIA is defined as an episode of focal visual, motor, or sensory loss that generally lasts only 2 to 15 minutes, but may last up to 24 hours. If these symptoms persist after 24 hours and then eventually subside, the episode is called a reversible ischemic neurologic deficit. After the attack, the patient returns to the preattack status with no apparent evidence of permanent damage. If the neurologic symptoms continue to evolve, the condition is called a stroke in progress or a stroke in evolution. It is after the neurologic deficits become permanent that a completed stroke is diagnosed.

CLINICAL PEARL

A TIA is defined as an episode of focal visual, motor, or sensory loss that generally lasts only 2 to 15 minutes, but may last up to 24 hours. After the attack, the patient returns to the preattack status with no apparent evidence of permanent damage.

The symptoms experienced by the patient will vary depending on the artery occluded, and therefore the area of the brain affected. If an embolus from a carotid plaque should lodge in the ophthalmic artery, the patient frequently notices a TMB, and classically describes the episode as "a shade being pulled down over my vision." Only one eye is affected, because the embolus results from the ipsilateral carotid plaque. Several minutes later, the "shade" is raised.

CLINICAL PEARL

If an embolus from a carotid plaque should lodge in the ophthalmic artery, the patient frequently notices a TMB, and classically describes the episode as "a shade being pulled down over my vision."

Wray has described four types of amaurosis fugax based on the cause of the vision loss.[61] Type 1 is caused by transient retinal ischemia due to embolism of fresh thrombus, cholesterol crystals (Hollenhorst plaques), calcific emboli, or emboli composed of platelets associated with thrombocytosis. The latter type of emboli occurs especially in association with heart disease, including myocardial infarction, mitral stenosis, and vegetative valvular lesions.[61] Additionally, mitral-annulus calcification,[62-64] mitral valve prolapse,[64-66] and myxoma of the heart[68] have been demonstrated to produce emboli with resultant amaurosis fugax. Other types of nonarteriosclerotic vasculopathies as well as altered states of blood viscosity and coagulation can be associated with type 1 amaurosis fugax.

Type 2 amaurosis fugax is caused by retinal vascular insufficiency. These temporary attacks of vision loss precede permanent loss of vision due to chronic hypoperfusion of the eye. Because of the nature of the change, the onset of vision loss is more gradual than in type 1 amaurosis fugax, and the episodes are of longer duration. Vision may not be lost totally, but contrast acuity is significantly affected. The chronic hypoperfusion state of the retina results in dilatation of the retinal venules, venous wall irregularity, fluorescein leakage from the venules, and peripheral microaneurysms and blot hemorrhages.[68] A case of temporal fossa sarcoid granulomata with transient obscurations of vision similar to type 2 amaurosis fugax has recently been described.[69]

Although type 3 amaurosis fugax also results from a decrease in perfusion to the eye, there is no persistent impairment of retinal perfusion.[61] In this case, the visual disturbances mimic those noted in type 2 cases, but they are most likely due to a spasm of the ophthalmic, retinal, or posterior ciliary arteries, as occurs in ocular migraine (see Chapter 9).

Idiopathic cases of amaurosis fugax are classified as type 4 cases. Younger patients, generally less than 30 years of age, have been noted to experience numerous episodes of sudden unilateral loss of vision without evidence of any detectable pathology. These episodes lasted from 30 to 60 minutes, or for a matter of seconds only.[61] No significant permanent loss of vision or other significant sequelae are expected in this group of patients experiencing amaurosis fugax.

Although TMB can result from any temporary reduction in blood flow to the ophthalmic artery,[70-76] the finding is frequently an indication that the patient has extensive cardiovascular disease.[12,77-79] It should be remembered that the risk for stroke after an episode of TVL is approximately 40%.[10,11,80] In a study of 34 cases presenting with TVL, 41% of the patients suffered a stroke in progress or a completed stroke within 7 days after the episode of TMB.[7,11] It is therefore imperative that noninvasive carotid testing be ordered on an emergency basis when a patient presents with TVL. The Amaurosis Fugax Study Group[81] had proposed appropriate management guidelines of patients presenting with TVL (Figure 7-5).

When embolization from a carotid plaque and subsequent occlusion of a cerebral artery occur, the patient can suffer a hemispheric TIA. The vessel that is affected will dictate whether or not the patient experiences motor, sensory, or speech deficits. Carotid artery disease

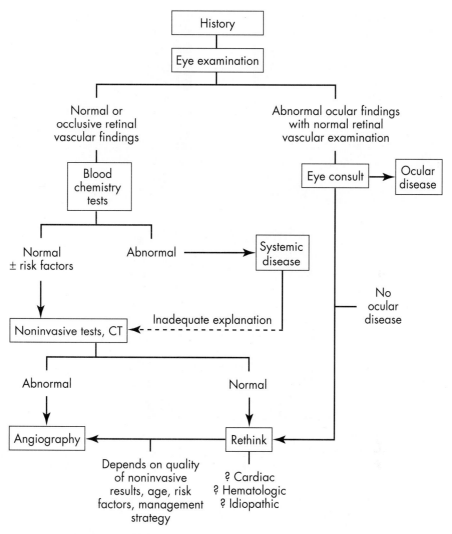

FIGURE 7-5 Scheme for workup of patients with transient visual loss. (From The Amaurosis Fugax Study Group: Amaurosis fugax (transient monocular blindness): a consensus statement. In Bernstein EF, ed: *Amaurosis fugax,* New York, 1988 Springer-Verlag, 290. Reprinted by permission of Springer-Verlag, 1988.)

may result in ocular symptoms and signs other than TVL. A Hollenhorst plaque is a cholesterol embolus from a carotid plaque that may be seen in the retina as an intra-arterial, yellow, glistening lesion that generally lodges at a bifurcation of a retinal arteriole (Figure 7-6). Central retinal artery occlusion, branch retinal artery occlusion, recurrent and chronic retinal ischemia, and retinal telangiectasia may be due to carotid arterial disease.

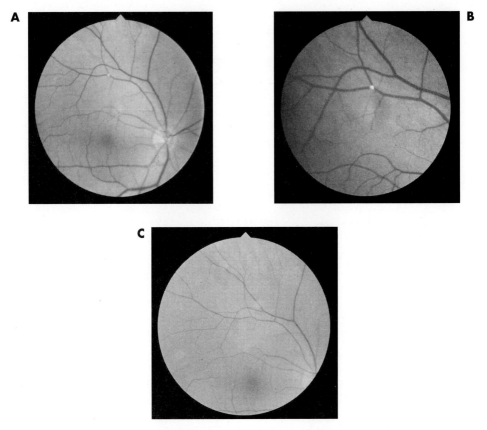

FIGURE 7-6 **A**, Hollenhorst plaque in the superior temporal branch of the central retinal artery. **B**, Magnified view. **C**, One week later, the plaque has broken up, and there is no ophthalmoscopic evidence of it.

CLINICAL PEARL

A Hollenhorst plaque is a cholesterol embolus from a carotid plaque that may be seen in the retina as an intra-arterial, yellow, glistening lesion that generally lodges at a bifurcation of a retinal arteriole.

When bilateral symptoms are noted, the cause is most likely an occlusion of the vertebrobasilar system, because the basilar artery branches supply both hemispheres. The anterior circulation is more commonly affected by emboli than the posterior circulation. It is estimated that the posterior circulation receives approximately 20% of the intracranial blood flow and, therefore, also receives about 20% of the emboli.[82] Occlusive disease or the heart may be the source of emboli to the posterior circulation.[83-87] The vertebral artery, the distal basilar bifurcation, and the posterior cerebral artery and its branches may be affected by embolic occlusion within the posterior circulation. Furthermore, atherosclerosis may affect the origin of the vertebral arteries, the distal vertebral artery, the proximal 2 cm of the basilar artery, and the proximal posterior cerebral arteries, although occlusion of branches of the posterior cerebral artery is usually secondary to embolization.[88] Interestingly, proximal vertebral artery lesions are rare in black patients but common in whites.[88] However, black patients demonstrate a propensity for atherosclerosis at the proximal posterior cerebral arteries.[83]

Unfortunately, there are few pathognomonic individual symptoms associated with posterior circulation ischemia.[90] The patient may complain of dizziness or vertigo, weakness or numbness of the limbs on both sides, diplopia, and bilateral loss of vision. The transient loss of vision associated with vertebrobasilar disease is not as classically described as that in TVL. The patient may find it difficult to explain the symptoms, except that an overall loss of vision occurred that lasted a few seconds to a few minutes. The patient frequently states that it is "as if looking through a fog," and there may be associated flashes of light in the involved field of vision.[74] Because the primary striate visual cortex is supplied by the posterior cerebral arteries, a bilateral visual loss is noted when both posterior cerebral arteries are affected. When only one posterior cerebral artery is occluded, the symptoms will be noted only in the contralateral visual field. It is interesting to note that patients will develop visual neglect and will not pay attention to objects in the contralateral visual field when the entire posterior cerebral artery territory is infarcted; however, when only the striate visual field cortex or the banks of the calcarine fissure are affected, this phenomenon does not occur.[90]

It is not uncommon for patients who demonstrate vertebrobasilar occlusive disease to also demonstrate carotid artery disease.[91,92] Patients with the subclavian steal syndrome also may note visual symptoms associated with vertebrobasilar insufficiency. In this syndrome, atherosclerosis with resultant hemodynamically significant stenosis or complete obstruction of the subclavian artery occurs proximal to the origin to the vertebral artery. Blood therefore cannot flow into the subclavian artery on the ipsilateral side. As blood flows up the contralateral vertebral artery, it is siphoned into the ipsilateral vertebral artery, where retrograde flow occurs (Figure 7-7).[93] Although blood flow to the arm becomes sufficient, ischemia to the vertebrobasilar territory results. Exertion of the ipsilateral arm results in increased metabolic demands, and subsequently the patient experiences increased symptoms typical of those involving the posterior circulation of the brain. It is estimated that approximately 4% of patients presenting with cerebrovascular disease demonstrate the subclavian steal syndrome, which also constitutes 17% of extracranial vascular disease.[94]

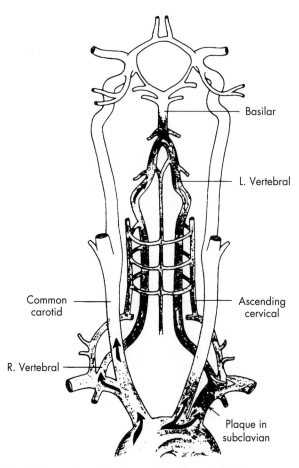

Basilar

L. Vertebral

Common carotid

Ascending cervical

R. Vertebral

Plaque in subclavian

FIGURE 7-7 Atherosclerotic plaque in the subclavian artery producing a subclavian steal syndrome. Note the blood flow up the opposite vertebral artery and then retrograde in the other vertebral artery to enter the stenosed subclavian artery. (From Blaustein B: The subclavian steal syndrome, *Clin Eye Vision Care* 3:25-28, 1991. Reprinted by permission of Butterworth-Heinemann, 1991.)

It must be remembered that there are several causes for stroke. Transient ischemic attacks are associated with either cerebral thrombosis or embolic events. When small infarctions occur in the deeper parts of the brain, in the internal capsule and basal ganglia of hypertensive patients, four clinical syndromes can occur associated with this type of lacunar stroke. The patient may demonstrate either pure motor hemiparesis, a purely sensory stroke, ataxic hemiparesis, or dysarthria–clumsy hand syndrome. Hypertensive patients also may demonstrate intracerebral hemorrhage or subarachnoid hemorrhage resulting in stroke. The terminology for symptoms and signs noted in various types of strokes is given in Table 7-2. When a patient

TABLE 7-2
Definitions of Common Neurologic Deficits

Neurologic Deficit	Definitions
Agnosia	Even though a given sense is intact, the patient is unable to use it for recognition of objects. Visual, tactile, or auditory agnosias are possible.
Agraphia	Inability to write.
Akinesia	Total absence or reduction of movement.
Alexia	Inability to read.
Aphagia	Patient does not eat. Does not have to be of neurologic origin.
Aphasia	Inability to express or comprehend spoken or written language, due to disease or trauma affecting the brain. Considered an outdated term, and more specific terminology should be used.[89]
Apraxia	Inability to perform purposeful, skilled, and complex movements, in the absence of paralysis or disturbed motor coordination or abnormalities in the sensory neurologic pathways.
Ataxia	Muscle coordination is absent or deficient. The muscles involved will be determined by the part of the brain or spinal cord affected by the neurologic disease.
Dysarthria	Difficulty articulating speech, due to incoordination of the muscles used in speaking, secondary to a neurologic deficit.
Dyskinesia	Involuntary abnormal movements. Voluntary movements are impaired.
Dysphagia	Inability to swallow, due to diseases (including but not limited to neurologic entities), trauma, or mechanical etiologies.
Dysphasia	While *aphasia* implies a total inability to express or comprehend language, *dysphasia* implies a partial loss of the language function, usually a single aspect of language. *Expressive dysphasia* implies the patient's inability to communicate with written or spoken words. *Cognitive dysphasia* prohibits the patient from understanding what is meant by language, and he or she is therefore unable to make the connection between sensory association areas and motor areas.[89] *Receptive dysphasias* prevent the patient from converting vision or hearing into language, so that, for example, reading may be impossible, even though the patient's vision is not affected.
Dysphonia	Difficulty or impairment of speech.
Hemiplegia	Paralysis of the arm and leg on one side.
Paresthesias	Abnormal sensations of numbness, burning, tingling, or general discomfiture, which is frequently seen in association with a loss of tactile sensibility.[35]

presents with suspected stroke, minimal physical examination should include palpation of radial and carotid pulses, bilateral brachial blood pressures, auscultation for carotid bruits and cardiac murmurs, and a brief neurologic examination. Appropriate referral then should be made for further diagnostic testing.

Testing for Carotid Artery and Vertebrobasilar Disease

When the devastating consequences of a stroke are considered, it is obvious that identifying potential stroke victims, determining the extent of their disease, and instituting appropriate prophylactic therapy are imperative. Noninvasive cerebrovascular examination procedures are intended to find treatable lesions in the extracranial carotid arteries so that occurrence of a stroke can be prevented. Before the availability of noninvasive tests for studying the carotid and cerebral circulation, the only means of doing so was an arteriogram. Although the goal of noninvasive test procedures is not the total elimination of arteriography,[95] the capability of anticipating the results of arteriography and thereby reducing the unnecessary studies certainly adds to the usefulness of the noninvasive diagnostic procedures.[96-99] Furthermore, clarification of those patients in whom arteriography is mandatory further increases the utility of these procedures. Studies indicate that approximately 65% of patients without disease may be spared unnecessary arteriographic testing[100,101] when noninvasive tests are performed first. Consequently it has become the standard of care to obtain noninvasive test results in many cases of suspected carotid atherosclerotic disease. Before referring the patient for noninvasive testing, the optometrist should perform several tests in the office to aid in the diagnosis of carotid or vertebrobasilar occlusive disease.

A gross inspection of the neck should be made for prominent pulsations to rule out pulsatile masses,[102,103] carotid aneurysm, thyrotoxicosis, and aortic insufficiency.[86] However, the neck will not demonstrate pulsation with carotid atherosclerotic disease. The carotid pulses should be auscultated in the anterior triangle of the neck. Standing to either the side or the back of the patient, the three middle fingers of the right hand can be used to auscultate the carotid pulse on the right side, and the three middle fingers of the left hand can be used for the left side. Alternatively, the left thumb can be used to palpate the right carotid pulse and the right thumb used for the left carotid pulse while standing in front of the patient. Pressure on the artery is slowly increased until a maximum pulsation is felt, and then the pressure is slowly released. The carotid pulsations are best felt when palpating at approximately the level of the thyroid cartilage. One side should be palpated at a time, and pressure should never be placed on both carotid vessels simultaneously. The pulses should be equal between the two sides, and graded according to the following published grading scale:[104]

Grade 0—No carotid pulse present
Grade TR—Trace pulse present
Grade 1+—Decreased pulse from normal
Grade 2+—Normal carotid pulse
Grade 3+—Pulsations increased from normal
Grade 4+—Greatly increased pulsations (clonus)

Normal blood flow through the vessels is silent. When a partial occlusion occurs in an artery, turbulence develops in the pattern of blood flow. Vibrations in the vessel walls subsequently occur, and those vibrations are transmitted through the skin to the stethoscope as "noise." If this noise is transmitted along larger arteries from the heart or from the heart itself, it is called a *murmur.* If the noise is heard in association with noncardiac vessels, it is called a *bruit.* By using a stethoscope to auscultate for carotid arterial bruits, it is possible to hear a soft, early systolic bruit when the carotid vessel is approximately 50% stenosed. The greater the occlusion, the greater the velocity of blood flowing through the stenosis. For that reason, if the artery is 70% to 80% stenosed, a bruit will be heard through both systole and diastole. It is unlikely that an occluded artery may have any associated bruit.

CLINICAL PEARL

When a partial occlusion occurs in an artery, turbulence develops in the pattern of blood flow. Vibrations in the vessel walls subsequently occur, and those vibrations are transmitted through the skin to the stethoscope as "noise."

The vaulted trumpet bell of the stethoscope should be used to auscultate the vessels of the neck. The chest piece is first placed in the supraclavicular fossa so that the subclavian artery can be auscultated (Figure 7-8). The vaulted trumpet bell then is used to auscultate the common carotid artery in the low position on the neck (Figure 7-9). At the midlevel position, the carotid bifurcation can be auscultated (Figure 7-10). At the high position on the neck, it is the internal carotid artery that is being auscultated (Figure 7-11). A bruit may be heard either at the sight of the stenosis or distal to it. Therefore if a bruit is noted at the low position on the neck, the sound must be emanating from the heart or large vessels proximal to the common carotid artery on the ipsilateral side. If, however, no bruit is noted in the common carotid artery, but a bruit is noted at the midposition and high positions on the neck, the stenosis must be present at the carotid bifurcation, and the sound is being transmitted distally along the vessel to be heard at the high position in the neck. Not only should the presence or absence of a bruit be recorded, but moreover it should be noted as to whether or not the bruit is systolic only or extends into diastole as well.

Orbital bruits may be heard in carotid-cavernous fistula,[105] thrombosis of the ipsilateral internal carotid artery,[106] narrowing of the ipsilateral internal carotid artery, and in states of marked anemia or hyperthyroidism.[107,108] Orbital bruits are auscultated by placing the bell of the stethoscope on the forehead at the midline and listening for bruits, as well as above the eyebrow and at the temple. The bell also

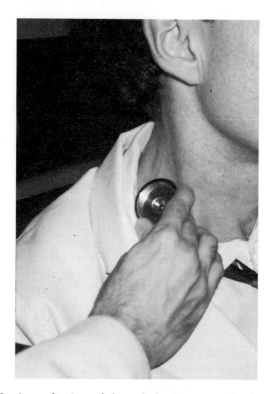

FIGURE 7-8 Auscultation of the subclavian artery in the supraclavicular fossa.

should be placed over the closed superior eyelid. No bruit should be heard in the normal patient in any of these positions.

Two broad types of noninvasive tests are available for study of extracranial carotid atherosclerotic disease. Direct testing studies the effects of the disease process at the site of the lesion. Direct tests diagnose carotid artery disease either by analysis of bruits or through ultrasonic analyses. Indirect evaluations analyze the effects that the lesion causes in the vasculature distal to the carotid bifurcation; therefore some inference is necessary to draw conclusions about carotid artery disease. Although auscultation for bruits should be performed on a routine basis during clinical examination, many patients will demonstrate stenotic lesions angiographically but not stethoscopically,[109] whereas some patients with audible bruits will not demonstrate stenosis on angiography.[110] These inconsistencies lead to the development of methods to electronically enhance the sounds created by stenotic lesions.

Carotid phonoangiography (CPA), a direct test of carotid stenosis, uses the time-honored clinical knowledge of bruit examination and interpretation and increases the evaluation capabilities by using engineering techniques to enhance the detection of bruits.[111,112] The bruit

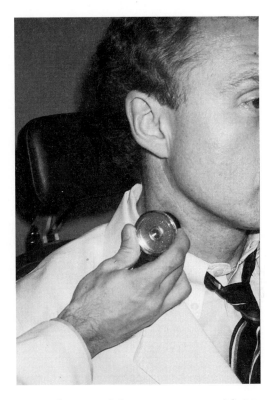

FIGURE 7-9 Auscultation of the common carotid artery in the low position on the neck.

is amplified by a microphone held directly over the vessels in the neck. The same three positions on the neck are studied with CPA as on carotid auscultation with a stethoscope. The examiner listens to the audible sounds through the electronic stethoscope and views the oscilloscopic projection of the audio frequency waveforms of the sounds. Either Polaroid photographs of the time series displayed on the cathode ray tube can be taken, or the instrument may provide a heat-sensitive paper printout as a permanent record. Several studies have demonstrated that CPA testing alone is neither highly sensitive nor specific;[3,113-121] however, the accuracy, sensitivity, and specificity of the technique is increased when it is used in combination with ocular plethysmography (OPG) testing. Many of the progressive, more active noninvasive vascular clinics have abandoned the use of CPA testing.[122]

Ultrasound technology provides a safe and noninvasive method of detecting blood flow, visualizing arterial wall motion, and examining vessel walls and stenosis. The brightness modulation mode, or B-mode, produces an image of the structure being visualized. The principles of carotid ultrasonography are exactly the same as those of

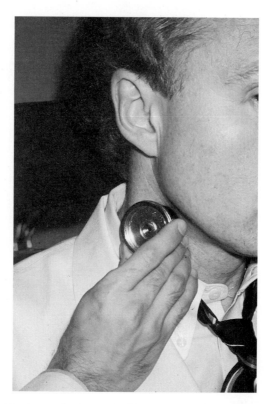

FIGURE 7-10 Auscultation of the carotid bifurcation at the midpoint on the neck.

ophthalmic ultrasonography. Each point in the field being studied corresponds to a dot on the oscilloscope screen. The amplitude of the reflected echo at that particular point is projected onto the screen as a dot whose brightness is proportional to the amplitude of the echo. Each point in the field is analyzed, and the relative brightness is projected onto the oscilloscope screen; thus an image of the area being scanned is produced with brighter and darker dots. This mode of ultrasonic study is especially helpful in visualizing anatomy, both normal and abnormal. The extracranial carotid vasculature can be examined noninvasively using B-mode ultrasound, and plaque formation can be visualized (Figures 7-12 and 7-13). Ultrasound diagnostic studies are safe for the patient, and create no physical damage or harm to the tissues through which the sound waves pass. Destructive cavitation of soft tissues can occur if sufficient intensity ultrasound is used for significant periods;[123] however, the diagnostic instruments currently available do not produce the intensity necessary for such damage to occur.

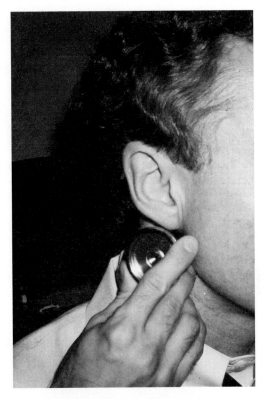

FIGURE 7-11 Auscultation of the internal carotid artery at the high position on the neck.

CLINICAL PEARL

Ultrasound technology provides a safe and noninvasive method of detecting blood flow, visualizing arterial wall motion, and examining vessel walls and stenosis. The brightness modulation mode, or B-mode, produces an image of the structure being visualized.

Duplex ultrasonography not only allows B-mode scanning of the vessels, but moreover allows the examiner to study blood flow patterns by performing Doppler evaluations. Sound emitted by a moving object is perceived as higher than the transmitted frequency if that object is moving toward the listener, and conversely will be perceived as being lower than the transmitted frequency if the source is moving away from the listener. The faster the object moves, the greater the change in frequency. In performing Doppler studies of the carotid vessels, the red blood cells act as the moving objects in the Doppler

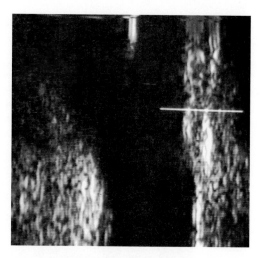

FIGURE 7-12 B-mode longitudinal view on carotid ultrasonography demonstrating the common carotid bifurcation and internal and external carotid arteries. The cursor is pointing to the bifurcation.

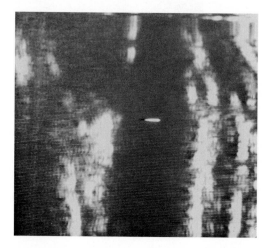

FIGURE 7-13 Atherosclerotic plaque at the carotid bifurcation seen on B-mode ultrasound imaging. The cursor is in the bifurcation, and the plaque is to the left of it.

principle. The velocity of blood flow can be determined, and therefore physiologic patterns of blood flow through a vessel can be "mapped."

There are several ways in which the Doppler results can be processed, displayed, and analyzed. The examiner may use an amplifier with or without earphones, or stethoscope-type earpieces to audibly analyze the signals. The extracranial carotid arteries have different flow patterns because of the degree of resistance distally;

thus the signals from the individual vessels can be differentiated audibly with some practice. Furthermore, abnormalities in blood flow produce characteristic sounds, thereby allowing the examiner to make a differential diagnosis with an accuracy exceeding 90%.[124] Sound spectrum analysis is a more accurate means of signal processing and display.[125] In this case, the various frequencies in amplitudes of the Doppler shift spectrum are plotted against time. A waveform is created, which demonstrates both the systolic and diastolic heartbeat. Normative data are available for each vessel in the neck, against which abnormal findings can be compared. With increasing degrees of stenosis, the velocity of red blood cells will necessarily be increased at the point of maximum stenosis; therefore a significant increase in blood cell velocity can be measured at that point. Furthermore, the degree of turbulence can be noted by examining the waveform itself to determine the range of velocities at which blood cells are traveling.

In color flow Doppler analysis, the echoes are displayed as colors that indicate the direction of blood flow according to the Doppler shifts represented. The brightness of the color can also represent the intensity of the echoes received by the transducer. In this way, a two-dimensional view of the vessels, with colors representing either forward blood flow or flow away from the transducer, are obtained.

Carotid duplex scans are performed with the patient in a supine position. The scan can take up to 30 minutes with an experienced technologist. A liberal amount of acoustic gel is applied to the patient's neck. The probe is placed above the clavicle in a longitudinal plane. The examiner scans the neck longitudinally in three different positions. Each position may provide entirely different ultrasonic information about the carotid arteries. An anteroposterior view, lateral-medial view, and posteroanterior view are obtained, in addition to a transverse view of all three vessels. During the entire study, the examiner wears a microphone, which allows a constant commentary as to the position of the probe.

In a normal artery, the lumen appears dark on B-mode ultrasonography. Disease is seen as echoes within the lumen. An impression of plaque composition can be obtained through B-mode scanning. The greater the density of the plaque, the greater the acoustical impedance, and therefore the brighter the echo noted on the image. When the plaque is calcified, it is highly echogenic and demonstrates a bright echo on the screen, with shadowing deep to the calcium, because the ultrasound beam cannot penetrate the calcium deposit. A soft plaque demonstrates low acoustic impedance, and, as such, will present as a subtle gray area. The clinical implications of the plaque description are such that the stability of the atheroma may correlate with its ultrasonic characteristics. A small, fibrous plaque may be more stable than a complicated plaque demonstrating calcification. Ulceration of the intimal lining can be visualized on real time B-mode scan. Most ulcerations occur at the proximal or middle portion of the plaque. An intraplaque hemorrhage may appear to be a crater within the atheroma, because the intima overlying it will not be seen, and the dark hemorrhage can mimic the darkly echogenic characteristics of an ulceration.

The degree of stenosis of the vessel also can be determined on B-mode ultrasonography. B-mode imagers have a cursor that allows an accurate measurement of the size of the lumen and the plaque itself. Appropriate measurements can be made on the videotape, and the degree of stenosis is easily calculated. Whether the degree of stenosis is calculated on a diameter or an area basis should be noted with any calculation. A lesion is not considered to be hemodynamically significant unless it creates a 50% or greater stenosis by diameter, or a 75% or greater stenosis by area.

One of the most important capabilities of real time B-mode imaging is the ability to differentiate stenosis from total occlusion of the vessel. A total occlusion of the lumen is characterized by soft gray echoes that fill the lumen of the vessel entirely. The vessel does not pulsate laterally distal to the area of occlusion. When the examiner attempts to obtain a Doppler flow pattern at the occlusion and distally, the signal is absent, because no blood is moving through the occluded area; furthermore, there will be an attenuated Doppler signal immediately proximal to the lesion.

Carotid duplex scans are indicated in several clinical situations. Most patients presenting with TIAs ultimately will have an arteriogram performed. If the patient has normal or completely occluded vessels, an arteriogram is not indicated, because surgical intervention is inappropriate. If a duplex scan can better define those patients in whom an arteriogram is not warranted, an unnecessary invasive procedure may be avoided. Duplex scanning therefore can be used as a screening procedure before ordering arteriography. The box below lists indications for carotid duplex scan studies.

Indications for Carotid Duplex Scans

Patients with cervical bruits

Patients with hemispheric symptoms

In conjunction with carotid arteriography to indicate areas for concentration of the study

Before surgery in patients at risk for stroke (carotid endarterectomy, cardiovascular procedures)

Postoperative monitoring of patients

Diagnosis of carotid atherosclerosis in patients with allergies to contrast agents used in arteriography

Both CPA and carotid duplex evaluations are examples of direct tests of the carotid circulation. In contrast, ocular plethysmography (OPG) is an indirect test of carotid vessel disease and records changes in the volume of the eye. OPG assesses the physiologic function of the ipsilateral carotid artery. Because the ophthalmic artery is the first major branch of the internal carotid artery, analysis of blood flow to that vessel yields indirect information with respect to the patency of the ipsilateral internal carotid artery.

When the left ventricle contracts, outflow from the heart is greater than inflow. The left ventricle expands when inflow is greater than outflow. Pulse plethysmography studies the periodic changes in volume of any part of the body as a result of left ventricular activity.[126] The volume changes in the eye that occur with the heartbeat can be measured by pulse plethysmography. As the heart contracts, blood surges through the ophthalmic arteries. The globe will expand slightly because of the increased volume of blood circulating through the ocular vessels. Pulse-delay OPG measures this change in volume, or flow patterns in the eye. Theoretically, if a hemodynamically significant stenosis exists, the decrease in volume may be explained either by a decrease in the velocity of the pulse wave beyond the stenosed vessel, or the decreased arterial flow may result in a slower increase in volume of the eye, and hence a delay in the pulse wave as compared with the opposite eye.[116] A comparison of the pulse arrival times between the right and left eyes is the basis of the OPG instrument of Kartchner and McRae,[127-129] also known as OPG/KM. The internal carotid arteries must be patent and void of any hemodynamically significant stenosis for the pulse arrival times to be equal between the eyes. A differential tracing produced on the instrument results from electronic amplification of the ocular pulses, and helps to detect very small phase shift differences in ocular volume that would not be obvious on visual examination of the tracings. In cases in which there are no significant stenotic lesions, the pulsations should be equal between the two eyes, and they should arrive at the eyes and ears at the same time. The ear pulse, an indirect measurement of external carotid artery function, is used as a reference point not only to detect external carotid stenoses, but moreover to aid in diagnosis of bilateral internal carotid stenoses. When all pulses arrive at the eyes and ears at the same time, all recorded pulse waveforms demonstrate a simultaneous rise, and a flat tracing is seen in the differential.[128,130]

The pulse-delay OPG instruments must not be confused with the pressure OPG instruments originally described by William Gee and his associates in 1974.[131] The OPG/Gee instrument uses the ophthalmic artery systolic pressure to help diagnose internal carotid artery stenosis. Just as a blood pressure cuff is used to increase pressure above the brachial systolic arterial pressure, the pressure ocular plethysmograph increases intraocular pressure to a point above the ophthalmic arterial systolic pressure. After suction cups are placed on the eyes, a vacuum is induced to 300 or 510 mm Hg. This negative pressure causes an increase in intraocular pressure to the extent that it is elevated above that of the ophthalmic artery. Pulsations of the artery then cease. As the vacuum is reduced, the intraocular pressure then falls below that of the ophthalmic systolic pressure, and the pulsations of the artery return. These pulsations are strictly a function of systolic blood pressure, in contrast to the volumetric changes measured in the OPG/KM. In both animal and human experimental studies, Gee demonstrated the correlation between the amount of negative pressure applied to the eye, the corresponding intraocular pressure, and the associated ophthalmic artery pressure.[131-133] Other research has demonstrated that, in fact, the ophthalmic artery pressure does reflect the ipsilateral internal carotid artery pressure.[134-136] Not only are the absolute ophthalmic artery systolic pressures important, but moreover the ratio between the ophthalmic systolic and brachial systolic pressures can detect bilateral internal carotid stenosis. Furthermore, the amplitude of the pulsations may give additional information. The side with the reduced ophthalmic pulse amplitude may have a significant stenosis, causing decreased pressure as well as decreased amplitude of the pulsation.

The distinction between pulse and pressure plethysmographic testing is an extremely important one. Hemodynamically significant stenosis resulting in a reduced distal arterial systolic blood pressure is a well-documented physiologic principle, whereas the physiologic basis for the pulse-delay method of OPG is still not well understood, and as such, its use in clinical studies remains somewhat controversial.[137] Therefore although OPG/Gee testing is routinely used in noninvasive vascular clinics, OPG/KM is rarely used.

The ocular blood flow rate can be calculated using OPG/Gee findings. The pulse rate, calibrated ocular pulse amplitude, and a constant (0.00149) are multiplied.[138] Because ocular blood flow is an indication of cerebral blood flow and consequent alterations in brain compliance due to cerebral edema, the reduction of ocular blood flow below 0.53 ml/minute bilaterally may be incompatible with cerebral survival.[139] When serial OPG studies are performed on comatose patients with head injuries, documentation of ocular blood flow and therefore cerebral blood flow may aid in making decisions as to appropriate therapy for the patient.[140] Ocular plethysmography testing also has been demonstrated to be helpful in differentiating giant cell arteritis as a cause of anterior ischemic optic neuropathy, as opposed to the nonarteritic cause of anterior ischemic optic neuropathy.[141] Patients demonstrating an abnormal temporal artery biopsy also had an average calculated ocular blood flow rate less than 0.60 ml/minute in patients with giant cell arteritis. Conversely, only one patient with a normal temporal artery biopsy demonstrated ocular blood flow rates in that range. Patients with normal temporal artery

biopsies demonstrated a mean ocular blood flow rate of 1.27 ml/
minute, with a standard deviation of 0.35 ml/minute. Ocular blood
flow was demonstrated to be a remarkably sensitive tool in diagnosing giant cell arteritis as a cause of anterior ischemic optic neuropathy
(see Chapter 6).

Other noninvasive tests study blood flow through the carotid and
ocular vasculature. The box below lists other procedures that may be
included in a noninvasive vascular examination.

Techniques for Noninvasive Cerebrovascular Evaluation

I. Indirect tests
   A. Periorbital Doppler survey (ophthalmosonometry)
      1. Supraorbital Doppler
      2. Frontal artery Doppler
      3. Complete periorbital Doppler
      4. Provocative maneuvers
   B. Photoplethysmography
   C. Ophthalmodynamometry
   D. Ocular plethysmography
      1. Pulse wave delay
      2. Ophthalmic systolic pressure
   E. Cerebrovascular thermography
II. Direct tests
   A. Carotid auscultation
   B. Carotid phonoangiography
      1. Qualitative visual analysis
      2. Quantitative frequency analysis
         (spectral phonoangiography)
   C. Doppler velocity waveform analysis
      1. Continuous wave Doppler
      2. Pulsed/gated Doppler
   D. Carotid imaging
      1. Ultrasonic Doppler arteriography
      2. Real-time B-mode
      3. Color-coded Doppler imaging
   E. Duplex scanning

Periorbital Doppler evaluations (ophthalmosonometry) use compression of collateral vessels feeding the ophthalmic artery to help
identify abnormal flow patterns resulting from internal carotid artery
obstruction.[142-145] Flow through the ophthalmic artery and its
branches is usually antegrade (Figure 7-14); however, if occlusion of
the ipsilateral internal carotid artery should occur, the external carotid

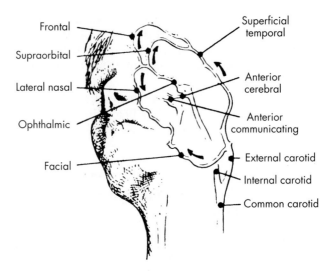

FIGURE 7-14 Arteries of significance to periorbital Doppler test. Normal flow pattern is shown by arrows. (From Brockenbrough EC: Periorbital Doppler velocity evaluation of carotid obstruction. In Bernstein EF, ed: *Noninvasive diagnostic techniques in vascular disease,* ed 3, St Louis, 1985 Mosby, 336. Reprinted by permission of Mosby.)

artery will provide collaterals, and the blood flow will therefore be reversed. A directional Doppler, which indicates forward or reversed blood flow, can therefore indicate whether antegrade or retrograde flow is present in the branches of the ophthalmic artery. By compressing various branches of the external carotid artery, the effect the compression has on retrograde flow through the ophthalmic artery branches is assessed. This technique is highly dependent on the experience and skill of the technician.[146] It is also time-consuming, because several compressive maneuvers must be performed on both sides. Consequently, ophthalmosonometry is no longer commonly performed in noninvasive vascular laboratories.

Supraorbital photoplethysmography also studies the periorbital collateral circulation but uses an infrared transducer instead of a Doppler velocity meter.[145] The results are somewhat less specific than those of Doppler ultrasonometry[147,148] but are generally similar. This test, like the periorbital survey, is not frequently performed.

Blood from the ophthalmic artery branches supplies the supraorbital region of the forehead. This area of the face generally demonstrates a slightly higher temperature than other areas. As a result, temperature differences on the face can be measured by using infrared thermography,[149] which measures infrared energy emissions from the skin of the face. The sensitivity of this test has been shown to be only around 57%, although the specificity is approximately 92%.[150] Provocative compression or cooling maneuvers increased both the sensitivity and specificity of the test. Although cerebrovascular thermography can correlate with occlusion of the extracranial carotid arteries, the expense of the equipment and the relatively low accuracy do not make it a very useful test for noninvasive diagnosis of carotid occlusive disease.

Phonoangiographic spectral analysis combines the theories of CPA and spectral analysis previously discussed. In this technique, phonoangiographic spectra produced are quantitatively analyzed, and the residual diameter of the arterial lumen is determined.[151-153] This technique has been demonstrated to be quite accurate,[151,154] although bruits arising from external carotid artery stenoses may confound the results. As with most noninvasive tests, a combination of this test with another noninvasive test would be most advantageous in diagnosing stenoses. In patients that do present with carotid bruits, spectral phonoangiography could be an effective means of monitoring the progression of the stenosis.

The field of noninvasive evaluation of carotid arterial disease is rapidly evolving. As a result, improved instrumentation is constantly being developed. Numerous techniques such as carotid compression tonography,[155,156] pneumatictonometry,[157,158] transcranial Doppler examination,[159,160] and pulsed Doppler arteriography[161,162] may be favored by specific noninvasive testing clinics over other techniques. It is generally desirable to perform both a direct and indirect assessment of carotid arterial function to enhance the accuracy of diagnosis, so that individual laboratories may perform any combination of these techniques.

Angiography

Angiography remains the gold standard for diagnosis of atheromatous disease, in spite of the numerous noninvasive tests available. This procedure involves inserting a catheter transfemorally and threading it retrograde through the aorta to the major vessels. A bolus of contrast dye is injected and fluoroscopic pictures are taken. The presence of atheromatous plaques, which can be displaced, constitutes a major risk factor with standard angiography. However, angiography provides information that will influence the therapeutic decision.[163,36] Surgical intervention is expected when a patient is referred for angiography.

CLINICAL PEARL

Angiography remains the gold standard for diagnosis of atheromatous disease, in spite of the numerous noninvasive tests available.

Arteriography demonstrates stenosis and occlusion when present (Figure 7-14) but does involve some risks (see the box below).[164-175] Those risks have been reduced with the digital subtraction arteriography (DSA) procedure.[177-179] Contrary to standard angiography, the catheter is advanced through a percutaneous femoral vein or antecubital vein access point to the superior vena cava. A fluoroscopic image of the neck is taken before injection of the contrast media, which is stored in a video processor. At a rate of 12 to 14 ml/second, 40 to 50 ml of contrast medium is injected. Fluoroscopic images are taken at 1-second intervals for 6 to 10 seconds when the contrast media enter the carotid arteries. The computer then digitally summates the images and subtracts them from the image of the neck taken before the injection, projecting the resultant image onto a television monitor. Digital subtraction arteriography provides images that are not as clear as those seen with standard arteriography, but the results obtained usually are diagnostically sufficient. There are indications for each type of study.[163]

Adverse Reactions to Arteriography

Histologic changes
  Reversible blood vessel endothelial damage[164,165]
  Reversible red blood cell hemolysis[164,165]
  Crenation[165,166]
  Impaired circulation due to intravascular sludging of red cells[164,165]
  Chemotoxic effect on the brain due to breakdown of the tight junctions in the brain capillary endothelial cells[166,167]
Signs and symptoms
  Nausea
  Hot flush
  Hematoma or posttraumatic fistula at puncture site
  Anaphylactic reactions, including urticaria, angioedema, rhinitis, hypotension, bronchospasm
  Embolization to distal vessels
  Acute renal dysfunction[169-172,175]
  Dehydration[173,174]
  Convulsions[167,168]
  Neurologic sequelae[167,168]
  Bradycardia
  Systemic hypotension, not associated with anaphylaxis

In a study of more than 1000 patients with TVL who underwent arteriography, Harrison notes that atheromatous disease of the ipsilateral internal carotid artery is present in 75% of cases[179] (Table 7-3).[9,10,12,51,53,76,180-191] It is interesting to note that carotid atheromatous disease at the bifurcation was less frequently seen in patients

TABLE 7-3
Angiographic Findings in Transient Visual Loss

Report	Number of Cases	Normal	Wall Irregularity	Stenosis	Occlusion	Wall Irregularity or Stenosis	Wall Irregularity, Stenosis, or Occlusion[†]	Normal
Harrison, Marshall[180]	19	6	6	4	3	10	13	0
Hooshmand, Vines, Lee et al[181]	34	2	18	12	2	30	32	0
Pessin, Duncan, Mohr et al[53]	33	8	5	15	5	20	25	0
Wilson, Ross Russell[182]	67	32	8	16	7	24	31	4
Eisenberg, Mani[183]	40	5	7	19	9	26	35	0
Thiele, Young, Chikos et al[51]	28	2	10	16	0	26	26	0
Parkin, Kendall, Marshall et al[10]	38	1	12	20	4	32	36	1
Adams, Putman, Corbett[184]	59	20	8	15	10	23	33	6
Marshall, Meadows[9]	21	10	—	—	4	7	11	0
Ramirez-Lassepas, Sandok, Burton[185]	27	1	—	—	6	20	26	0
Sandok, Trautmann, Ramirez-Lassepas[186]	43	1	—	—	12	30	42	0
Lemak, Fields[187]	234	51	—	—	33	150	183	0
Poole, Ross Russell[12]	60	35	—	—	6	15	21	4
Mungas, Baker[188]	107	12	—	—	—	—	95	0
Hurwitz, Heyman, Wilkinson et al[77]	90	22	—	—	—	—	68	0
Harrison, Marshall[189]	55	8	—	—	—	—	39	8
Bogousslavsky, Hachinski, Barnett[190]	55	21	—	—	—	—	34	0
Hedges, Giliberti, Margargal (DSA)[191]	17	6	—	—	—	—	11	0
Total	1027	243	74/318	117/318	101/703	413/703	761/1027	251/1027
Percent		24	23	37	14	59	74	2

*Modified from Harrison MJG: Angiography in amaurosis fugax. In Bernstein EF, ed: *Amaurosis fugax,* New York, 1988, Springer-Verlag, 288-289.
†Not all studies reported specific findings on angiography. Thus some would report vessel wall irregularity and stenosis separately, while others would report all vessel wall irregularity and stenosis in one category. The same holds true for those studies that combined wall irregularity, stenosis, and occlusion and did not delineate them as separate entities. A dash in a column indicates that the entity was not specifically reported in the paper.

209

with TVL.[189] It is likely that the emboli that cause TVL most frequently arise from atheromas at the carotid plaque, whereas hemispheric TIAs and completed stroke result more often from embolization from the heart.

Magnetic Resonance Angiography

Because magnetic resonance imaging is a noninvasive procedure without significant side effects, it is an ideal method for studying vascular disease. It has the ability to differentiate signals between stationary tissue (i.e., the vessel wall) and the moving blood column. Magnetic resonance imaging has the advantage over ultrasound studies because it is capable of imaging deeper vessels, such as the intracranial vessels, the basilar artery, and the origins of both the common carotid and vertebral arteries.[192] Because of the potential advantages of this modality, several studies have attempted to generate angiographic-type magnetic resonance images.[193-197] The stationary tissue in the blood vessel has insufficient time to recover strength between the rapid radiofrequency pulses to which it is subjected,[193] and consequently a low signal strength is obtained on the image. The moving column of blood is constantly providing new "tissues" moving from outside the plane of excitation into it, and it therefore possesses full magnetization strength. The image of the moving blood column therefore demonstrates high signal strength. The moving blood column appears bright, whereas the surrounding tissue, the vessel wall, appears as a low signal image. Magnetic resonance angiography (MRA) is the result. The images obtained on MRA testing are very similar to those of conventional contrast angiography and have been shown to be precise in delineating lesions of the extracranial carotid arteries.[198] The patency of the vessel or the site of stenosis are accurately determined with MRA, and ulceration of the intimal lining can be seen. Blood flow velocities and patterns also can be monitored with MRA,[196,199-207] which has been shown to be extremely accurate (Figure 7-15).[194,208] The fact that MRA allows three-dimensional reconstruction of the site yields further weight in favor of this procedure, because the optic viewing angle can be chosen.

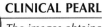

CLINICAL PEARL

The images obtained on MRA testing are very similar to those of conventional contrast angiography and have been shown to be precise in delineating lesions of the extracranial carotid arteries.

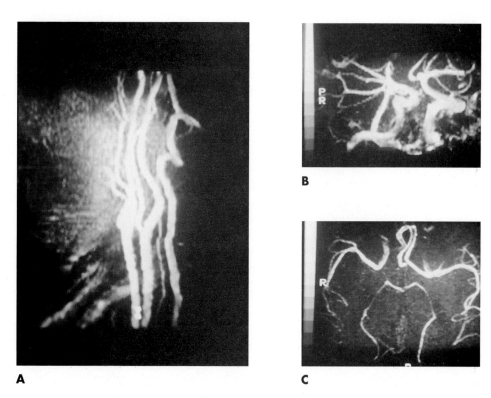

FIGURE 7-15 A, Longitudinal view of the extracranial carotid arteries on magnetic resonance angiography. The vertebral arteries are also seen. **B**, Looking at the base of the cranium, the basilar artery is seen on the left. Compare with Figure 7-3. **C**, The circle of Willis. The brightest vessels on each side are the middle cerebral arteries. Compare with Figure 7-2.

Treatment

The decision as to the appropriate treatment of patients with TVL or hemispheric TIAs, whether medical or surgical, can be made only after the type and degree of stenosis or occlusion are determined. The results of both noninvasive vascular screening tests and invasive examinations must be considered. Consideration must be made as to whether the plaque results in hemodynamically significant stenosis, the presence of ulceration of the plaque, and the patient's general well-being.

Medical treatment of patients with transient symptoms or permanent disability may include anticoagulant therapy or platelet antiaggregation therapy.

Anticoagulation treatment is not a useful therapy for patients with completed stroke. It is intended to prevent the progression of thrombotic stroke by preventing clotting at several points in the normal coagulation process. Heparin, coumadin, and protamine sulfate are anticoagulants used to retard the progression of thrombotic stroke. Transient visual loss and hemispheric TIAs may be caused by platelet thromboemboli.[209-211] Unfortunately, several studies using small sample sizes have each demonstrated that patients presenting with TIAs do not demonstrate a significant reduction in the incidence of stroke or death when treated with anticoagulants as opposed to placebo drugs.[213-216] Most clinicians, however, prefer immediate heparinization of patients presenting with a stroke in progress[216] after intracranial hemorrhage has been ruled out. A recently available thrombolytic agent, tissue plasminogen activator (t-PA), acts on plasminogen only in the presence of fibrin, which effectively limits its activity to the accessible surface of the clot.[217,218] There is subsequently less systemic depletion of fibrinogen and other clotting factors than occurs with other thrombolytic therapy, and therefore t-PA may decrease the risk of cerebral hemorrhage in these patients,[219-225] a major concern when prescribing other thrombolytic agents.

Aspirin, a platelet aggregation inhibitor, has been shown to reduce the incidence of TIAs and stroke, as well as the death rate in patients presenting with impending stroke. The Aspirin in Transient Ischemic Attacks (AITIA) Study, reported in 1977[226] and 1978,[227] studied the effectiveness of aspirin in preventing stroke in patients with TVL or hemispheric TIAs. Aspirin prevents platelet aggregation at the site of ulcerated atherosclerotic plaque by inhibiting cyclooxygenase, thereby preventing conversion of arachidonic acid to cyclic endoperoxides and subsequently thromboxane A_2, a platelet proaggregation agent. The AITIA Study demonstrated that patients receiving aspirin had more favorable outcomes than those patients randomized into the placebo group (Table 7-4).[226] Other studies also have demonstrated that aspirin is an effective form of treatment for patients with TIAs.[227-229]

TABLE 7-4

Results of the Medical Group in the Aspirin in Transient Ischemic Attacks (AITIA) Study

Outcome	Aspirin	Placebo
Unfavorable		
Death—cerebral infarction	0	2
Death—cardiovascular	1	4
Death—intracerebral hemorrhage	1	0
Nonfatal cerebral infarction	4	8
Retinal infarction	1	0
Excessive ratio of transient ischemic attacks	8	20
Favorable	63	43
Less than 6 months follow-up	10	13
Total	88	90

From Fields WS, Lemak NA, Frankowski RF, et al: Controlled trial of aspirin in cerebral ischemia, *Stroke* 8:301-316, 1977. Reprinted by permission of the American Heart Association, 1977.

Interestingly, aspirin also has been demonstrated to increase the risk of hemorrhagic infarction when used as the sole source of antiplatelet therapy or in conjunction with t-PA.[225] The usual dose of aspirin is 100 to 325 mg per day.[206,209,230,231] Dypyridamole (Persantine [Boehringer Ingelheim, Ridgefield, CT]) and ticlopidine are other platelet antiaggregation agents used to treat stroke or impending stroke.

CLINICAL PEARL

Aspirin, a platelet aggregation inhibitor, has been shown to reduce the incidence of TIAs and stroke, as well as the death rate in patients presenting with impending stroke.

Ticlopidine is a relatively new platelet-aggregation inhibitor that inhibits platelet aggregation by selectively interfering with adenosine diphosphate on the platelet membrane.[232] The effect of ticlopidine on stroke and cardiovascular events was studied in two multicenter randomized double-blind trials involving over 4000 patients.[233,234] The North American Ticlopidine Aspirin Stroke Study showed ticlopidine to be significantly more effective than aspirin in reducing the incidence of fatal and nonfatal stroke than aspirin in patients with TIA or minor stroke. The Canadian American Study showed that ticlopidine reduced overall stroke risk by 24% compared with a placebo in patients who had suffered a recent thromboembolic stroke.[235]

Other forms of medical treatment are being studied. For example, there is great promise in reducing low-density lipoproteins by both medical therapy and extracorporeal plasma exchange, with proven resultant regression of carotid atherosclerotic plaque.[236]

Surgical intervention is considered in patients with symptoms of TVL and proven stenosis of the ipsilateral carotid artery of at least 50%, but it is not considered in patients with complete occlusion of the vessel.[81]

Carotid endarterectomy is considered the appropriate surgical procedure for carotid atherosclerosis. In this procedure, the extracranial carotid artery is incised, and the atherosclerotic plaque is dissected and removed. A new procedure using argon laser to cleave the atheroma from the media has been described and shows much promise.[237] Because the associated mortality for carotid endarterectomy is approximately 1.8% and the perioperative stroke rate is 5.2%,[196] careful consideration must be made as to appropriate surgical candidates. Attention to detail in both the neurologic monitoring of the patient, as well as the surgeon's technique of arterial reconstruction, has been shown to be of paramount importance when considering the safety of carotid endarterectomy procedures.[238]

The North American Symptomatic Carotid Endarterectomy Trial (NASCET) was designed to compare the efficacy of medical therapy with that of carotid endarterectomy in patients with a history of recent hemispheric TIA or a mild, nondisabling stroke and ipsilateral narrowing of the internal carotid artery.[239] A preliminary review of the data showed that patients with a high-grade stenosis (70% to 99%) had significantly better outcomes with surgical intervention.[240,241] The results were skewed so positively in favor of surgical intervention that patients were no longer enrolled in the medical treatment group. The NASCET study continues to examine the role surgery should play in the symptomatic patient with a lower degree of stenosis.

While the NASCET study involved symptomatic patients, the Asymptomatic Carotid Atherosclerosis Study (ACAS) enrolled only asymptomatic patients with a demonstrated carotid stenosis resulting in greater than 60% reduction in diameter of the vessel.[242] The patients all received daily doses of aspirin and underwent aggressive management of any modifiable risk factors. Additionally, they were randomized to surgical or nonsurgical intervention groups. In September 1994, the National Institutes of Neurological Disorders and Stroke issued a clinical advisory notifying the medical community that the trial had reached statistical significance at an early stage and that all patients were to be reevaluated for the possibility of undergoing surgery.[243] In the study of asymptomatic patients, it was determined that carotid endarterectomy resulted in a statistically significant absolute reduction of 5.8% for stroke within 5 years, with a relative risk reduction of 55%.[243] It is important to note that the study design only included surgeons with documented perioperative morbidity and mortality rates of less than 3%,[244] an important consideration in interpretation of the results.

While obviously beneficial to many patients, problems with recurrent stenosis[245,246] following carotid endarterectomy as well as cerebrovascular hemodynamic changes resulting from the surgery[247] still need to be addressed.

REFERENCES

1. Gowers WR: *A manual of diseases of the nervous system,* Philadelphia, 1893, Blakiston.
2. McDowell F: Transient cerebral ischemia: diagnostic considerations, *Prog Cardiovasc Dis* 22:309-324, 1980.
3. Abernathy M, Brandt MM, Robinson C: Noninvasive testing of the carotid system, *Am Fam Physician* 29:157-168, 1984.
4. American Heart Association: *Heart facts 1984,* Dallas, 1982, American Heart Association.
5. Kurtzke JF: Epidemiology and risk factors in thrombotic brain infarction. In Harrison MJG, Dyken ML, eds: *Cerebral vascular disease,* London, 1983, Butterworths International Medical Review, 27-45.
6. Wolf PA, Kannel WB, Verter J: Current status of risk factors for stroke, *Neurol Clin* 7:317-343, 1983.

7. Gautier JC: Clinical presentation and differential diagnosis of amaurosis fugax. In Bernstein EF, ed: *Amaurosis fugax,* New York, 1988, Springer-Verlag, 24-42.

8. Ross Russell RW: Natural history of amaurosis fugax. In Bernstein EF, ed: *Amaurosis fugax,* New York, 1988, Springer-Verlag, 174-182.

9. Marshall J, Meadows SP: The natural history of amaurosis fugax, *Brain* 91:419-434, 1968.

10. Parkin PJ, Kendall BE, Marshall J, et al: Amaurosis fugax: some aspects of management, *J Neurol Neurosurg Psychiatry* 45:1-6, 1982.

11. Morax PV, Aron Rosa D, Gautier JC: Symptomes et signes ophthalmologique des stenoses et occlusions cartidiennes, *Bull Soc Ophthalmol Fr* 1:169, 1970 (suppl).

12. Poole CJM, Ross Russell RW: Mortality and stroke after amaurosis fugax, *J Neurol Neurosurg Psychiatry* 48:902-903, 1985.

13. Howard RS, Ross Russell RW: Prognosis of patients with retinal embolism, *J Neurol Neurosurg Psychiatry* 50:1142-1147, 1987.

14. Mohr JP, Caplan LR, Melski JW, et al: The Harvard cooperative stroke registry: a prospective registry, *Neurology* 106:754-762, 1978.

15. Kannel WB, Dawber TR, Cohen MS, et al: Vascular disease of the brain: epidemiologic aspects: the Framingham study, *Am J Public Health* 55:1355-1366, 1965.

16. Matsumoto N, Whisnant JP, Kurland LT, et al: Natural history of stroke in Rochester, Minn, 1955 through 1969: an extension of a previous study, 1945 through 1954, *Stroke* 4:20-29, 1973.

17. Mohr JP, Kase CS, Adams RD: Cerebrovascular diseases. In Petersdorf RG, Adams RD, Braunwald E, et al, eds: *Harrison's principles of internal medicine,* ed 10, New York, 1983, McGraw-Hill, 2028-2060.

18. McDonald FH: Transient cerebral ischemia: diagnostic considerations. In McDowell FH, Sonnonblick EH, Lesch M, eds: *Current concepts in cerebrovascular disease,* New York, 1980, Grune & Stratton, 309-324.

19. Culicchia F, Mohr JP: Morbidity and mortality of stroke. In Moore WS, ed: *Surgery for cerebrovascular disease,* New York, 1987, Churchill Livingstone, 35-39.

20. Soltero I, Liu K, Cooper, et al: Trends in mortality from cerebrovascular diseases in the United States, 1960 to 1975, *Stroke* 9:549-558, 1978.

21. Sacco RL, Wolf PA, Kannel WB, McNamara PM: Survival and recurrence following stroke: the Framingham study, *Stroke* 13:290-295, 1982.

22. Dyken ML: Risk factors predisposing to stroke. In Moore WS, ed: *Surgery for cerebrovascular disease,* New York, 1987, Churchill Livingstone, 79-93.

23. Wolf PA, Kannel WB, Verter J: Current status of risk factors for stroke, *Neurol Clin* 1:317-343, 1983.

24. Caplan LR, Cooper ES: Cerebrovascular disease in blacks, *J Natl Med Assoc,* 79:33-36, 1987.

25. Klatsky AL, Armstrong MA, Friedman GD: Racial differences in cerebrovascular disease hospitalizations, *Stroke* 22:299-304, 1991.

26. Kannel WB, Wolf PA, Verter J, McNamara PM: Epidemiologic assessment of the role of blood pressure in stroke: the Framingham study, *JAMA* 214:301-310, 1970.

27. Veterans Administration Cooperative Study Group on Antihypertensive Agents: Effects of treatment on morbidity in hypertension. II. Results in patients with diastolic blood pressures averaging 90 through 114 mm Hg, *JAMA* 213:1143-1152, 1970.

28. Taguchi J, Freis ED: Partial reduction of blood pressure and prevention of complications in hypertension, *N Engl J Med* 291:329-331, 1974.

29. Management Committee: The Australian therapeutic trial in mild hypertension, *Lancet* 1:1261-1267, 1980.

30. Hypertension Detection and Follow-up Program Cooperative Group: Five-year findings of the hypertension detection and follow-up program. III. Reduction in stroke incidence among persons with high blood pressure, *JAMA* 247:633-638, 1982.

31. Wolf PA, Abbott RD, Kannel WB: A trial fibrillation as an independent risk factor for stroke: the Framingham study, *Stroke* 22:983-988, 1991.
32. Cairns, JA, Connally SJ: Nonrheumatic atrial fibrillation: risk of stroke and role of antithrombotic therapy, *Circulation* 84:469-481, 1991.
33. Stroke Prevention in Atrial Fibrillation Investigators: Stroke prevention in atrial fibrillation study: final results, *Circulation* 84:527-539, 1991.
34. Wolf PA, D'Agostino RB, Belanger AJ, Kannel WB: Probability of stroke: a risk profile from the Framingham study, *Stroke* 22:312-318, 1991.
35. Carpenter MB, Sutin J: Blood supply of the central nervous system. In *Human neuroanatomy,* ed 8, Baltimore, 1983, Williams & Wilkins, 707-742.
36. Pansky B, House EL: *Review of gross anatomy,* ed 3, New York, 1975, Macmillan, 92.
37. Hillen B: The variability of the circulus arteriosus (Willisii): order or anarchy? *Acta Anat (Basel)* 129:74-80, 1987.
38. van der Zwan A, Hillen B: Review of the variability of the territories of the major cerebral arteries, *Stroke* 22:1078-1084, 1991.
39. Whisnant JP, Fitzgibbon JP, Kurland LT, et al: Natural history of stroke in Rochester, Minnesota 1945 through 1954, *Stroke* 2:11-22, 1971.
40. Kannel MB, Wolf PA, Verter J, et al: Epidemiologic assessment of the role of blood pressure and stroke: the Framingham study, *JAMA* 214:301-310, 1970.
41. Sherman DG, Easton JD: Spectrum of pathology responsible for ischemic stroke. In Moore WS, ed: *Surgery for cerebrovascular disease,* New York, 1987, Churchill Livingstone, 43-49.
42. Lusby RJ: Lesions, dynamics, and pathogenetic mechanisms responsible for ischemic events in the brain. In Moore WS, ed: *Surgery for cerebrovascular disease.* New York, 1987, Churchill Livingstone, 51-76.
43. Bierman EL: Atherosclerosis and other forms of arteriosclerosis. In Petersdorf RG, Adams RD, Braunwald E, et al, eds: *Harrison's principles of medicine,* ed 10, New York, 1983, McGraw-Hill, 1465-1475.
44. DePalma RG, Lowes AW: Interventions in atherosclerosis: a review for surgeons, *Surgery* 84:175-189, 1978.
45. Hata Y, Hower J, Insull WJ: Cholesterol ester-rich inclusions from human aortic fatty streak and fibrous plaque lesions of atherosclerosis, *Am J Pathol* 75:423-456, 1974.
46. Haust MD: The morphogenesis and fate of potential and early atherosclerotic lesions in man, *Hum Pathol* 2:1-29, 1971.
47. O'Connor RAJ: The anatomy and pathophysiology of extracranial atherosclerotis cerebrovascular disease. In Hershey FB, Barnes RW, Sumner DS, eds: *Noninvasive diagnosis of vascular disease,* Pasadena, Calif, 1984, Appleton Davies, 157-177.
48. Lusby RJ, Ferrell LD, Ehrenfeld WK: Carotid plaque hemorrhage: its role in the production of cerebral ischaemia, *Arch Surg* 117:1479-1488, 1982.
49. Erskine JM, Tierney LM Jr: Blood vessels & lymphatics: occlusive cerebrovascular disease. In Krupp MA, Schroeder SA, Tierney LM Jr, eds: *Current medical diagnosis and treatment,* Norwalk, Conn, 1987, Appleton & Lange, 291-341.
50. Lusby RF, Ferrell LD, Wylie EJ: The significance of intraplaque hemorrhage in the pathogenesis of carotid atherosclerosis. In Bergan JJ, Yao ST, eds: *Cerebrovascular insufficiency,* New York, 1983, Grune & Straton, 41-55.
51. Thiele BL, Young JV, Chikos PM, et al: Correlation of arteriographic findings and symptoms of cerebrovascular disease, *Neurology* 30:1041-1046, 1980.
52. Eisenberg RL, Nemzek WR, Moore WS, et al: Relationship of transient ischaemic attacks and angiographically demonstrable lesions of the carotid artery, *Stroke* 8:483-486, 1977.
53. Pessin MS, Duncan GW, Mohr JP, et al: Clinical and angiographic features of carotid transient ischaemic attacks, *N Engl J Med* 296:358-362, 1977.
54. Houser OW, Baker HL, Sandok BA, Holley KE: Cephalic arterial fibromuscular dysplagia, *Radiology* 101:605-611, 1971.

55. Shahar A, Sadeh M: Severe anemia associated with transient neurological deficits, *Stroke* 22:1201-1202, 1991.

56. Sauer CM: Recurrent embolic stroke and cocaine-related cardiomyopathy, *Stroke* 22:1203-1205, 1991.

57. Olszewski J: Subcortical arteriosclerotic encephalopathy, *World Neurol* 3:359-375, 1962.

58. DeReuck J, Crevits J, Coster WD, et al: Pathogenesis of Binswanger chronic progressive subcortical encephalopathy, *Neurology* 30:920-928, 1980.

59. Nichols FT, Mohr JP: Binswanger's subacute arteriosclerotic encephalopathy. In Barnett HMJ, Mohr JP, Stein BM, Yatsu FM, eds: *Stroke: pathophysiology, diagnosis and management,* New York, 1986, Churchill Livingstone, 875-885.

60. Jacobson DM: Systemic cholesterol microembolization syndrome masquerading as giant cell arteritis, *Surv Ophthalmol* 36:23-27, 1991.

61. Wray SH: Visual aspects of extracranial internal carotid artery disease. In Bernstein EF, ed: *Amaurosis fugax,* New York, 1988, Springer-Verlag, 72-80.

62. D'Cruz IA, Cohen HC, Prabhu R, et al: Clinical manifestations of mitral-annulus calcification, with emphasis on its echocardiographic features, *Am Heart J* 94:367-377, 1977.

63. Guthrie J, Fairgrieve J: Aortic embolism due to myxoid tumor associated with myocardial calcification, *Br Heart J* 25:137-140, 1963.

64. diBono DP, Warlow CP: Mitral-annulus calcification and cerebral or retinal ischemia, *Lancet* 2:383-385, 1979.

65. Barnett HJM: Transient cerebral ischemia pathogenesis, prognosis and management, *Annual Rev College Physicians Surgeons Canada* 7:153-173, 1974.

66. Barnett HJM: Delayed cerebral ischemic episodes distal to occlusion of major cerebral arteries, *Neurology* 28:769-774, 1978.

67. Barnett HJM, Boughner DR, Cooper PF, et al: Further evidence relating mitral valve prolapse to cerebral ischemic events, *N Engl J Med* 302:139-144, 1980.

68. Kearns TP, Hollenhorst RW: Venous stasis retinopathy of occlusive disease of the carotid artery, *Mayo Clin Proc* 38:304-312, 1963.

69. Katz B: Disc edema, transient obscurations of vision, and a temporal fossa mass, *Surv Ophthalmol* 36:133-139, 1991.

70. Safran AB: Neuro-ophthalmology in the recent European literature: III. Heredo-degenerations, stroke, pain and diagnostic techniques, *J Clin Neuro Ophthalmol* 4:275-284, 1984.

71. Fisher CM: Transient monocular blindness associated with hemiplegia, *Transactions Am Neurol Assoc* 47:154-157, 1951.

72. Witmer R, Schmid A: Cholesterinkristall als retinaler arterieller embolus, *Ophthalmologica* 135:432-433, 1958.

73. Hollenhorst RW: Significance of bright plaques in the retinal arterioles, *JAMA* 178:23-29, 1961.

74. Hepler RS, Yee RD: Ophthalmic manifestations of cerebrovascular disease. In Moore WS, ed: *Surgery for cerebrovascular disease,* New York, 1987, Churchill Livingstone, 147-160.

75. Weinberger J, Bender AN, Yang WC: Amaurosis fugax associated with ophthalmic artery stenosis: clinical simulation of carotid artery disease, *Stroke* 11:290-293, 1980.

76. Burger SK, Saul RF, Selhorst JB, Thurston SE: Transient monocular blindness caused by vasospasm, *N Engl J Med* 325:870-873, 1991.

77. Hurwitz BJ, Heyman A, Wilkinson WE, et al: Comparison of amaurosis fugax and transient cerebral ischemia: a prospective clinical and arteriographic study, *Ann Neurol* 18:698-704, 1985.

78. Pfaffenbach DD, Hollenhorst RW: Morbidity and survivorship of patients with embolic cholesterol crystals in the ocular fundus, *Am J Ophthalmol* 75:66-72, 1973.

79. Cazzato G, Torre P: Amaurosis fugax, *Clin Neurol (Italy)* 51:1-26, 1981.

80. Hollenhorst RW: The neuro-ophthalmology of strokes. In Lawton-Smith J, ed: *Neuro-ophthalmology,* St Louis, 1965, Mosby, 109-121.

81. Barnett HJM, Bernstein EF, Callow AD, et al: The Amaurosis Fugax Study Group. Amaurosis fugax (transient monocular blindness): a consensus statement. In Bernstein EF, ed: *Amaurosis fugax*, New York, 1988, Springer-Verlag, 286-303.
82. Caplan LR, Hier DB, D'Cruz I: Cerebral embolism in the Michael Reese Stroke Registry, *Stroke* 14:530-536, 1983.
83. Castaigne P, L Hermitte F, Gautier JC, et al: Arterial occlusions in the vertebro-basilar system. A study of 44 patients with post-mortem data, *Brain* 96:133-154, 1973.
84. Caplan L: Occlusion of the vertebral or basilar artery, *Stroke* 10:277-282, 1979.
85. George B, Laurian C: Vertebrobasilar ischemia with thrombosis of the vertebral artery: report of two cases with embolism, *J Neurol Neurosurg Psychiatry* 45:91-93, 1982.
86. Caplan L, Rosenbaum A: Role of cerebral angiography in vertebrobasilar occlusive disease, *J Neurol Neurosurg Psychiatry* 38:601-612, 1975.
87. McCusker E, Rudick R, Honch G, et al: Recovery from the locked-in syndrome, *Arch Neurol* 39:145-147, 1982.
88. Gorelick P, Caplan L, Hier D, et al: Racial differences in the distribution of posterior circulation occlusive disease, *Stroke* 16:785-790, 1985.
89. Curtis BA: Cerebrum. In *Neurosciences: the basics*, Philadelphia, 1990, Lea & Febiger, 92-120.
90. Caplan LR: Transient ischemic attacks and stroke in the distribution of the vertebrobasilar system: clinical manifestations. In Moore WS, ed: *Surgery for cerebrovascular disease*, New York, 1987, Churchill Livingstone, 103-129.
91. Humphries AW, Young JR, Beven EG, et al: Relief of vertebrobasilar symptoms by carotid endarterectomy, *Surgery* 57:48-52, 1965.
92. Thiele BL, Strandness DE Jr: Distribution of intracranial and extracranial arterial lesions in the patients with symptomatic cerebrovascular disease. In Bernstein EF, ed: *Noninvasive diagnostic techniques in vascular disease*, ed 3, St Louis, 1985, Mosby, 316-322.
93. Blaustein BH: The subclavian steal syndrome, *Clin Eye Vision Care* 3:25-28, 1991.
94. Fields WS, Lemak NA: Joint study of extracranial arterial occlusion: subclavian steal, a review of 168 cases, *JAMA* 222:1139-1143, 1972.
95. McRae LP, Kartchner MM: Pressure and volume measurements from the eye for detecting possible arterial obstruction, *Ann Biomed Eng* 12:63-78, 1984.
96. McRae LP, Cadwallader JA, Kartchner MM: Oculoplethysmography and carotid phonoangiography for the noninvasive detection of extracranial carotid occlusive disease, *Med Instrument* 13:87-91, 1979.
97. Kirkpatrick JF, Phillips AW: Comparison of carotid phonoangiography, oculo-plethysmography, angiography, and surgical findings in carotid artery occlusive disease, *J Med Assoc Ga* 70:491-493, 1981.
98. O'Leary DH, Persson AV, Clouse ME: Noninvasive testing for carotid artery stenosis: I. Prospective analysis of three methods, *Am J Radiol* 137:1189-1194, 1981.
99. Perry HA, Morros CD: Predicting significant atherosclerosis of the carotid artery, *Am Surg* 49:21-25, 1983.
100. Sumner DS, Russell JB, Miles RD: Are noninvasive tests sufficiently accurate to identify patients in need of carotid arteriography? *Surgery* 91:700-706, 1982.
101. Pollak EW: Noninvasive cerebrovascular evaluation: a prerequisite for angiography? *Am J Surg* 144:203-205, 1982.
102. Bates B: *A guide to physical examination and history taking*, ed 4, Philadelphia, 1987, JB Lippincott.
103. Myers JD: The mechanisms and significances of continuous murmurs. In Leon DF, Shaver JA, eds: *Physiologic principles of heart sounds and murmurs*, New York, 1975, American Heart Association.
104. Judge RD, Zuidema GD, Fitzgerald FT: *Clinical diagnosis: a physiologic approach*, ed 4, Boston, 1982, Little, Brown.

105. Troost BT, Glaser JS: Aneurysms, arteriovenous communications, and related vascular malformations. In Duane TD, ed: *Clinical ophthalmology,* vol 2, ch 17, Philadelphia, 1981, Lippincott.
106. Merritt HH: Neurological aspects of internal carotid obstruction, *Bull NY Acad Med* 37:151-155, 1961.
107. Roy FH: *Ocular differential diagnosis,* ed 2, Philadelphia, 1975, Lea & Febiger.
108. Cohen JH, Miller S: Eyeball bruits, *N Engl J Med* 255:459-464, 1956.
109. Ziegler DK, Zileli T, Dick A, et al: Correlation of bruits over the carotid artery with angiographically demonstrated lesions, *Neurology* 21:860-865, 1971.
110. David TE, Humphries AW, Young TR, et al: A correlation of neck bruits and arteriosclerotic carotid arteries, *Arch Surg* 107:729-731, 1973.
111. Fronek A: Impact of bioengineering on noninvasive diagnostics, *Ann Biomed Eng* 12:51-54, 1984.
112. Lees RS, Dewey CF: Phonoangiography: a new noninvasive diagnostic method for studying arterial disease, *Proceed National Acad Science USA* 67:935-942, 1970.
113. Aburahma AF, Diethrich EB: The yield and reliability of oculoplethysmography and carotid phonoangiography in stroke screening and the diagnosis of extracranial carotid occlusive disease: our experience in 1650 patients, *W V Med J* 75:254-260, 1979.
114. Blackshear WM, Thiele BL, Harley JD, Chikos PM, et al: A prospective evaluation of oculoplethysmography and carotid phonoangiography, *Surg Gynecol Obstet* 148:201-205, 1979.
115. Keagy BA, Pharr WF, Thomas DD, Bowes DE: Oculoplethysmography/carotid phonoangiography, *Arch Surg* 115:1199-1202, 1980.
116. Walden R, L'Italien G, Megerman J, Bouchier-Hayes D, et al: Complementary methods for evaluating carotid stenosis: a biophysical basis for ocular pulse wave delays, *Surgery* 88:162-167, 1980.
117. Keagy BA, Pharr WF, Thomas D, Bowes DE: Comparison of oculoplethysmography/carotid phonoangiography with duplex scan/spectral analysis in the detection of carotid artery stenosis, *Stroke* 13:43-45, 1982.
118. House SL, Mahalingam K, Hyland LJ, Ferris EB, et al: Noninvasive flow techniques in the diagnosis of cerebrovascular disease, *Surgery* 87:696-700, 1980.
119. Dietzen CD, Batson RC, Hollier LH: Carotid phonoangiography and oculoplethysmography for noninvasive evaluation of carotid occlusive disease, *South Med J* 74:796-798, 1981.
120. Miller A, Lees RS, Kistler JP, Abbott WM: Spectral analysis of arterial bruits (phonoangiography): experimental validation, *Circulation* 61:515-520, 1980.
121. Satiani B, Copperman M, Clark M, Evans WE: Assessment of carotid phonoangiography and oculoplethysmography in the detection of carotid artery stenosis, *Am J Surg* 136:618-621, 1978.
122. Turnipseed WD, Archer CW: The diagnostic interface between noninvasive cerebral vascular testing and digital arteriography, *J Vasc Surg* 3:486-492, 1986.
123. Leopold GR: Pulse echo ultrasonography for the noninvasive imaging of vascular anatomy. In Bernstein EF, ed: *Noninvasive diagnostic techniques in vascular disease,* ed 3, St Louis, 1985, Mosby, 219-228.
124. Barnes RW: Continuous-wave Doppler ultrasound. In Bernstein EF, ed: *Noninvasive diagnostic techniques in vascular disease,* ed 3, St Louis, 1985, Mosby, 19-24.
125. Rittgers SE, Putney WW, Barnes RW: Real-time spectrum analysis and display of the directional Doppler ultrasound blood velocity signals, *IEEE Transactions Biomed Engineering* 27: 723-728, 1980.
126. Sumner DS: Volume plethysmography in vascular disease: an overview. In Bernstein EF, ed: *Noninvasive diagnostic techniques in vascular disease,* ed 3, St Louis, 1985, Mosby, 97-118.
127. Kartchner MM, McRae LP, Morrison FD: Noninvasive detection and evaluation of carotid occlusive disease, *Arch Surg* 106:528-535, 1973.

128. Kartchner MM, McRae LP: Noninvasive evaluation and management of the "asymptomatic" carotid bruit, *Surgery* 82:840-847, 1977.

129. Kartchner MM, McRae LP, Crain V, et al: Oculoplethysmography: an adjunct to arteriography in the diagnosis of extracranial carotid occlusive disease, *Am J Surg* 132:728-732, 1976.

130. McRae LP, Crain V, Kartchner MM: *Oculoplethysmography and carotid flow angiography, OPG/CPA: interpretation manual,* ed 2, Tucson, 1978, Tucson Medical Center.

131. Gee W, Smith CA, Hinson CE, et al.: Ocular pneumoplethysmography in carotid artery disease, *Med Instrument* 8:244-248, 1974.

132. Gee W, Mehigan JT, Wylie EJ: Measurement of collateral cerebral hemispheric blood pressure by ocular pneumoplethysmography, *Am J Surg* 130:121-127, 1975.

133. Gee W, Oller DW, Homer LD, Bailey RC: Simultaneous bilateral determination of the systolic pressure of the ophthalmic arteries by ocular pneumoplethysmography, *Invest Ophthalmol Vis Sci* 16:86-89, 1979.

134. Johnston GG, Bernstein EF: Quantitation of internal carotid artery stenosis by ocular plethysmography, *Surg Forum* 26:290-291, 1975.

135. Eikelboom BC: *Evaluation of carotid artery disease and potential collateral circulation by ocular pneumoplethysmography,* thesis, State University of Leiden, Netherlands, 1981.

136. Ricotta JJ: Definition of extracranial carotid disease: comparison of oculopneumoplethysmography continuous wave Doppler angiography and measurement at operation. In Greenhalgh RM, Clifford RF, eds: *Progress in stroke research,* ed 2, London, 1983, Pitman, 91-102.

137. Kempczinski RF: Indirect cerebrovascular testing. In Kempczinski RF, Yao JST, eds: *Practical noninvasive vascular diagnosis,* ed 2, Chicago, 1987, Year Book Medical Publishers, 262-285.

138. Gee W, Madden AE, Perline RK, Smith CA: Ocular pneumoplethysmography. In Moore WS: *Surgery for cerebrovascular disease,* New York, 1987, Churchill Livingstone, 305-338.

139. Gee W, Rhodes M, Denstman FJ, et al: Ocular pneumoplethysmography in head-injury patients, *J Neurosurg* 59:46-50, 1983.

140. Eikelboom BC: Ocular pneumoplethysmography. In Bernstein EF, ed: *Noninvasive diagnostic techniques in vascular disease,* ed 3, St Louis, 1985, Mosby, 91-96.

141. Bosley TM, Savino PJ, Sergott RC, et al: Ocular pneumoplethysmography can help in the diagnosis of giant-cell arteritis, *Arch Ophthalmol* 107:379-381, 1989.

142. Maroon JC, Pieroni DW, Campbell RL: Ophthalmosonometry, an ultrasonic method for assessing carotid blood flow, *J Neurosurg* 30:238-246, 1969.

143. Machleder HI, Barker WF: Stroke on the wrong side: use of the Doppler ophthalmic test in cerebral vascular screening, *Arch Surg* 105:943-947, 1972.

144. Barnes RW, Wilson MR: *Doppler ultrasonic evaluation of cerebrovascular disease,* Iowa City, 1975, University of Iowa Press.

145. Barnes RW, Russell HE, Bone GE, et al: The Doppler cerebrovascular examination: improved results with refinements in techniques, *Stroke* 8:468-471, 1977.

146. Brockenbrough EC: Periorbital Doppler velocity evaluation of carotid obstruction. In Bernstein EF, ed: *Noninvasive diagnostic techniques in vascular disease,* ed 3, St Louis, 1985, Mosby, 335-351.

147. Kempczinski RF: Clinical application of noninvasive testing in cerebrovascular arterial occlusive disease. In Kempczinski RF, Yao JST, eds: *Practical noninvasive vascular diagnosis,* ed 2, Chicago, 1987, Year Book Medical Publishers, 364-390.

148. Barnes RW: Other noninvasive techniques in cerebrovascular disease. In Bernstein EF, ed: *Noninvasive diagnostic techniques in vascular disease,* ed 3, St Louis, 1985, Mosby, 442-447.

149. Wood EH: Thermography in the diagnosis of cerebrovascular disease, *Radiology* 85:270-283, 1965.

150. Capistrant TD, Gumnit RJ: Detecting carotid occlusive disease by thermography, *Stroke* 4:57-64, 1973.

151. Kistler JP, Lees RS, Miller A: Correlation of spectral phonoangiography and carotid angiography with gross pathology in carotid stenosis, *N Engl J Med* 305:417-419, 1981.

152. Duncan GW, Gruber J, Dewey CF Jr, et al: Evaluation of carotid stenosis by phonoangiography *N Engl J Med* 293: 1124-1128, 1975.

153. Baker JD: Diagnosis of carotid stenosis by bruit spectral analysis, *Am J Surg* 144:207-210, 1982.

154. Knox R, Breslau P, Strandness DE Jr: Quantitative carotid phonoangiography, *Stroke* 12:798-803, 1981.

155. Barrios RR, Solis C: Carotid-compression tonographic test: its application in the study of carotidartery occlusions, *Am J Ophthalmol* 62:116-125, 1966.

156. Cohen DN, Wangelin R, Trotta C, et al: Carotid compression tonography: correlation with bilateral carotid arteriography in the diagnosis of extracranial carotid occlusive disease, *Stroke* 6:257-262, 1975.

157. Langham ME, Toomey KF, Preziosi TJ: Carotid occlusive disease: effect of complete occlusion of internal carotid artery on intracular pulse/pressure relation and on ophthalmic arterial pressure, *Stroke* 12:759-765, 1981.

158. Oculocerebrovasculometry: a new procedure for the measurement of the ophthalmic artery pressure, *Bruit* 4:34, 1980.

159. Otis SM: Noninvasive vascular examination in amaurosis fugax. In Bernstein EF, ed: *Amaurosis fugax,* New York, 1988, Springer-Verlag; 183-199.

160. Spencer M, Whisler D: Transorbital Doppler diagnosis of ultracranial arterial stenosis, *Stroke* 17:916-920, 1986.

161. Russell JB: Pulsed-Doppler ultrasound arteriography. In Hershey FB, Barnes RW, Sumner DS, eds: *Noninvasive diagnosis of vascular disease,* Pasadena, Calif, 1984, Appleton Davies; 268-280.

162. Bernstein EF: The clinical spectrum of ischemic cerebrovascular disease. In Bernstein EF, ed: *Noninvasive diagnostic techniques in vascular disease,* ed 3, St Louis, Mosby, 1985, 301-315.

163. Moore WS: Indications for angiography and basis for selecting the type of angiographic study. In Moore WS, ed: *Surgery for cerebrovascular disease,* New York, 1987, Churchill Livingstone, 377-382.

164. Haugen OD, Brindle MJ: Effects of contrast media on blood coagulation, *J Can Assoc Radiol* 21:146-148, 1970.

165. Bjork L: Effect of angiocardiography on erythrocyte aggregation in the conjunctival vessels, *Acta Radiol* 6:459-464, 1967.

166. Rapaport S: Reversible opening of blood brain barrier by osmotic shrinkage of the cerebro-vascular and endothelium: opening up the tight junctions as related to carotid arteriography. In Hilal S, ed: *Small vessel angiography: imaging, morphology, physiology and clinical applications,* St Louis, 1973, Mosby 137-151.

167. Levitan H, Rapaport SI: Contrast media: quantitative criteria for designing compounds with low toxicity, *Acta Radiol* 1F:81-92, 1976.

168. Hilal S: Hemodynamic responses in the cerebral vessels to angiographic contrast media, *Acta Radiol* 5:211-231, 1966.

169. Port FK, Wagoner RD, Fulton RE: Acute renal failure after angiography, *Am J Roentgenol Radium Ther Nucl Med* 121:544-550, 1974.

170. Older RA, Miller JP, Jackson DC, et al: Angiographically induced renal failure and its radiographic detection, *Am J Roentgenol* 126:1039-1045, 1976.

171. Pillay VK, Robbins PC, Schwartz FD, et al: Acute renal failure following intravenous urography in patients with long standing diabetes mellitus and azotemia, *Radiology* 95:633-636, 1970.

172. Gomes AS, Baker JD, Martin-Paredero V, et al: Acute renal dysfunction following major arteriography, *AJR* 145:1249-1253, 1985.

173. Eisenberg RL, Bank WO, Hedgcock MW: Neurologic complications of angiography in patients with critical stenosis of the carotid artery, *Neurology* 30:892-895, 1980.

174. Talner LB: Does hydration prevent contrast material renal injury? [editorial] *AJR* 136:1021-1022, 1981.

175. Shafi T, Chou SY, Porush JG, Shapiro WB: Infusion intravenous pyelography and renal failure, *Arch Intern Med* 138:1218-1221, 1978.

176. Turski PA, Strother CM, Turnipseed WD, et al: Evaluation of extracranial occlusive disease by digital subtraction angiography, *Surg Neurol* 16:349-348, 1981.

177. Strother CM, Sackett JF, Crummy AB, et al: Clinical applications of computerized fluoroscopy: the extracranial carotid arteries, *Radiology* 136:781-783, 1980.

178. Turnipseed WD: Digital subtraction angiography: intravenous and intra-arterial routes. In Moore WS, ed: *Surgery for cerebrovascular disease*, New York, 1987, Churchill Livingstone, 383-397.

179. Harrison MJG: Angiography in amaurosis fugax. In Bernstein EF: *Amaurosis fugax*, New York, 1988, Springer-Verlag, 227-235.

180. Harrison MGJ, Marshall J: Indicators for angiography and surgery in carotid artery disease, *Br Med J* 1:616-617, 1975.

181. Hooshmand H, Vines FS, Lee HM, et al: Amaurosis fugax: diagnostic and therapeutic aspects, *Stroke* 5:643-647, 1974.

182. Wilson LA, Ross Russell RW: Amaurosis fugax and carotid artery disease: indications for angiography, *Br Med J* 2:435-437, 1977.

183. Eisenberg RL, Mani RL: Clinical and arteriographic comparison of amaurosis fugax with hemispheric transient ischemic attacks, *Stroke* 9:254-255, 1978.

184. Adams HP, Putman SF, Corbett JJ, et al: Amaurosis fugax: the results of arteriography in 59 patients, *Stroke* 14:742-744, 1983.

185. Ramirez-Lassepas M, Sandok BA, Burton RC: Clinical indicators of extracranial carotid artery disease in patients with transient symptoms, *Stroke* 4:537-540, 1973.

186. Sandok BA, Trautmann JC, Ramirez-Lassepas M, et al: Clinical angiographic correlations in amaurosis fugax, *Am J Ophthalmol* 79:137-142, 1974.

187. Lemak NA, Fields WS: The reliability of clinical prediction of extracranial artery disease, *Stroke* 7:377-379, 1976.

188. Mungas JE, Baker WH: Amaurosis fugax, *Stroke* 8:232-235, 1977.

189. Harrison MJG, Marshall J: Arteriographic comparison of amaurosis fugax and hemispheric transient ischaemic attacks, *Stroke* 16:795-797, 1985.

190. Bogousslavsky J, Hachinski VC, Barnett HJM: Causes cardiaques et arterielles de cecite monoculaire transitoire, *Rev Neurol* 141:774-779, 1985.

191. Hedges TR, Giliberti OL, Margargal LE: Intravenous digital subtraction angiography and its role in ocular vascular disease, *Arch Ophthalmol* 103:666-669, 1985.

192. Tsuruda JS, Saloner D, Anderson C: Noninvasive evaluation of cerebral ischemia: trends for the 1990s, *Circulation* 83(suppl I):176-189, 1991.

193. Masaryk TJ, Modic MT, Ross JS, et al: Intracranial circulation: preliminary results with three-dimensional (volume) MR angiography, *Radiology* 171:793-799, 1989.

194. Nishimura D, Macovski A, Jackson H, et al: Magnetic resonance angiography by selective inversion recovery using a compact gradient echo sequence, *Magn Reson Med* 8:96-103, 1988.

195. Ruggieri PM, Laub GA, Masaryk TJ, Modic MT: Intracranial circulation: pulse sequence considerations in three-dimensional (volume) MR angiography, *Radiology* 171:785-791, 1989.

196. Dumoulin C, Souza S, Walker M, Yoshitome E: Time-resolved magnetic resonance angiography, *Magn Reson Med* 6:275-286, 1988.

197. Dumoulin C, Souza S, Walker M, Wagle W: Three-dimensional phase contrast angiography, *Magn Reson Med* 9:139-149, 1989.

198. Mattle HP, Kent KC, Edelman RR, et al: Evaluation of the extracranial carotid arteries: correlation of magnetic resonance angiography, duplex ultrasonography, and conventional angiography, *J Vasc Surg* 13:838-845, 1991.

199. Moran P: A flow velocity zeugmatographic interlace for NMR imaging in humans, *Magn Reson Imaging* 1:197-203, 1983.
200. Firmin D, Nayler G, Klipstein R, et al: In vivo dilation of MR velocity imaging, *J Comput Assist Tomogr* 11:751-756, 1987.
201. Meier D, Maier S, Boesiger P: Quantitative flow measurements on phantoms and on blood vessels with MR, *Magn Reson Med* 8:25-34, 1988.
202. Walker M, Souza S, Dumoulin C: Quantitative flow measurement in phase contrast MR angiography, *J Comput Assist Tomogr* 12:304-313, 1988.
203. Gunter B, Cranney G, Lotan C, et al: Assessment of carotid flow using nuclear magnetic resonance phase velocity mapping, *Proc Eighth Ann Meeting, Soc Mag Res Med Amsterdam*, 163, 1989.
204. Matsuda T, Shimizu K, Sakurai T, et al: Measurement of aortic blood flow with MR imaging: comparative study with Doppler US, *Radiology* 162:857-861, 1987.
205. Hennig J, Mueri M, Brunner P, Friedburg H: Quantitative flow measurement with the fast Fourier technique, *Radiology* 166:237-240, 1988.
206. Saloner D, Anderson CM: Flow velocity quantitation by inversion tagging, *Magn Reson Med* 16:269-279, 1990.
207. Edelman R, Mattle H, Kleefield J, Silver M: Quantification of blood flow with dynamic MR imaging and presaturation bolus tagging, *Radiology* 171:551-556, 1989.
208. Gunter B, Cranney G, Lotan C, et al: Assessment of carotid flow using nuclear magnetic resonance phase velocity mapping, *Proc Eighth Ann Meeting, Soc Mag Res Med, Amsterdam*, 163, 1989.
209. Gunning AJ, Pickering GW, Robb-Smith AHT, et al: Mural thrombosis of the internal carotid artery and subsequent embolism, *Q J Med* 33:155-195, 1964.
210. Turpie AG, Hirsh J: Thromboembolic cerebral vascular diseases. In Kwaan HC, Bowie EJW, eds: *Thrombosis*, Philadelphia, 1982, WB Saunders, 154-167.
211. Whisnant JP, Matsumoto N Elveback LR: Transient cerebral ischemic attacks in a community: Rochester, Minn, 1955 through 1969, *Mayo Clin Proc* 48:194-198, 1973.
212. Report of the Veterans Administration: Cooperative study of atherosclerosis, neurology section. An evaluation of anticoagulant therapy in the treatment of cerebrovascular disease, *Neurology* 11:132-138, 1961.
213. Baker RN, Broward JA, Fang HC, et al: Anticoagulant therapy in cerebral infarction, *Neurology* 12:823-835, 1962.
214. Pierce JMS, Gubbey SS, Walton JN: Long-term anticoagulant therapy in transient ischemic attacks, *Lancet* 1:6-9, 1965.
215. Baker RN, Schwartz W, Rose AS: Transient ischemic attacks: a report of a study of anticoagulant treatment, *Neurology* 16:841-847, 1966.
216. Easton JD, Sherman DG: Medical management of territorial transient ischemic attacks. In Moore WS, ed: *Surgery for cerebrovascular disease*, New York, 1987, Churchill Livingstone, 419-425.
217. Garabedian M, Gold H: Dose dependent thrombolysis, pharmacokinetics, and hemostatic effects of rTPA for coronary thrombosis, *Am J Cardiol* 58:673-679, 1986.
218. Del Zoppo G, Zeumer H, Harker L: Thrombolytic therapy in stroke: possibilities and hazards, *Stroke* 17:595-607, 1986.
219. Zivin JA, Fisher M, DeGirolami U, et al: Tissue plasminogen activator reduces neurological damage after cerebral embolism, *Science* 230:1289-1292, 1985.
220. Lyden PD, Zivin JA, Clark WM, et al: TPA mediated thrombolysis of cerebral emboli and its effect on hemorrhagic infarction on rabbits, *Neurology* 39:703-708, 1989.
221. Lyden PD, Madden KP, Clark WM, et al: Incidence of cerebral hemorrhage after antifibrinolytic treatment for embolic stroke in rabbits, *Stroke* 21:1589-1593, 1990.
222. Kissel P, Chehrazi B, Seibert JA, Wagner FC: Digital angiographic quantification of blood flow dynamics in embolic stroke treated with TPA, *J Neurosurg* 67:399-405, 1987.

223. Del Zoppo GJ, Copeland BR, Anderchek K, et al: Hemorrhagic transformation following tissue plasminogen activator in experimental cerebral infarction, *Stroke* 21:596-601, 1990.

224. Phillips D, Fisher M: The angiographic efficacy of TPA in a cerebral embolization model, *Ann Neurol* 23:391-394, 1988.

225. Clark WM, Madden KP, Lyden PD, Zivin JA: Cerebral hemorrhagic risk of aspirin on heparin therapy with thrombolytic treatment in rabbits, *Stroke* 22:872-876, 1991.

226. Fields WS, Lemak NA, Frankowski RF, et al: Controlled trial of aspirin in cerebral ischemia, *Stroke* 8:301-316, 1977.

227. Fields WS, Lemak NA, Frankowski RF, et al: Controlled trial of aspirin in cerebral ischemia: part II. Surgical group, *Stroke* 9:309-319, 1978.

228. Canadian Cooperative Study Group: A randomized trial of aspirin and sulfinpyrazone in threatened stroke, *N Engl J Med* 299:53-59, 1978.

229. Bousser MG, Eschwege E, Haguenau M, et al: "AICLA" controlled trial of aspirin and dipyridamole in the secondary prevention of atherothrombotic cerebral ischemia, *Stroke* 14:5-14, 1983.

230. Fields WS, Lemak NA: Aspirin trials in the United States. In Bernstein EF, ed: *Amaurosis fugax*, New York, 1988, Springer-Verlag, 236-250.

231. Dale J, Myhre E, Storstein O, et al: Prevention of arterial thromboembolism with acetylsalicylic acid: a controlled clinical study in patients with aortic ball valves, *Am Heart J* 94:101-111, 1977.

232. Savi P, Laplace MC, Maffrand JP, Herbert JM: Binding of [3H]-2-methylthio ADP to rat platelets—effect of clopidogrel and ticlopidine, *J Pharmacol Exp Ther* 269 (2): 772–777, 1994.

233. Hass WK, Kamm B: The North American Ticlopidine Aspirin Study: structure, stratification variables, and patient characteristics, *Agents, actions* 15(suppl):273-278, 1984.

234. Gent M, Ellis D: Canadian American Ticlopidine Study (CATS) in thromboembolic stroke, *Agents, actions* 15(suppl):283-296, 1984.

235. Verry M, Panak E, Cazenave JP: Antiplatelet therapy in the prevention of ischemic stroke, *Nouv Rev Fr Hematol* 36(3):213-228, 1994.

236. Hennerici M, Kleophas W, Gries FA: Regression of carotid plaques during low density lipoprotein cholesterol elimination, *Stroke* 22:989-992, 1991.

237. Eugene J, Ott RA, Nudelman KL, et al: Initial clinical evaluation of carotid artery laser endarterectomy, *J Vasc Surg* 12:499-503, 1990.

238. Fode NC, Sundt TM: The safety of carotid endarterectomy for amaurosis fugax. In Bernstein EF, ed: *Amaurosis fugax*, New York, 1988, Springer-Verlag, 264-272.

239. North American Symptomatic Carotid Endarterectomy Trial (NASCET) Steering Committee: North American symptomatic carotid endarterectomy trial, *Stroke* 22:711-720, 1991.

240. National Institute of Neurological Disorders and Stroke: *Clinical alert news*, Washington, DC, 1991, National Library of Medicine.

241. Reinmuth OM, Dyken ML Jr: Carotid endarterectomy: bright light at the end of the tunnel, *Stroke* 22:835-836, 1991.

242. The Asymptomatic Carotid Atherosclerosis Study Group (Toole JF, Howard VJ, Chambless LE): Study design for randomized prospective trial of carotid endarterectomy for asymptomatic atherosclerosis, *Stroke* 20:844-9, 1989.

243. National Institute of Neurological Disorders and Stroke: Clinical advisory: carotid endarterectomy for patients with asymptomatic internal carotid artery stenosis, Washington, DC, 1994, National Institutes of Health.

244. Moore WS, Vescera CL, Robertson JT, Baker H, Howard VJ, Toole JF: Selection process for participating surgeons in the Asymptomatic Carotid Atherosclerosis Study (ACAS), *Stroke* 22:1353-7, 1991.

245. Callow AD, Mackey WC: Optimum results of the surgical treatment of carotid territory ischemia, *Circulation* 83(suppl I):1190-1195, 1991.

246. O'Donnell TF Jr, Callow AD, Scott G, et al: Ultrasound characteristics of recurrent carotid disease: hypothesis explaining the low incidence of symptomatic recurrence, *J Vasc Surg* 2:26-41, 1985.

247. Araki CT, Babikian VL, Cantelmo NL, Johnson WC: Cerebrovascular hemodynamic changes associated with carotid endarterectomy, *J Vasc Surg* 13:854-860, 1991.

8

Visual Field Deficit

Bernard H. Blaustein
Gerald Selvin

Key Terms

optic chiasm	central scotoma	homonymous
papillomacular bundle	arcuate scotoma	hemianopsia
	nasal step	noncongruent
arcuate bundles	bitemporal	quadrantanopsia
nasal radial bundle	hemianopsia	macular sparing
knee of Wildebrand	pituitary adenoma	optokinetic
Meyer's loop	junction scotoma	nystagmus

No area in clinical optometry better exemplifies the intimate relationship between anatomy and clinical manifestation than does the visual field deficit. The visual fibers are laid down in a very specific architecture as they course their way from the retina to the occipital cortex. During their circuitous route, they pass through a significant portion of the temporal lobe, parietal lobe, and occipital lobe. Indeed, it has been estimated that the visual fibers constitute approximately 38% of the total number of nerve fibers within the brain.[1]

Pathologies within the cortices are apt to impact the visual fibers, causing specific visual field defects. The configuration of these defects is often very characteristic and may lead to the precise localization of the lesion as well as to an understanding of its cause. Thus an analysis of the visual field is an integral component of the neuro-ocular evaluation.

This chapter correlates the anatomic considerations with the clinical manifestations of visual field defects. Kinetic and static visual field plots are displayed to clarify specific points. In addition, simple chairside procedures are described to assist the clinician in predicting the presence of a visual field deficit before a formal visual field evaluation is performed.

Anatomic Considerations

The neural visual pathway can be divided into four functional territories. Each territory has distinct characteristics and is well demarcated.

Territory 1 encompasses the outer retina and includes the photoreceptors and their connections to the bipolar, amacrine, and horizontal cells by the outer plexiform layer. Territory 1 arbitrarily ends between the inner plexiform layer and the ganglion cell layer.

Territory 2 consists of the inner retina and includes the ganglion cell layer and its axons, the nerve fiber layer. The nerve fiber layer enters the optic nerve and becomes the first part of the long chain of visual fibers that terminates in the occipital cortex. Territory 2, then, may be thought of as the optic nerve. Territory 2 ends at that point where the optic nerve joins the optic chiasm.

The nerve fiber layer is further divided into three distinct bundle groups: the papillomacular bundle, the superior and inferior arcuate bundles, and the nasal radial bundle (Figure 8-1).

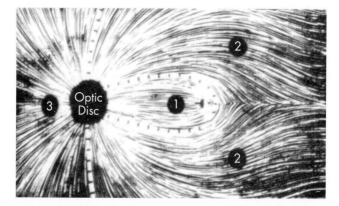

FIGURE 8-1 The retinal nerve fiber layer. **1,** The papillomacular bundle. **2,** The arcuate bundles. **3,** The nasal radial bundle.

The papillomacular bundle consists of axons (nerve fibers) from the ganglion cells in the macula as well as ganglion cells between the macula and optic nerve head. This bundle essentially represents cones, and as such, conveys sensory information about visual detail, color, and light brightness. This bundle also includes the bulk of the afferent fibers for the pupillomotor system (see Chapter 3). The fibers within the bundle run a relatively straight course, enter the temporal half of the optic nerve head, and subsequently occupy the central core of the optic nerve.

CLINICAL PEARL

The papillomacular bundle consists of axons (nerve fibers) from the ganglion cells in the macula as well as ganglion cells between the macula and optic nerve head. This bundle essentially represents cones, and as such, conveys sensory information about visual detail, color, and light brightness.

The arcuate bundles originate temporal to the macula and are so called because they arch above and below the papillomacular bundle and enter the superior and inferior poles of the optic nerve head (Figure 8-1). An important anatomic characteristic of this bundle is that the fibers in the superior and inferior divisions do not comingle. Rather, they are segregated by the temporal horizontal raphe of the retina.

The nasal radial bundle (cuneate bundle) originates from the ganglion cells nasal to the optic disc and fans into the disc radially in a wedgelike pattern. These fibers are not segregated into upper and lower compartments and consequently do mix as they cross the horizontal midline.

Potts and his coworkers[2] analyzed the nerve fibers that coursed through the optic nerve and found that the total number of nerve fibers numbered approximately 1 million. They also discovered that most of the fibers subserved macular cones. At first, these data were puzzling, because it was known that the nerve fiber layer represented ganglion cell axons from the entire retina. Furthermore, it was known that the retina consisted of approximately 125 million rods and 6 million cones.[3] They explained this apparent discrepancy in the following way:

The macula is a very dense area of receptors, most of which are cones. Within the macula, the retinal area in which the receptors innervate any one ganglion cell (the receptive field) is very small. Thus each ganglion cell in the macula essentially subserves cones. In areas away from the macula, the rods increase in number and the receptive fields become larger. Thus in the peripheral retinal area, each ganglion cell subserves thousands of rods. The net effect of this neural confluence is that the optic nerve is predominantly composed of fibers subserving macular cones, and may be thought of as a structure for macular projection, i.e., a cone structure.[2]

CLINICAL PEARL

The optic nerve is predominantly composed of fibers subserving macular cones, and may be thought of as a structure for macular projection, i.e., a cone structure.

Territory 3 consists of the visual fibers within the optic chiasm from the point where the optic nerve ends to that point where the optic tract begins. The chiasm consists of crossed and uncrossed fibers. Nerve fibers from the nasal retina of each eye cross and subsequently enter the contralateral optic tract. The temporal retinal fibers from each eye do not cross and enter the ipsilateral optic tract. An important anatomic consideration is that the inferior nasal fibers from each eye sweep into the contralateral optic nerve for a short distance (von Willebrand's loop) before traversing the chiasm (Figure 8-2).

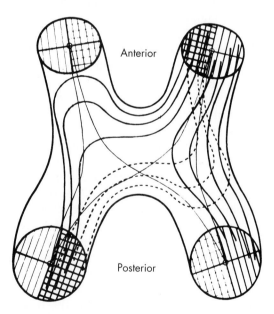

FIGURE 8-2 The optic chiasm. The temporal retinal fibers pass into the ipsilateral optic tract; the nasal retinal fibers cross into the contralateral optic tract. Note that the inferior nasal fibers sweep into the contralateral optic nerve for a short distance.

In a classic histologic study, Hoyt and Luis[4] demonstrated that the crossing system of the chiasm is composed predominantly of fibers from the macula and thus represents cones. Thus, like the optic nerve, the chiasm may functionally be considered a macular structure.

Territory 4 consists of the postchiasmal visual fibers from the ipsilateral temporal retina and the contralateral nasal retina and runs from the optic tract to the occipital cortex. Within the cortices, the fibers are known as the optic radiations.

The postchiasmal fibers are configured such that the superior and inferior visual fibers remain in their respective positions throughout the pathway.[5] Thus after synapsing in the lateral geniculate body, the inferior fibers loop around the anterior aspect of the temporal horn of the lateral ventricle (Meyer's loop) and course through the temporal lobe. The superior fibers do not negotiate this loop and proceed instead through the parietal lobe to their terminus in the occipital lobe (see Figure 1-2).

Additionally, fibers in the optic tract, lateral geniculate body, and temporal lobe are relatively separated. As the fibers exit the temporal lobe to travel within the parietal lobe, they approximate each other more closely. Nerve fibers within the occipital lobe are packed tightly together.[5]

Clinical Correlates

Territory 1

Lesions in territory 1 are caused by pathologies that are either congenital or acquired. The congenital pathologies affecting this territory are numerous but most commonly include the hereditary dystrophies (e.g., rod-cone dystrophy, retinitis pigmentosa, fundus albipunctatis, Best's disease, Stargardt's disease).[6] The acquired pathologies include entities that originate in the choroid, Bruch's membrane, and retinal pigment epithelium and subsequently affect the photoreceptors.

Most of the lesions in territory 1 are visible by ophthalmoscopy and create discrete, dense, and frequently absolute scotomas that correspond to the ophthalmoscopic location. Unless the pathologies are bilateral, the visual field defects present monocularly. The most significant feature of the visual field defects that affect this territory is the "lack of respect" for the vertical and nasal horizontal meridians. Thus field defects may straddle the vertical meridian and do not cut off nasally in a sharp step. The following case is illustrative.

A patient presented with a history of reduced vision in dim illumination. Ophthalmoscopy showed bone-spicule pigment formations clustered around blood vessels in the midperiphery of the retina. The resultant visual field showed ring scotomas that crossed the vertical midline and did not cut off nasally in a sharp step (Figure

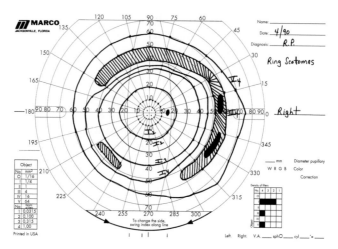

FIGURE 8-3 Territory 1 defect. Note the ring scotomas straddling the vertical meridian and not cutting off nasally in a sharp step.

8-3). Subsequent electrodiagnostic testing led to the diagnosis of retinitis pigmentosa.

Territory 2

The configuration of the visual field defects from lesions in this territory depends on which nerve fiber bundle or bundles are implicated. If the pathology involves the papillomacular bundle and specifically impacts on the macular ganglion cells or their fibers, a central scotoma results (Figure 8-4). If the ganglion cells or fibers between the macula and optic nerve head are also impacted, the resulting scotoma extends from the point of fixation to the blind spot and is referred to as a centrocecal scotoma (Figure 8-5).

Because macular ganglion cells subserve macular cones, papillomacular bundle defects result in reduced visual acuity, decreased sensitivity to color, decreased sensitivity to light, and an afferent pupil defect. (See Chapter 3 for a complete description of afferent pupil defects.) The following case is illustrative:

CLINICAL PEARL

Papillomacular bundle defects result in reduced visual acuity, decreased sensitivity to color, decreased sensitivity to light, and an afferent pupil defect.

A 24-year-old woman presented with a sudden reduction in visual acuity in the right eye and pain on extreme lateral gaze. Neither a refraction nor a pinhole improved the vision. She reported a decrease

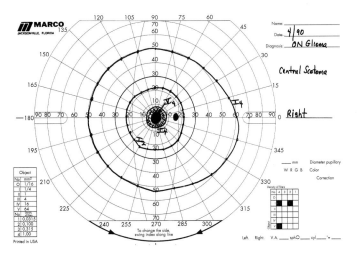

FIGURE 8-4 Central scotoma. There is damage to fibers coming from ganglion cells in the macula.

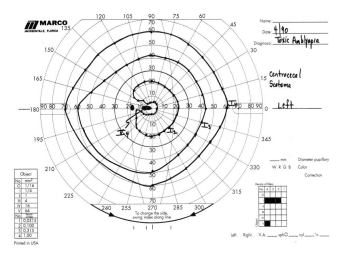

FIGURE 8-5 Centrocecal scotoma. There is damage to fibers coming from ganglion cells in the macula and in the retina between the macula and the optic disc.

in the saturation of a red target when comparing her right eye with her left. She also reported a decrease in the brightness of a light source when viewed with her right eye. Finally, she manifested a definite afferent pupil defect in the right eye. Ophthalmoscopy did not show any abnormality in the right optic nerve. The resultant visual field disclosed a centrocecal scotoma (Figure 8-5). Retrobulbar optic neuritis was diagnosed.

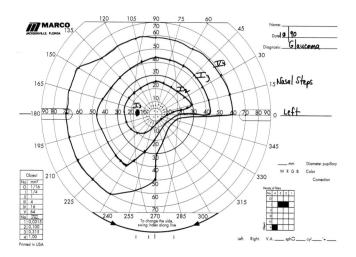

FIGURE 8-6   Nasal steps from a large arcuate bundle defect.

The special anatomy of the arcuate bundles creates the characteristic field defects that result from arcuate bundle pathology. The discrete separation of the superior and inferior arcuate bundles by the temporal raphe of the retina results in a corresponding division along the nasal horizontal meridian of the visual field. Thus a scotoma from a significant arcuate bundle defect does not cross the nasal horizontal meridian. Rather, the defect takes the form of a steplike depression that is aligned along the nasal horizontal meridian (Figure 8-6).

It is the nasal step that characterizes the arcuate bundle and differentiates field defects in territory 2 from those in territory 1. Consider the following case.

A myopic man presented with slightly elevated intraocular pressures and suspicious optic nerve heads. Glaucoma was suspected. A visual field screening showed a discrete arcuate scotoma that crossed the nasal horizontal meridian (Figure 8-7). Such a scotoma does not represent a defect in the arcuate bundles and is not representative of glaucoma. Indirect ophthalmoscopy showed a splitting of the outer and inner retina (retinoschisis), a territory 1 lesion.

Not all lesions of the arcuate bundles are large enough to produce a nasal step within the visual field. If the lesion impacts fibers close to the disc, a partial arcuate scotoma results (Figure 8-8). Lesions involving a small number of fibers are apt to produce a paracentral scotoma (Figure 8-9).

Pathologies that affect the nasal radial bundle do not result in field defects that align along the temporal horizontal meridian. Rather, the comingling of the superior and inferior fibers within this bundle results in a wedgelike defect with no steplike characteristics (Figure 8-10). The nasal radial bundle is less frequently affected than the papillomacular or arcuate bundles.[6]

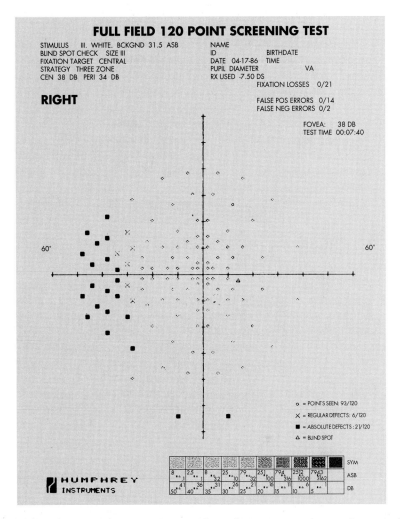

FIGURE 8-7 Arcuate scotoma that does not respect the nasal horizontal meridian. Such a defect represents a territory 1 defect.

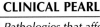

CLINICAL PEARL

Pathologies that affect the nasal radial bundle do not result in field defects that align along the temporal horizontal meridian. Rather, the comingling of the superior and inferior fibers within this bundle results in a wedgelike defect with no steplike characteristics.

It should be noted that most pathologies that affect the optic nerve impact the papillomacular bundle and arcuate bundles.[7] A notable exception is glaucoma, which preferentially affects the arcuate

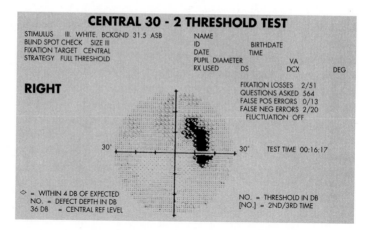

FIGURE 8-8 Partial arcuate scotoma from damage to fibers located near the optic disc.

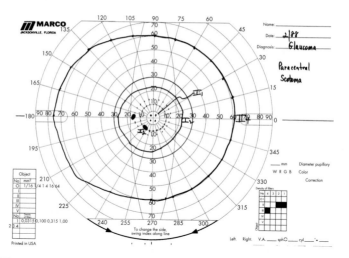

FIGURE 8-9 Paracentral scotoma from damage to a small number of fibers located in the midzone of the superior arcuate bundle.

bundles and spares the papillomacular bundle until late in the course of the disease.

Territory 3

At the chiasm, all afferent nerve fibers from both eyes are segregated into crossed and uncrossed systems. As a result, the visual system becomes functionally divided vertically through the fixation point such that the fibers from the hemifields of each eye blend and course to the contralateral occipital lobe. Chiasmal as well as postchiasmal lesions produce hemianopic defects, i.e., defects with a border aligned

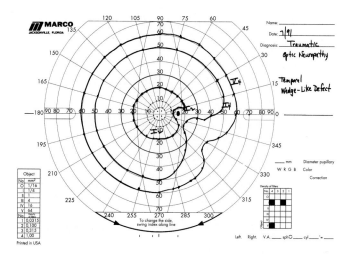

FIGURE 8-10 Temporal wedgelike defect from damage to the nasal radial bundle.

along the vertical meridian that extends through the fixation point. The defect does not cross this vertical meridian. It should be noted that the entire hemifield need not be involved. Some of the isopters, however, always will be aligned along this vertical meridian.

CLINICAL PEARL

Chiasmal as well as postchiasmal lesions produce hemianopic defects, i.e., defects with a border aligned along the vertical meridian that extends through the fixation point. The defect does not cross this vertical meridian.

The hallmark of classic chiasmal compression is bitemporal hemianopsia. Typically, the most common cause of the chiasmal compression is a pituitary tumor that initially impacts the chiasm from below.[8] As a result, the early field deficit is often a superior bitemporal defect. In advanced cases, a total bitemporal hemianopsia may result (Figure 8-11). Additionally, 45% of pituitary tumors are secretory and result in provocative clinical manifestations.[9] Consider the following case.

A 33-year-old woman presented with chronic recurring headaches and indicated that she was constantly bumping into the sides of hallways. She also indicated that she was being treated by her gynecologist for amenorrhea (absence of menstruation) and galactorrhea (a discharge of milk from the breasts). A visual field showed a bitemporal hemianopsia (Figure 8-11). A secretory pituitary tumor was suspected. Subsequent neuroimaging showed a large suprasellar mass impinging on the chiasm. Blood tests disclosed an elevated

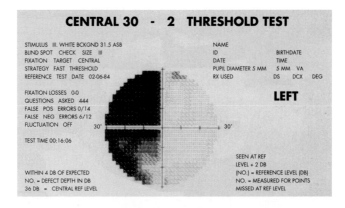

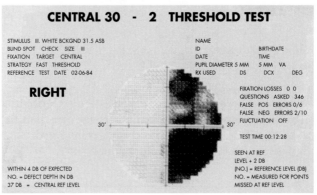

FIGURE 8-11 Bitemporal hemianopsia from chiasmal compression.

serum prolactin level. After surgery, the diagnosis of a prolactin-secreting pituitary adenoma was confirmed.

In 25% to 30% of the cases, the compressing tumor impacts the anterior aspect of the chiasm at the point where the inferior nasal fibers sweep into the contralateral optic nerve.[10,11] Such a lesion impacts on territory 2 ipsilaterally and on territory 3 contralaterally. Thus the ipsilateral eye manifests nerve fiber bundle defects and the contralateral eye manifests a superior temporal field defect. This characteristic visual field configuration is known as a junction scotoma (Figure 8-12).

Finally, in 10% of patients, the body of the chiasm is either anterior (prefixed) or posterior (postfixed) to the pituitary gland.[12] If the chiasm is prefixed, an enlarging pituitary tumor might compress the optic tract, resulting in homonymous hemianopsia. (Hemianopsia will be discussed in the next section.) If the chiasm is postfixed, an enlarging pituitary tumor might encroach on the optic nerve, resulting in territory 2 field defects. Thus the clinician should consider pituitary tumor in any patient who presents with visual field defects suggestive of territory 2 lesions or optic tract lesions.

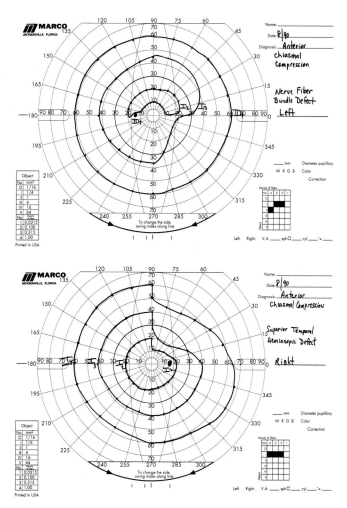

FIGURE 8-12 Junction scotoma from a lesion at the junction of the left optic nerve and the chiasm.

Territory 4

Lesions that impact the postchiasmal fibers result in contralateral hemianopic defects that are homonymous, i.e., occupy the same side of the visual field in each eye. Moreover, the hemianopsias have no effect on visual acuity even in patients with complete, fixation-splitting homonymous hemianopsias. The configuration and congruity of the field defects, however, depend on the specific location of the postchiasmal lesion.

Lesions of the optic tract and lateral geniculate body constitute approximately 2% of those that affect territory 4.[13,14] The resultant field defects are markedly noncongruent, i.e., do not extend to the same angular meridian in each eye and are dissimilar as to size, shape, or depth.

CLINICAL PEARL

Lesions of the optic tract and lateral geniculate body constitute approximately 2% of those that affect territory. The resultant field defects are markedly noncongruent.

Pathologies in the temporal lobe constitute approximately 25% of those that affect the postchiasmal area.[16] The lesions are 90% neoplastic and 10% vascular and are most apt to impact the inferior postchiasmal fibers[15] (see Figure 1-2). The resultant visual field deficit is a contralateral superior quadrantanopsia, often called a "pie in the sky" defect (Figure 8-13). The defects are usually noncongruous, although

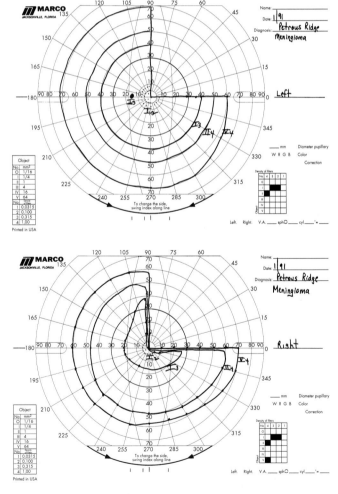

FIGURE 8-13 Right superior quadrantanopsia ("pie in the sky" defect) from a left temporal lobe neoplasm.

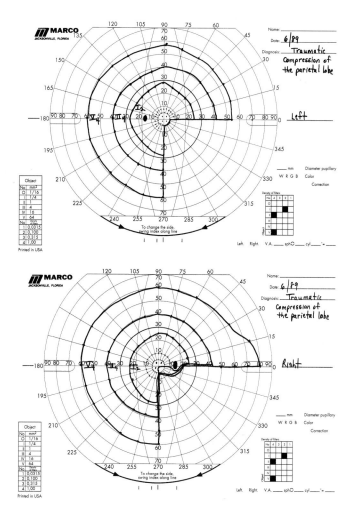

FIGURE 8-14 Right inferior quadrantanopsia from compression to the left parietal lobe.

not as marked as those from optic tract lesions. Additionally, temporal lobe lesions may cause olfactory and gustatory hallucinations (uncinate fits), seizures, formed hallucinations, and aphasia (if the dominant side is involved).

Lesions in the parietal lobe constitute approximately 35% of the postchiasmal lesions and are 50% neoplastic.[15] Most are apt to impact the postchiasmal superior fibers (see Figure 1-2 in Chapter 1). The resultant field deficit is a relatively congruent, contralateral inferior quadrantanopsia or a hemianopsia that is denser below the horizontal meridian (Figure 8-14). Other clinical manifestations of parietal lobe pathology may include acalculia, agraphia, left–right confusion, dressing apraxia, finger agnosia, motor impersistence, and ipsilateral pursuit function.

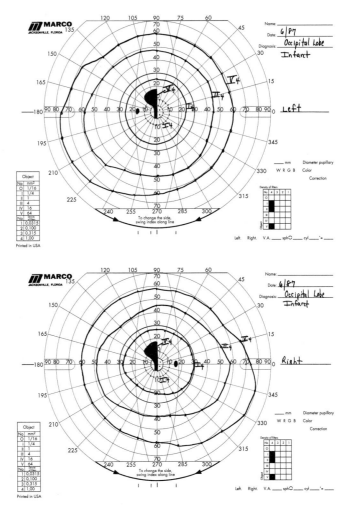

FIGURE 8-15 Left homonymous paracentral scotomas from a small infarct in the right occipital cortex.

Lesions in the occipital lobe constitute approximately 43% of the postchiasmal lesions and are caused by vascular infarct 80% of the time.[15] The resultant field deficit is usually a complete hemianopsia. Small infarcts within the occipital cortex may produce incomplete hemianopsias, but their congruity is striking (Figure 8-15).

A pathognomonic feature of the hemianopsias produced by occipital lobe lesions is the presence of macular sparing[16,17] (Figure 8-16). One explanation for the sparing of the central 20° (i.e., the macula) in these hemianopsias is as follows: the macular representation in the occipital cortex receives a dual blood supply—the posterior cerebral artery and the middle cerebral artery. Should one of the vascular supplies be compromised, the other vascular source would be sufficient to

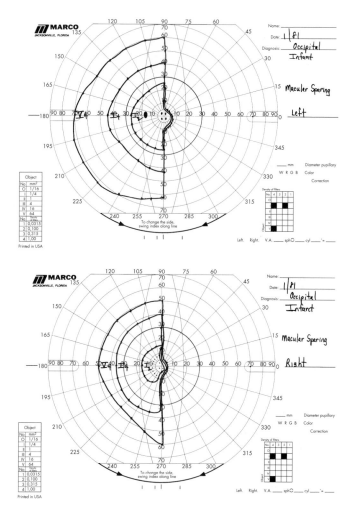

FIGURE 8-16 Right homonymous hemianopsia with macular sparing. The sparing of the fixational area signifies occipital cortical disease.

retain neural function, and the central 20° would be spared. The rest of the visual cortex, representing the midperipheral and far peripheral visual field, does not receive this dual blood supply. In the event of infarct, that portion of the cortex would be irreversibly damaged, resulting in a hemianopic field cut.[16,17]

Occasionally, infarcts in the occipital lobe spare a small portion of the anterior mesial portion of the occipital cortex and result in retention of the temporal crescent[18,19] (Figure 8-17). The temporal crescent is an area within the temporal periphery that extends from approximately 50° to 90°. This extreme peripheral field is only subserved by the nasal retinal fibers of the ipsilateral eye. The

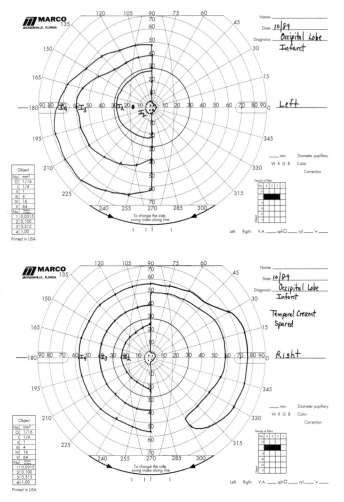

FIGURE 8-17 Right homonymous hemianopsia with sparing of the temporal crescent. The spared crescent represents a spared portion of the anterior mesial visual cortex.

nose blocks the temporal retinal fibers of the contralateral eye from perceiving the image. The nasal retinal fibers cross and course back to the anterior mesial aspect of the occipital cortex.

CLINICAL PEARL

Occasionally, infarcts in the occipital lobe spare a small portion of the anterior mesial portion of the occipital cortex and result in retention of the temporal crescent.

Finally, occipital lobe lesions do not result in neurologic stigmata other than hemianopic defects. The occipital cortex only subserves vision.

Practical Adjuncts to Predict Visual Field Deficit

Territory 2

As was previously indicated, the central core of the optic nerve is occupied primarily by the papillomacular nerve fiber bundle. This bundle conducts visual information from the center of the visual field and is also responsible for pupillomotor function, light brightness determination, and color perception. By evaluating these physiologic attributes at the chairside, the clinician can detect optic nerve deficit and predict the presence of a central scotoma.

The sine qua non of optic nerve disease is the presence of a relative afferent pupil defect.[20] This can be detected by the swinging light test. (See Chapter 3 for a complete discussion.) If the swinging light test is equivocal, the patient can be asked to compare the brightness of a light source when viewed with either eye. A suggested protocol is to ask the patient to place a dollar value on the brightness of the light. ("If the light is worth 1 dollar when viewed with your good eye, how much is it worth when viewed with your bad eye?") A decreased sensitivity to light brightness in one eye implies optic nerve disease.[20]

The perception that colors are desaturated, particularly red, is a sensitive barometer of optic nerve disease.[20] The clinician may present a red target and ask the patient to compare the "redness" with each eye. Alternatively, color vision plates can be used for comparison. Another chairside maneuver is to have the patient view two red targets simultaneously with each eye. One target is placed centrally and the other eccentrically. The patient is asked to compare the color intensity. If the patient states that the eccentric target is more intensely red than the central target, optic nerve disease is suspect.

CLINICAL PEARL

The perception that colors are desaturated, particularly red, is a sensitive barometer of optic nerve disease.

The clinician can explore the fixational area and the centrocecal area with a relatively large red target. The patient is asked to indicate when the color brightens as the clinician moves the target throughout the areas. In optic nerve disease, the patient will state that the color brightens as the target moves out of the scotoma. The patient will not

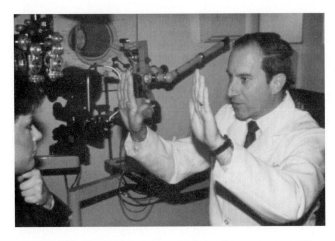

FIGURE 8-18 Simultaneous presentation of targets on either side of the midline increases the sensitivity of the confrontation test.

report a color change across the vertical meridian, however, unless the chiasm (territory 3) is involved.

Territory 3

Inasmuch as the main crossing bar of the chiasm is composed of fibers from macular cones, qualitative color comparison across the vertical meridian can be used. A red target may be moved across the vertical meridian while having the patient fixate a central point, or two red targets can be presented simultaneously on either side of the vertical midline. If the patient reports that the nasal stimulus looks brighter or redder with each eye, bitemporal hemianopsia is suspect.

Confrontation techniques are easily performed at the chairside and are useful in eliciting chiasmal defects. The patient is asked to count fingers in the temporal and nasal fields of each eye. An inaccurate count in the temporal fields of each eye implies a chiasmal defect. Simultaneous presentation of fingers or simultaneous hand comparison in the nasal and temporal fields may increase the sensitivity of the procedure and uncover a subtle defect (Figure 8-18).

Territory 4

Confrontation techniques are useful in eliciting hemianopic defects from postchiasmal pathologies. An inability to correctly count fingers in the same hemifield of each eye signifies a contralateral postchiasmal lesion. Asking the patient to compare clarity above and below the horizontal in the defective hemifield may lead to detection of a hemianopsia that is denser above or below.

Finally, the clinician may suspect the presence of a parietal lobe lesion by noting an asymmetric optokinetic nystagmus (OKN).[23-25] Normally, when an optokinetic tape is passed before the eyes, there is a slow following phase toward the side of the target movement, and a rapid jerk return in the opposite direction. The slow pursuit movement originates in the occipital lobes; the rapid refixation originates in the contralateral frontal lobe.[23]

CLINICAL PEARL

The clinician may suspect the presence of a parietal lobe lesion by noting an asymmetric optokinetic nystagmus (OKN).

The normal OKN response is dependent on intact optomotor fibers descending from the occipital lobes to the frontal lobes. The fibers descend in the internal sagittal striatum and are medial to the visual radiation fibers, which course through the deep parietal lobe on their way to the visual cortex. Parietal lobe lesions may interrupt these descending fibers. A defective OKN may result.

Typically, the OKN response is used in the following manner: a patient presents with a homonymous hemianopsia that signifies a contralateral postchiasmal lesion. The optokinetic tape is moved away from the lesion, eliciting an OKN. The tape then is moved toward the side of the lesion. If the resultant OKN is of diminished amplitude and frequency (i.e., asymmetric), the patient is said to exhibit a positive OKN sign. Such asymmetry is pathognomonic of parietal lobe lesions. Defective OKN does not occur with lesions of the optic tract, temporal lobe, or occipital lobe.[21-23]

References

1. Hoyt WF: The human optic chiasm: a neuroanatomical review of current concepts, recent investigations, and unresolved problems. In Smith JL, ed: *The University of Miami Neuroophthalmology Symposium.* Springfield, 1964, Charles C Thomas, 64-111.
2. Potts AM, Hodges D, Shelman CB, et al: Morphology of the primate optic nerve, Parts I and II, *Invest Ophthalmol* 11:980, 1972.
3. Dowling JE: Organization of the vertebrate retina, *Invest Ophthalmol* 9:655, 1970.
4. Hoyt WF, Luis O: The primate chiasm: details of visual fiber organization studied by silver impregnation techniques, *Arch Ophthalmol* 70:69, 1963.
5. Glaser JS, Sadun A: Anatomy of the visual sensory system. In Glaser JS, ed: *Neuro-ophthalmology,* Philadelphia, 1990, Lippincott, 72-73.
6. Trobe JD, Glaser JS: *The visual fields manual,* Gainesville, 1983, Triad, 29-44.
7. Burde RM, Savino PL, Trobe JD eds: *Clinical decisions in neuro-ophthalmology,* St Louis, 1985, Mosby, 29.
8. Hollenhorst RW, Young BR: Ocular manifestations produced by tumors of the pituitary gland: analysis of 1000 cases. In Kohler PO, Ross GT eds: *Diagnosis and treatment of pituitary tumors,* New York, 1973, American Elsevier, 53-64.
9. Wilson CB: A decade of pituitary microsurgery: the Herbert Olivecrona lecture, *Ophthalmology* 61:1265, 1983.

10. Chamiln M, Davidoff LM, Feiring EH: Ophthalmoscopic changes produced by pituitary tumors, *Am J Ophthalmol* 40:353, 1955.
11. Wilson P, Falconer MA: Patterns of visual failure with pituitary tumors: clinical and radiological correlation, *Br J Ophthalmol* 52:94, 1968.
12. Bergland RM, Ray BS, Torack R: Anatomical variations in the pituitary gland and adjacent structures in 225 human autopsy cases, *J Neurosurg* 28:93, 1968.
13. Bender MB, Bodis-Wollner I: Visual dysfunctions in optic tract lesions, *Ann Neurol* 3:187, 1978.
14. Savino PJ, Paris M, Schatz NJ, et al: Optic tract syndrome: a review of 21 patients, *Arch Ophthalmol* 96:656, 1978.
15. Smith J: Homonymous hemianopia: a review of one hundred cases, *Am J Ophthalmol* 616:623, 1962.
16. Smith CG, Richardson WFG: The course and distribution of the arteries supplying the visual (striate) cortex, *Am J Ophthalmol* 1391:1396, 1966.
17. Hoyt WF, Newton TH: Angiographic changes with occlusion of arteries that supply the visual cortex, *N Z Med J* 72:310, 1970.
18. Benton S, Levy I, Swash M: Vision in the temporal crescent in occipital infraction, *Brain* 103:83, 1980.
19. Walsh TJ: Temporal crescent or half-moon syndrome, *Ann Ophthalmol* 6:501, 1974.
20. Thompson HS, Montague P, Cox TA, Corbett JJ: The relationship between visual acuity, pupillary defect, and visual field loss, *Am J Ophthalmol* 3:681, 1982.
21. Balch RW, Yee RD, Honrubia V: Optokinetic nystagmus and parietal lobe lesions, *Ann Neurol* 7:269, 1979.
22. Gay AJ, Newman J, Keltner JL, Stroud M, eds: *Eye movement disorders,* St Louis, 1974, Mosby, 50.
23. Smith JL: *Optokinetic nystagmus,* Springfield, 1963, Charles C Thomas, 55–67.

9

Chronic Recurring Headache

Bernard H. Blaustein

Key Terms

vascular headaches	migraine	cranial neuralgia
serotonin	equivalents	traction headaches
classic migraine	sumatriptan	brain tumor
scintillating scotoma	cluster headaches	intracranial
common migraine	muscle contraction	hematomas
complicated	headache	
migraine		

Headache is a common complaint of optometry patients and may be one of the most common grievances of the civilized world. Patients with chronic, recurring headache are apt to present to the optometrist because the headaches frequently localize in and around the eyes. Thus patients assume that the head pain represents eyestrain or ocular disease.

Certain types of refractive errors, incipient presbyopia, poorly compensated phorias, or accommodative-convergence dysfunctions may indeed produce generalized asthenopia and eyeache. The patient generally presents with a vague feeling of visual fatigue and discomfort rather than true head pain, however. Moreover, the eyestrain is usually associated with a specific visual task such as reading or prolonged viewing of a computer screen.

Recurrent ocular pathology such as episcleritis, scleritis, keratitis, uveitis, chronic intermittent angle closure attacks, retrobulbar optic neuritis, orbital cellulitis, orbital pseudotumor, nonspecific granulomatous cavernous sinus inflammation, or ischemic ocular inflammation may also produce periocular head pain. These diagnoses, however, are usually self-evident by gross observation or with the slit lamp and ophthalmoscope. A complete description of the visual anomalies and ocular diseases that cause pain is beyond the scope of this chapter. Moreover, headaches of ocular origin do not represent the vast majority of chronic recurring headaches.[1]

CLINICAL PEARL

Headaches of ocular origin do not represent the vast majority of chronic recurring headaches.

This chapter concentrates on chronic recurrent headaches that are not of ocular origin. Cause and pathophysiology are addressed, and clinical evaluation and management approaches are emphasized.

Anatomic Substrate of Head Pain

In 1940, Ray and Wolff[2] defined the pain-sensitive structures of the head (Table 9-1). Extracranial pain-sensitive structures include the skin, fascia, subcutaneous fat, head and neck muscles, arteries, and veins. Intracranial pain-sensitive structures include the mucosa lining

TABLE 9-1
Pain-Sensitive Structures of the Head

Intracranial	Extracranial
Bony sinuses	Skin
Dura mater at the base of the brain	Fascia
Dura mater around large vessels	Subcutaneous fat
Arteries of the dura mater	Muscles
Arteries at the base of the brain	Arteries
Great venous sinuses	Veins
Intracerebral arteries	
Cranial nerves V, VII, IX, X	
Upper cervical nerves	

the bony sinuses, the dura mater at the base of the brain and around the large blood vessels, dural arteries and arteries at the base of the brain, the great venous sinuses, the intracerebral arteries, and trigeminal, facial, glossopharyngeal, and vagus cranial nerves, as well as the upper cervical nerves. The bony skull, parenchyma of the brain, much of the dura and pia matter, the lining of the ventricles, and the choroidal plexus are not sensitive to pain.

In general, pain sensation from structures above the tentorium cerbelli is referred to the frontal, temporal, or parietal regions of the skull. Pain sensation from structures below the tentorium cerebelli is referred to the occipital region of the head. There must be pressure, traction, inflammation, or irritation of pain-sensitive structures, however, for a patient to feel pain. Thus chronic recurring headache should be considered a symptom and not an entity unto itself.

CLINICAL PEARL

There must be pressure, traction, inflammation, or irritation of pain-sensitive structures, however, for a patient to feel pain. Thus chronic recurring headache should be considered a symptom and not an entity unto itself.

Classification of Headaches

Headache classification may be very complex; some writers divide headaches into multiple categories.[3-5] This approach taxes the memory and is clinically unwieldly. Dividing headaches into four main groups is recommended: vascular, muscle contraction, inflammatory and traction, and headaches due to other factors.

Vascular Headaches

Vascular headaches include migraine headaches, cluster headaches, toxic vascular headaches, and hypertensive headaches. Dilation and distension of branches of the external carotid artery are common findings in all of these headaches.

CLINICAL PEARL

Vascular headaches include migraine headaches, cluster headaches, toxic vascular headaches, and hypertensive headaches. Dilation and distension of branches of the external carotid artery are common findings in all of these headaches.

Migraine headaches

Researchers have estimated that 10% of the general population experiences migraine.[6] The clinician must be careful when making this diagnosis, however, because many patients will describe any recurring headache as a migraine. Patients with migraine headaches usually present with a stereotypical symptom complex; the clinical features of migraines follow. The head pain is described as a throbbing, pulsating, and pounding that is unilateral in onset but may become generalized. The headache usually is accompanied by a variety of symptoms that often include anorexia, nausea, vomiting, diarrhea and cramping, photophobia, hyperacussis leading to sonophobia, hyperosmia, excessive sweating (diaphoresis), and vertigo. Indeed, migraineurs may be quite sick and often refer to their headaches as being "sick headaches." When in the throes of a headache, patients often retire to a dark room and lie down with a wet cloth across the brow.

Characteristics of the migraineur. Most patients note that their migraines began in the early teens or, less commonly, in childhood. The onset of migraine headaches is not common after the age of 40 and is rare after the age of 65.[7]

CLINICAL PEARL

The onset of migraine headaches is not common after the age of 40 and is rare after the age of 65.

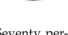

Migraine headaches have a strong familial tendency. Seventy percent to eighty percent of migraineurs indicate that other members of their families have experienced similar headaches.[7]

Migraines occur in both sexes, but are two to three times more common in women than in men.[7] Hormonal factors influence migraine attacks in these women; they often report an increase in the intensity and frequency of their headaches during menstruation. In addition, the use of oral contraceptives appears to increase the incidence and severity of migraines, whereas pregnancy tends to lessen the frequency of the headaches. Menopause may cause the migraine headaches to cease.[8,9]

Approximately 30% of migraine patients report that the ingestion of certain foods will trigger a headache.[10] These foods contain vasoactive substances that result in vasodilation of the extracranial vessels.[11] Red wines and other alcoholic beverages, as well as caffeine-rich drinks and foods such as coffee, tea, cola, or chocolate are noteworthy in this regard. Other foods that may precipitate headaches in susceptible individuals include hot dogs, bacon, ham, and salami, which contain sodium nitrite; tyramine-rich foods such as aged cheeses, pickled herring, chicken livers, canned figs, and pods of broad beans; or foods containing monosodium glutamate.[12]

Many migraineurs note that undue mental stress or fatigue precipitates headaches. Other triggering events include bright light reflected off shiny metal surfaces, excessive exertion, head trauma, or high altitude. The box below summarizes the characteristics of the migraineur.

═══ Characteristics of the Migraineur

Migraines begin in childhood or early teens
Migraines have a strong family history
Migraines are more common in females
Migraines increase in frequency during menstruation
Migraines increase in frequency with birth control pills
Migraines decrease in frequency during pregnancy
Migraines decrease in frequency after menopause
Migraines may be triggered by foods containing tyramine, nitrites, or monosodium glutamate
Migraines may be triggered by mental stress, exertion, dazzling light, or high altitude

---

Pathophysiology of migraine. The pathophysiology of migraine has been under intense study for many years, and several conflicting theories have been put forth.[13-17] The precise underlying cause is still unknown, but the following is a likely scenario.

Subsequent to some stress or nonspecific stimulus, platelets tend to aggregate and release serotonin. The serotonin causes vasoconstriction of certain blood vessels that supply the posterior portions of the brain. The resultant regional reduction in blood flow causes a spread of cortical depression that proceeds anteriorly. The relative reduction in local cerebral blood flow probably results in the prodromal signs and symptoms that often precede the headache.

The consequent local tissue abnormalities from the reduced blood supply include hypoxia, acidosis, and carbon dioxide buildup. The parenchymal arteries dilate in response to the carbon dioxide increase and to the local metabolic demands, and pain fibers within the trigeminovascular system at the base of the brain are activated. If vasodilation is sufficiently great, the cranial arteries on the outside of the head also expand.

The alteration in tone of the extracranial arteries provokes the liberation of multiple local and chemical vasoactive substances including prostaglandins, histamine, peptide kinins, and other sterile inflammatory substances. These products produce edema, sensitize cranial pain receptors, lower the pain threshold, and ultimately result in the characteristic pounding headache.

Finally, interesting studies by Anselmi et al.[18] indicate that migraineurs may not possess adequate amounts of endogenous beta-endorphins and other pain-modulating substances that are necessary to tolerate pain. Thus nonmigraineurs as well as migraineurs may undergo the same central and peripheral vascular processes. The migraineur, however, lacking the analgesic capabilities, suffers the severe headache.

CLINICAL PEARL

Nonmigraineurs as well as migraineurs may undergo the same central and peripheral vascular processes. The migraineur, however, lacking the analgesic capabilities, suffers the severe headache.

Migraine with aura (classic migraine). Classic migraine occurs in approximately 10% to 15% of migraine sufferers.[4,7] The classic migraine is characterized by visual prodromal symptoms that precede the headache by 10 to 20 minutes.[19] Visual symptoms usually include flickering, flashing, or scintillating positive scotomas that may surround an area of reduced vision—a negative scotoma. These auras may appear as sparkles, flashes of light, or heat waves and often have a zigzag appearance reminiscent of the picket posts in a fort (Figure 9-1). The scintillations often begin near the center of the visual field and expand slowly as they move outward toward the periphery. The scintillating scotomas are usually hemianopic in nature and occur contralateral to the subsequent headache. Other less experienced prodromes include hemianopsias or visual hallucinations such as macropsia or micropsia.

The intense, pounding headache with the attendant constitutional signs and symptoms usually lasts from 3 to 7 hours.[19] After the pulsatile head pain, the patient may report sustained muscle contractions in the neck and shoulders.

Migraine without aura (common migraine). Common migraine is characterized primarily by headache and gastrointestinal signs and symptoms but without specific, easily identifiable prodromes. The patient may state that she or he felt drowsy, depressed, or generally unwell, or experienced fluid retention or bouts of frequent yawning before the headache. The patient may not indicate any premonitory symptoms, however, and often will state that he or she awoke with the headache.

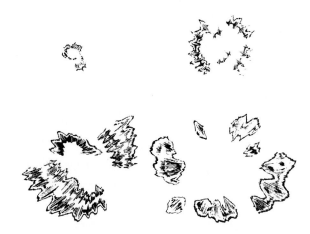

FIGURE 9-1 Migraine aura. These scintillations begin in the center of the field and expand slowly as they migrate toward the periphery.

The headache may last for hours or days with the patient seeking a secluded dark environment for relief.

It should be emphasized that migraine attacks with and without aura usually occur in the same individual at different times.[17] It is also important to note that any of the signs or symptoms occurring before or in association with the pain may be so mild that the patient may not appreciate their significance.

Complicated migraine. Complicated migraine is a broad category describing patients who develop paroxysmal, neurologic dysfunction. The neurologic signs and symptoms may precede or occur coincident with the headache and often last longer than the pain. Headache need not be an important component of complicated migraine, however. If headache is present, it may be shorter and less severe than in other forms of migraine.

The neurologic disturbance may include monocular visual loss, ophthalmoplegia, hemiplegia, hemiparesis, hemisensory loss, or disturbances of higher cortical function.[20] These neurologic phenomena are usually transient but may become permanent on rare occasions.[21]

Ocular migraine is a special type of complicated migraine in which there is vasospasm of the retinal arterioles, central retinal artery, or ciliary vasculature.[22-24] The resultant effect is a central scotoma, monocular vision loss, or an altitudinal field defect. The visual defect is usually short-lived but may become permanent following repeated attacks. Headache is an inconsistent accompaniment of ocular migraine, and, when present, may precede the visual deficit.

Migraine equivalents (migraine variants, migraine accompaniments, acephalgic migraines) refer to short-lived, episodic dysfunctions of an organ or an organ system that occur without the headache.[25] The patient usually has a history of typical migraine headaches or a strong family history of migraine. However, migraine equivalents may occur in persons who have never had a migraine attack.

CLINICAL PEARL

Migraine equivalents (migraine variants, migraine accompaniments, acephalgic migraines) refer to short-lived, episodic dysfunctions of an organ or an organ system that occur without the headache. Migraine equivalents may occur in persons who have never had a migraine attack.

Visual symptoms are the most frequently reported manifestations of migraine equivalents and usually affect patients older than age 40.[26] They usually take the form of the scintillating scotomas reported by classic migraineurs and have the characteristic buildup and movement across the visual field. The light patterns usually last from 15 to 20 minutes.[27] Other common symptoms include paresthesia that moves and spreads up and down the limbs, cyclical abdominal pain accompanied by nausea and vomiting, diarrhea, cyclical chest pain, or transient mood disturbances. The neurologic equivalents, however, can take almost any form and may confound the unwary practitioner. Characteristically, the patient is free of symptoms between attacks, and no offending lesion is ever noted. The various equivalent symptoms usually respond to various antimigrainous drugs. The salient points relevant to migraine equivalents may be summarized as follows:

Headaches replaced by equivalent systemic syndromes
No demonstrable systemic lesion
Absence of signs or symptoms between attacks
Relieved by antimigraine medications

Treatment of migraine. The treatment of migraine may be divided into three categories: general measures, abortive treatment of the acute attack, and prophylactic therapy to prevent recurrence (see the box below).

Treatment of Migraine Headaches

General measures
Avoid foods that trigger the headache
Refrain from using birth control pills
Minimize stress and fatigue

☰ Treatment of Migraine Headaches—cont'd

Abortive treatment
   Analgesics (aspirin, Tylenol)
   NSAIDS (Naprosyn, Motrin, Voltaren, Indocin)
   Ergotamine preparations (Ergomar, Ergostat, Cafergot, Cafergot PB)
   Midrin
   Sumatriptan (Imitrex)
   Massage of the superficial temporal arteries

Prophylactic treatment
   Beta-adrenergic blockers (Inderal)
   Methysergide maleate (Sansert)
   Tricyclic antidepressants (Elavil, Triavil)
   NSAIDS (aspirin, Naprosyn, Motrin, Voltaren, Indocin)
   Calcium channel blockers (Calan, Isoptin)

General measures include minimizing the conditions and agents that precipitate migraine attacks. In particular, the patient should attempt to avoid those dietary items that have been shown to have vasoactive properties. The patient should also refrain from using birth control pills. Finally, the patient should attempt to minimize mental stress and physical fatigue.

For mild migraines the most commonly used preparations are the simple analgesics (aspirin, Tylenol) and the nonsteroidal anti-inflammatory drugs (NSAIDS). The NSAIDS such as naproxyn (Naprosyn), ibuprofen (Motrin), diclofenac sodium (Voltaren), and indomethocin (Indocin) inhibit prostaglandin synthesis and thereby reduce pain induced by the trigemino-vascular system.[28-30]

The mainstay of abortive treatment for more severe migraines is the wide variety of ergotamine preparations (Ergomar, Ergostat). These compounds are derivatives of ergot alkaloids and are potent vasoconstrictors. They specifically counteract the episodic dilation of various branches of the external carotid artery, which are affected in migraine. If ergotamine is to be effective in migraine, it must be administered soon after headache onset. Because it does not affect intracranial circulation, the drug can be used during the painless, preheadache phase that may herald the onset of migraine. Ergotamine tartrate may be given parenterally, orally, sublingually, by inhalation, or rectally. The drug may be combined with caffeine (Cafergot), or caffeine, belladonna, and a short acting phenobarbital (Cafergot PB). For persons who cannot tolerate ergotamine compounds, a drug containing isometheptine mucate, dichloralphenazone, and acetaminophen (Midrin) is effective in aborting migraine.[28-30]

In 1992 a new migraine drug, sumatriptan (Imitrex), became available to the general public. Sumatriptan is a serotonin receptor agonist that inactivates receptors located on peripheral trigeminal nerve terminals that supply pain-sensitive vascular meningeal structures. Additionally, sumatriptan blocks the neuropeptide-mediated inflammatory response after trigeminal stimulation and may also block transmission in trigeminal neurons. Finally, sumatriptan constricts branches of the external carotid artery.[31-33]

CLINICAL PEARL

In 1992 a new migraine drug, sumatriptan (Imitrex), became available to the general public. Sumatriptan is a serotonin receptor agonist, and in some fashion, inactivates receptors located on peripheral trigeminal nerve terminals that supply pain-sensitive vascular meningeal structures.

Sumatriptan is administered subcutaneously by the patient by means of a special autoinjector syringe. Studies indicate that approximately 75% of patients report a reduction of head pain and gastrointestinal distress within 1 hour after injection, and 81% to 86% of patients had improvement after 2 hours.[31,32]

Another approach to migraine therapy is that of bilateral digital massage of the superficial temporal artery at the first sign of the visual aura. In one study, this technique was successful in aborting 81% of attacks in 15 patients.[34] It is speculated that the massage stimulates perivascular nerve fibers supplying the extracranial vasculature and, in some unknown fashion, stops the ensuing pain phase of the headache.

Prophylactic treatment is warranted when migraine attacks are frequent and the patient's lifestyle is disrupted. Among the most effective prophylactic drugs are the beta-adrenergic blockers, particularly propranolol (Inderal).[35] These drugs block arterial dilation of the branches of the external carotid artery, inhibit platelet aggregation, and reduce the liberation of prostaglandins and other sterile inflammatory substances that induce pain.

Other useful prophylactic medications include the following: methysergide maleate (Sansert), the tricyclic antidepressants (Elavil, Triavil), NSAIDS (aspirin, Indocin, Naprosyn, Motrin), and the calcium channel blockers (Calan, Isoptin).[36-38]

Methysergide maleate and the tricyclic antidepressants may prevent migraine by blocking the trigeminal nerve terminals that supply pain-sensitive vascular and meningeal structures. The tricyclic antidepressants are particularly useful for preventing migraine in patients who also have muscle contraction headaches caused by depression or tension. The calcium channel blockers may prevent intracranial vasoconstriction and spreading cortical depression.[39-41]

Cluster headaches

Cluster headaches are considered to be the most severe type of headache experienced by patients. These headaches occur in episodes or "clusters" that last from 2 to 12 weeks. Each headache is short-lived, lasting from 30 to 120 minutes, and may occur 1 to 5 times per day. After the cluster period, the patient may go into remission and be headache-free for months or years.

CLINICAL PEARL

Cluster headaches are considered to be the most severe type of headache experienced by patients. These headaches occur in episodes of "clusters" that last from 2 to 12 weeks.

The patient is usually awakened by the headache in the middle of the night. The pain is severe and burning and almost always one-sided in the oculotemporal or oculofrontal area. The patient tends to pace the floor in an attempt to mitigate the excruciating pain. The most common symptoms that accompany the head pain are ipsilateral facial sweating, lacrimation, nasal congestion, and a ptosis and miosis (Horner's syndrome). If the cluster attacks are numerous, the patient may be left with a permanent Horner's syndrome.

Characteristics of the cluster headache patient. Cluster headaches predominate in males by a ratio of 5:1 over females.[42] Typically, the male is between the ages of 20 and 40. Studies indicate that these patients are heavy smokers and heavy drinkers as compared with control subjects.[43-45] Graham[46] described patients with cluster headaches as having characteristic facial features including a leonine appearance, thick glabellar and nasolabial folds, telangiectasia, coarse cheek skin, broad chin, and a chiseled lower lip. It has also been found that these patients have a high incidence of peptic ulcer.[46] The box below summarizes the salient clinical features of cluster headaches.

Characteristics of the Cluster Headache Patient

A middle-aged man with a heavy, chiseled face who smokes and drinks heavily

Headaches awaken the patient at night and last 30 to 120 minutes

Headaches occur 1 to 5 times per day and occur in episodes lasting from 2 to 12 weeks

Accompanying symptoms include facial sweating, lacrimation, nasal congestion, and Horner's syndrome

Pathophysiology of cluster headaches. The etiology of cluster headaches remains obscure. Horton[47] suggested that they may be associated with an unusual sensitivity to histamine. Indeed, 0.35 mg of histamine injected subcutaneously induced headaches identical to those occurring spontaneously.

The sphenopalatine ganglion may play a significant role in the development of cluster headaches. Electric stimulation of the ganglion produces a syndrome much like that of cluster headaches, and local anesthetic applied to the ganglion has been successful in treating the cluster attacks.[48] Diamond and Dalessio[49] believe that heavy smokers consistently irritate the sphenopalatine ganglion, causing it to be hypersensitive to nonspecific stimuli.

The mechanism of the Horner's syndrome that accompanies the cluster headache is also speculative. The oculosympathetic paresis might be due to the repeated dilation and edema of the internal carotid artery. This would result in damage to the sympatheic plexus that surrounds that vessel.

Treatment of cluster headaches. Treatment of cluster headaches should be directed toward symptomatic relief during the attack and toward prophylactic treatment to prevent further cycles from occurring (see the box below).

Treatment of Cluster Headaches

Abortive Treatment

Sumatriptan
Ergotamine preparations (Ergomar, Ergostat)
Oxygen
Topical anesthesia of the sphenopalatine ganglion

Prophylactic Treatment

Prednisone
Lithium carbonate (Eskalith, Lithobid)
Histamine desensitization
Indomethacin (Indocin)
Methysergide maleate (Sansert)
Calcium-channel blockers (Isoptin, Calan, Procardia)

Sumatriptan appears to be an effective and well-tolerated treatment for acute attacks of cluster headaches. In a well-controlled study, the severity of the headache decreased in 74% of attacks within 15 minutes of treatment. Thirty-six percent of the patients were pain free in 10 minutes.[50]

Ergotamine tartrate compounds have some efficacy during the acute attack if taken at the onset of the headache. If the medication is not taken early enough, however, it will usually not abort the head pain. Inhalation of 100% oxygen has also been shown to be effective in aborting attacks.[51] A less commonly used abortive therapy for cluster headaches consists of topical anesthesia of the sphenopalatine ganglion using 4% lidocaine solution.[52]

Assuming no contraindication, prednisone is the drug of choice for prophylaxis of episodic cluster headaches when patients are in the acute cycle. Lithium carbonate (Eskalith, Lithobid) is the drug of choice for prophylactic treatment of cluster headaches when patients are in remission. Other useful prophylactic regimens include histamine desensitization, indomethacin (Indocin), methysergide maleate (Sansert), and calcium-channel blockers (Isoptin, Calan, Procardia).

Toxic vascular headaches

Toxic vascular headaches are evoked by a systemic vasodilation that may be produced by fever, abrupt cessation of coffee drinking, or inhalation of certain environmental toxins. The headaches are described as being throbbing in nature but without the intense severity that characterizes the migraine headache. There are usually no attendant constitutional signs or symptoms. The headaches will almost always disappear when the underlying etiology is addressed. Thus recovery from the febrile illness, adaptation to the cessation of caffeine, or avoidance of the environmental toxins is all that is required.

Hypertensive headaches

Hypertensive headaches are related to elevations in systemic arterial blood pressure. Sustained elevation in the diastolic component or sudden elevation in the systolic component may result in pulsatile headaches that increase in severity upon the patient's awakening. The headaches will usually remit upon appropriate treatment of the patient's hypertension.

Muscle Contraction Headaches (Tension Headaches)

The terms "muscle contraction headache" and "tension headache" have been used synonymously for almost 40 years to describe nonspecific, chronic headaches that are not vascular and are not associated with traction or inflammation. These headaches are thought to account for 90% of all chronic, recurrent headaches.[53]

The muscle contraction headache is a steady, nonpulsatile headache due to chronic contraction and subsequent spasm of the muscles of the head, neck, and face. The pain is usually diffuse and occurs in the forehead and temples or in the back of the head and neck. The patient often states that the head pain feels as if a band or vice is being tightened about the head. If the clinician palpates the diffusely aching muscle tissues, he may find one or more tender areas (nodules) that are sharply localized. Although tension headaches are often brief, they may be sustained with varying intensity for weeks, months, or even years.[54]

Characteristics of tension headache patients

There is no sexual predisposition for muscle contraction headaches, and there appears to be no familial tendency. There are also no associated or concurrent constitutional signs or symptoms. The majority of patients with muscle contraction headaches suffer from depression or anxiety or some other emotional conflict.[54,55] Moreover, there is usually an accompanying sleep disturbance in addition to the headache.[54] If the patient is anxious, he or she usually manifests difficulty in falling asleep. If the patient is depressed, there is frequent awakening during the middle of the night or early awakening. In some rare instances, the depressed patient may exhibit hypersomnia (excessive sleep).

CLINICAL PEARL

The majority of patients with muscle contraction headaches suffer from depression or anxiety or some other emotional conflict. Moreover, there is usually an accompanying sleep disturbance in addition to the headache.

Pathophysiology of muscle contraction headaches

The etiology of muscle contraction headaches is thought to stem from an underlying emotional conflict. In a classic study, Martin et al.[56] suggest that the muscle contraction is a physiological expression of the underlying psychoneurotic stress that is so prevalent in these patients. Anxiety, and especially depressive, symptoms undergo somatization resulting in prolonged muscle contraction in the head, neck, and face. The subsequent muscle spasms result in cramping and pain. Thus the psychological symptoms are converted into physical symptoms that are more acceptable to the patient.

Treatment of muscle contraction headaches

Antidepressant drugs such as amitryptyline hydrochloride (Elavil), imipramine hydrochloride (Tofranil), protriptyline hydrochloride (Vivactil), tranylcypromine sulfate (Parnate), or phenelzine sulfate provide the most effective treatment for the muscle contraction headache due to depression.[57] Other important treatment modalities include a drug containing aspirin, butalbital, and caffeine (Fiorinal), biofeedback training in an attempt to learn how to relax the contracted muscles, and psychological counseling.[57] For those patients whose headaches contain features common with migraine headaches, antimigrainous therapy may prove beneficial.

Inflammatory and Traction Headaches

Headaches from intracranial sources are most often produced by inflammation or traction of the pain-sensitive structures of the head. As a group, these headaches are known as organic headaches. They are evoked by organic diseases of the skull or its components, including the brain, meninges, arteries, veins, eyes, ears, teeth, nose, and paranasal sinuses. For clarification, inflammatory headaches and traction headaches will be discussed separately.

Inflammatory headaches

Inflammation of intracranial or extracranial pain-sensitive structures will often result in diffuse chronic head pain. Removing the inflammatory focus will result in a dramatic reduction in the quality and frequency of the head pain.

Brain abscess. Brain abscess is a relatively rare cause of intracranial inflammation.[58] It is most commonly found in association with cyanotic congenital heart disease, chronic sinusitis, or chronic otitis in an immunosuppressed child. The brain abscess results in a breakdown of parenchymous brain tissue and a walled-off cystic tumor. The subsequent head pain is caused by local traction of pain-sensitive structures as the abscess gradually increases in size. As brain tissue is displaced, the intracranial pressure rises and papilledema results. In addition, high fever, projectile vomiting, and convulsions usually accompany the severe headache. These patients require hospitalization and intensive antibiotic therapy or surgical drainage to effect a cure. Optometrists are not likely to evaluate these patients in the primary care setting.

A brain abscess is often associated with disease of the adjacent otologic structures or paranasal sinuses. In fact, it is common to have headaches from the latter sources long before the brain tissue becomes inflamed.[58]

Otologic inflammation. Recurrent otologic pain may be localized and directly related to disease of the external ear, external ear canal, tympanic membrane, or middle ear. The disease processes that affect the ear and result in primary, recurrent pain include trauma, infections, or neoplasms. Secondary or referred otalgia may result from involvement of nonotologic structures in the head and neck.[59] These pathologies may impact on branches of the fifth, seventh, ninth, or tenth cranial nerves as well as the second and third cervical nerves. All of these nerves provide sensory fibers to the regions of the auricle, external ear canal, tympanic membrane, and middle ear.

Recurrent pain in and around the ear should be referred to the otologist for appropriate evaluation. Pertinent laboratory studies include a complete blood count, and cultures and sensitivity testing of any infectious lesions. In addition, pathological evaluation of biopsy specimens, standard temporal bone radiographs, CT or MRI scans, and gallium scans may also be of benefit.

Sinusitis. Inflammation of the mucous membranes of the nose or paranasal sinuses may result in recurrent midface pain over the distribution of the first and second divisions of the trigeminal nerve.[60] The pain may be described as a burning sensation that is exacerbated when the patient bends over or blows his nose. There may be tenderness to palpation or percussion over the affected sinus. Pain may also be referred to contiguous facial structures. For example, maxillary sinusitis may result in pain in the teeth or gums. Frontal sinusitis has primary symptoms of frontal headaches, but the pain may radiate behind the eyes and to the vertex of the skull. In ethmoid sinusitis, the headache is located between or behind the eyes. The eyes may be exquisitely sensitive to pressure, and eye movement may accentuate the pain. Sphenoid sinusitis may result in headache that is localized to the orbit, frontal, or occipital regions.

CLINICAL PEARL

Inflammation of the mucous membranes of the nose or paranasal sinuses may result in recurrent midface pain over the distribution of the first and second divisions of the trigeminal nerve.

Recurrent head pain suggestive of rhinologic or sinus disease should be referred to the otolaryngologist for appropriate evaluation and treatment. Physical examination includes a complete evaluation of the head and neck. The patient's nose, paranasal sinuses, and nasopharynx should be examined both before and following shrinkage of the mucosa by appropriate vasoconstrictive agents. Radiologic studies of the skull and sinuses may reveal inflammatory changes or bone changes secondary to benign or malignant tumors.

Dental inflammation. Dental infections, particularly periapical abscesses of the maxillary teeth, may give rise to chronic recurrent headaches in the area of the maxillary sinus.[61] Temporomandibular joint (TMJ) dysfunction associated with dental malocclusions or arthritis may give rise to recurrent pain in and around the ear. Patients may complain of pain and a clicking or grinding sensation whenever they open and close their jaws.[62] This phenomenon can be substantiated by palpating the TMJ while having the patients open and close

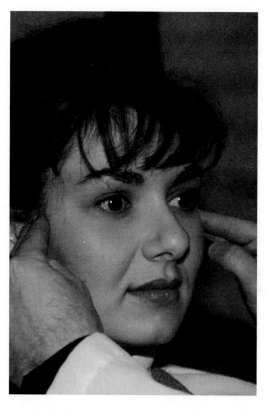

FIGURE 9-2 Temporomandibular joint dysfunction can be substantiated by palpating the temporomandibular joint while the patient opens and closes the mouth.

their mouths (Figure 9-2). Head pain thought to be due to dental disease or TMJ dysfunction should be referred to a dentist who is knowledgeable in this field.

Arteritis. Chronic recurrent headaches may result from inflammation of the cranial arteries. Several collagen-vascular autoimmune diseases such as primary granulomatous cerebral arteritis, polyarteritis nodosa, systemic lupus erythematosus, and giant cell arteritis may be associated with severe headaches. The cause of such headaches is usually ascribed to arterial inflammation.[63]

Giant cell arteritis (GCA) is probably the most commonly encountered vasculitis in optometric practice. It is a disease of the elderly; the diagnosis is rarely made in patients under the age of 50 years.[64] GCA affects the walls of medium and large arteries throughout the body. The arterial walls become infused with inflammatory cells, including giant cells. Subsequently, the internal elastic membrane becomes thickened, and the arterial lumen narrows.

The patient with GCA may manifest a variety of signs and symptoms (see the box below). Malaise, weakness, anorexia, low-grade fever, and joint and muscle pain have been reported. When the cranial arteries become inflamed (cranial arteritis), the patient may complain of deep, boring headaches, scalp tenderness, or claudication when chewing. The claudication becomes acute when the superficial temporal arteries become nodular and distended (temporal arteritis). Irreversible vision loss occurs in 50% of the untreated cases because of an inflammation of the ophthalmic artery and its derivatives, the short posterior ciliary arteries. The resultant anterior ischemic optic neuropathy is characterized by a pallid disk edema with adjacent, linear, flame-shaped hemorrhages and severe, irreversible visual deficit. (See Chapter 6 for a complete discussion.) It should be noted that an occult form of GCA exists with minimal or subclinical systemic manifestations. Patients with occult GCA present with acute vision failure as their first clinical manifestation.

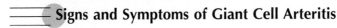

Signs and Symptoms of Giant Cell Arteritis

Headache and scalp tenderness
Claudication on chewing
Malaise
Anorexia and scalp tenderness
Weight loss
Recurrent low-grade fevers
Proximal joint and muscle pain
Transient ischemic attacks
Transient diplopia

CLINICAL PEARL

When the cranial arteries become inflamed (cranial arteritis), the patient may complain of deep, boring headaches, scalp tenderness, or claudication when chewing.

The diagnosis of GCA is made on the basis of an elevated erythrocyte sedimentation rate (ESR) (i.e., over 50 mm/hr) and the presence of the characteristic giant cells in the temporal artery biopsy.[64-66] Once the presumptive diagnosis is made, the patient is placed on large doses of systemic steroids until the ESR and serial biopsies indicate the disease is remitting.

Cranial neuralgia. Inflammation of the trigeminal (CN V) and glossopharyngeal (CN IX) nerves may produce recurrent, severe, throbbing, or stabbing pains in their course or distribution. Trigeminal neuralgia (tic douloureux) presents as an episodic, recurrent unilateral pain that usually occurs in female patients older than 50 years of age.[67] The pain usually occurs in the distribution of the maxillary and mandibular divisions. A very intense jab lasting less than 30 seconds, it has been likened to an electric shock. Between each pain attack, there is a period of relief lasting a few seconds to a minute. Then, another intense jab of pain occurs. When the patient is in the throes of an attack of tic douloureux, there are areas of increased sensitivity on the face about the nares and mouth. When these trigger zones are stimulated by touching or washing the face, or by chewing, the attack is precipitated.

The most common site of occurrence is in the distribution of the maxillary division of the trigeminal nerve.[67] The cause is thought to be vascular compression of the sensory root of CN V nerve as it enters the pons. A diagnosis of tic douloureux in a young person, however, particularly if the condition is bilateral, warrants a work-up for multiple sclerosis.

Glossopharyngeal neuralgia is a similar phenomenon to trigeminal neuralgia, but is seen much less frequently. The symptoms are related to CN IX with the stabbing pain usually being appreciated in the tongue, tonsils, and pharynx. The painful paroxyms often are initiated by eating, swallowing, or yawning, but the etiology is unknown.

The cranial neuralgias will often spontaneously go into periods of remission. If this does not occur, drugs such as carbamazepine (Tegretol), phenytoin (Dilantin), baclofen (Lioresal), and clonazepam (Klonopin) may be used to nudge the patient into remission.[68] Surgical treatments for trigeminal neuralgia include vascular decompression and a variety of percutaneous procedures to destroy the pain fibers of the trigeminal nerve.[69] The surgical treatment for glossopharyngeal neuralgia is the intracranial sectioning of the nerve fibers of CN IX.

Traction headaches

Headaches from intracranial masses are caused by traction on pain-sensitive structures or elevation of the intracranial pressure. The typical headache is intermittent and is usually described as being deep and aching rather than throbbing. Nausea and vomiting are often associated with the headache. Ten percent of adults and two thirds of children with brain tumors are awakened from sleep by headache.[70] The pain may be worse upon awakening and may be aggrevated by the Valsalva maneuver as in bending, lifting, coughing, or sneezing. The pain is frequently worse with a change of posture. Interestingly, the head pain is often mitigated by common analgesics or cold packs. In addition to the headaches, there is almost always some focal neurologic sign or symptom that is manifest. For example, the patient may experience episodic diplopia, tinnitus, aphasia, or dementia as well as papilledema. The box below summarizes the characteristics of traction headaches.

Characteristics of Traction Headaches

Headaches are intermittent
Headaches are nonpulsatile
Nausea and vomiting are frequent concomitants
Headaches are worse upon awakening
Headaches are exacerbated by the Valsalva maneuver
Headaches are exacerbated by changes in posture
Headaches may be mitigated by analgesics or cold packs
Patients manifest some focal neurologic sign or symptom

CLINICAL PEARL

Headaches from intracranial masses are due to traction on pain-sensitive structures or elevation of the intracranial pressure. Nausea and vomiting are often associated with the headache.

Brain tumor. Traction headache is an important symptom of brain tumor. The head pain occurs as an initial symptom in 20% to 25% of patients and in as many as 90% at some time during the course of their illness.[70] The headache overlies the tumor in approximately one third of these patients in the initial stages of the neoplasm.[70] As the tumor grows, the pain tends to spread and be referred to other areas. If the tumor is supratentorial, the pain tends to localize to the side of the tumor at the vertex or at the frontal area of the skull. If the tumor is below the tentorium, the pain is generally bilateral and is referred to the occipital portion of the skull. Additional manifestations of brain tumors include nausea or vomiting, hemianopsias, disorders of equilibrium, gait, and coordination, ataxia, motor weakness, seizures and hypoesthesias, reflex abnormalities, and disorders of speech or personality.

CLINICAL PEARL

Traction headache is an important symptom of brain tumor. The head pain occurs as an initial symptom in 20% to 25% of patients and in as many as 90% at some time during the course of their illness.

Cerebral aneurysms and arteriovenous malformations. Cerebral aneurysms are present in approximately 5% of the adult population.[71] These aneurysms are outpouchings of intracranial arteries that occur as a result of defects in the elastic and muscular coats. Most aneurysms are congenital, but factors such as hypertension and arterial wall degeneration play a role in the development of aneurysms.

Arteriovenous malformations (AVMs) are developmental abnormal communications between arterial and venous systems. The most common AVMs consist of a tortuous mass of abnormally sized arteries and veins. Blood is shunted directly from the arterial circulation to the venous circulation without passing through a capillary bed.

Blood vessels that are prone to develop aneurysms as well as those vessels that form AVMs do not possess the structural integrity of normal blood vessels and are prone to hemorrhage into the brain or the subarachnoid space. The most common manifestations of such hemorrhages include an extremely severe, excruciating headache, convulsions, progressive hemispheric neurologic deficit, and mental deterioration. The headache occurs as a result of three mechanisms: stretching and tearing of the involved blood vessel, chemical irritation of the pain-sensitive perivascular meninges by extravasated blood, and increased intracranial pressure from blood being discharged into the nonexpansile cranial vault.

Unruptured aneurysms and AVMs may also produce chronic recurring headaches in about 50% of patients.[72] These sentinel headaches occur in the days to weeks preceding the acute subarachnoid hemorrhage and are probably a consequence of a slow, intermittent leakage.

Of particular interest are those AVMs that involve the occipital lobe. These lesions may create symptoms that can be mistaken for classic migraine headaches. When there is partial leakage into the occipital lobe, the patient may report severe headaches and sensations of moving lights in the right or left homonymous fields. However, the auras are usually not similar to the angular, scintillating scotomas that are characteristic of the classic migraine. In addition, the light flashes often persist throughout the headache and may continue after the headache subsides. The headache itself is almost always localized to the same side of the head, a situation which does not occur with migraines.[73]

Intracranial hematomas. Intracranial hematomas are localized masses of extravasated blood that usually result from trauma to the blood vessels in the dura. These hematomas are divided into several subgroups, although it may not always be possible to differentiate between them clinically.

Epidural hematomas most frequently appear after significant blunt head trauma, although the injury is usually not severe enough to result in unconsciousness. Usually there is injury to the middle meningeal artery on the underside of the temporal bone.[74] The escaping blood separates the dura and its smaller blood vessels from their natural attachment to the bone. The subsequent traction on these pain-sensitive structures produces deep, aching head pain. As the mass lesion increases in size, the brain becomes compressed, resulting in restlessness, combativeness, and deteriorating consciousness.

Subdural hematomas occur between the dura and the brain. Acute subdural hematomas are those that become clinically significant within 48 hours of the head injury. The head injury is usually severe, resulting in unconsciousness. Headache is, therefore, not an important clinical symptom.

Subacute subdural hematomas are those that become clinically significant 2 to 14 days after the head injury.[74] Headache, when present, is similar to that described with epidural hematomas.

Chronic subdural hematomas are those that become clinically significant more than 14 days after head trauma.[74] The antecedent injury is usually mild, and the patient does not usually experience unconsciousness. Small rents in the tiny vessels within the dura result in a slow leakage of blood. The headache that results is presumed to be secondary to the stretching of the tributary veins that pass from the cerebral hemispheres to the sagittal sinus. Patients may indicate that the headache is accentuated by sudden head movements or by taps to the head.

All hematomas involving the dura can usually be diagnosed by nonenhanced CT scans.[74] Therapy includes drainage of the epidural or subdural collections by repeated taps or shunting procedures.

Pseudotumor cerebri. Pseudotumor cerebri is an entity in which there is increased intracranial pressure with no clearly identifiable underlying cause. As such, the diagnosis is one of exclusion. Recurrent, deep boring headaches are characteristic of this condition.

CLINICAL PEARL

Pseudotumor cerebri is an entity in which there is increased intracranial pressure with no clearly identifiable underlying cause. Recurrent, deep boring headaches are characteristic of this condition.

The syndrome of pseudotumor cerebri predominates in obese females from the teens through the 50s but is not exclusive to this group.[75] In addition to the headaches, florid disc edema, transient obscurations of vision, and sixth nerve palsy are among the most prevalent characteristics of this syndrome. (See Chapter 6 for a complete discussion of pseudotumor cerebri.)

Headaches Due to Other Factors

This classification includes all of those chronic recurrent headaches that do not easily fit into the aforementioned categories. However, it is probable that many have a vascular component.

Systemic medications

Any systemic medication may produce idiosyncratic side effects among which might be chronic recurrent headaches. Drugs that have a propensity to produce such headaches include ethyl alcohol, birth control pills, major tranquilizers, antihypertensives, antidepressants, caffeine, and aspirin.

Posttrauma

Most persons who injure their heads have pain and tenderness at the site of the impact for a short time thereafter. However, between one third and one half of patients have posttraumatic headaches that persist for more than 2 months.[76] The headache is characterized by a dull, aching sensation that tends to occur daily and may last for hours. It may also be throbbing and mimic a migraine. Other symptoms that accompany the posttraumatic headaches include vertigo, impairment of memory, inattentiveness, and variable degrees of emotional impairment.

Ischemic cerebrovascular disease

Chronic recurring headaches may precede ischemic cerebral vascular episodes whether they be transient ischemic attacks or completed cerebral infarcts. The cause of these ischemic headaches is not known, but the occurrence of chronic headaches in patients with signs and symptoms of impending stroke warrants a cerebrovascular investigation.

CLINICAL PEARL

Chronic recurring headaches may precede ischemic cerebral vascular episodes whether they be transient ischemic attacks or completed cerebral infarcts.

Exertion

There is a selected group of patients that experiences chronic recurring headaches that begin shortly after completion of an activity requiring physical exertion such as running or weightlifting. The headaches may last for hours and are migrainelike in character. In fact, many patients who experience these headaches report a family history of migraine.[77] Exertion headaches can often be prevented by daily treatment with indomethacin (Indocin).

Coitus

Benign coital cephalgia is related to exertion headache. The headache begins during sexual intercourse, often just before or at the time of orgasm, and usually resolves in minutes to several hours. Sudden increases in blood pressure or sudden rises in vasoactive substances have been implicated as the possible etiology. Both propranolol (Inderal) and indomethacin have been reported to be successful in the prophylaxis of these headaches.[78]

Optometric Workup

The optometrist should approach the patient with chronic recurring headache in a systematic fashion. The evaluation should consist of a careful history, ophthalmoscopy, sphygmomanometry, cranial nerve evaluation, and visual field analysis.

A detailed and relevant history is the most important factor in evaluating the headache patient. By carefully questioning and directing the inquiry, a particular headache profile may emerge that permits a diagnosis to be made. Specific points in the headache history should include onset, time of day, location, frequency, duration, quality and severity, prodromes, precipitating factors, associated symptoms, family history, medical history, and response to therapy. The clinician should be particularly concerned when an adult not prone to headaches suddenly presents with recurring headaches. If the headaches are accompanied by an atypical feature such as focal neurologic stigmata, a diagnosis of organic headaches should be considered.

Ophthalmoscopy is performed to rule out optic disc edema and to obtain some insight into the nature of the cerebral vasculature. Disc edema might imply that the intracranial pressure is elevated or that an arteritic diathesis is present. (See Chapter 6 for a complete discussion.)

Sphygmomanometry is performed in order to rule out hypertension, an accepted cause of chronic recurring headaches. These headaches are usually present upon awakening and often disappear as the day goes on.

Cranial nerve evaluation and visual field testing are integral parts of the optometric workup. These procedures may yield insight into the patient's general neurologic status. (See Chapters 1 and 8 for a complete discussion.)

References

1. Carlow TJ: Headache and the eye. In Dalessio DJ, ed: *Wolff's headache and other head pain*, New York, 1987, Oxford Press, 304.
2. Ray BS, Wolff HG: Experimental studies on headache: pain sensitive structures of the head and their significance in headache, *Arch Surg* 41:813-817, 1940.

3. Friedman AP, Finley KH, Grahm JR et al: Classification of headache, *Neurology* 12: 173-175, 1962.
4. Burde R, Savino P, Trobe JD: *Clinical decisions in neuro-ophthalmology,* St Louis, 1985, Mosby, 304-306.
5. Headache Classification Committee of the International Headache Society: Classification and diagnostic criteria for headache disorders, cranial neuralgias, and facial pain, *Cephalalgia* 7, 1988.
6. Goldor H: Headache and eye pain. In Gay AJ, Burde RM, eds: Clinical concepts in neuro-ophthalmology, *Ophthalmol Clin* 7(4):697, 1967.
7. Walsh FB, Hoyt WF: *Clinical neuro-ophthalmology,* ed 3, Baltimore, 1969, Williams & Wilkins, 1654-1689.
8. Waters WE, O'Connor PJ: Prevalence of migraine, *J Neurol Neurosurg Psychiatry* 38:613-616, 1975.
9. Dalton K: Migraine and oral contraceptives, *Headache* 15:247, 1975.
10. Raskin NH: Chemical headaches, *Annu Rev Med* 32:63, 1981.
11. Smith I, Kellow AH, Hanington E: Clinical and biochemical correlation between tyramine and migraine headache, *Headache* 10:43, 1970.
12. Schaumburg HH, Byck R, Gerstl R, Mashman JH: Monosodium glutamate: its pharmacology and role in the Chinese restaurant syndrome, *Science* 163:826-828, 1969.
13. Rossor M: Headache, stupor, coma. In Walton J, ed: *Brain's diseases of the nervous system,* ed 10, New York, 1993, Oxford University Press, 76-126.
14. Olsen J: Migraine and regional blood flow, *Trends Neurosci* 8:318-322, 1985.
15. Lauritzen M: Cortical spreading depression as a putative migraine mechanism, *Trends Neurosci* 10:8-13, 1987.
16. Milner PM: Note on the possible correspondence between the scotomas of migraine and spreading depression of Leao, *EEG Clin Neurophysiol* 10:705, 1958.
17. Sandy KR, Awerbuch GI: The co-occurrence of multiple sclerosis and migraine headache: the serotoninergic link, *Int J Neurosci* 76(3-4): 249-257, 1994.
18. Anselmi B, Baldi E, Cassaci F, Salmon S: Endogenous opioids in cerebrospinal fluid and blood in idiopathic headache sufferers, *Headache* 20:294-299, 1980.
19. Manzoni GC, Farina S, Lanfranchi M, Solari A: Classic migraine: clinical findings in 164 patients, *Eur Neurol* 24:163-169, 1985.
20. Kysersmith MJ, Warren FA, Chase NE: The non-benign aspects of migraine, *Neuro-ophthalmology* 7:1-10, 1987.
21. Bruyn GW: Complicated migraine. In Vinken PJ, Bruyn GW, eds: *Handbook of clinical neurology,* vol 5, *Headache and cranial neuralgias,* New York, 1968, American Elsevier, 10-40.
22. Katz B, Bramford C: Migrainous ischemic optic neuropathy, *Neurology* 35:112-114, 1985.
23. Katz B: Migrainous central retinal artery occlusion, *J Clin Neuro-Ophthalmol* 6:69-71, 1986.
24. Graveson CS: Retinal artery occlusion in migraine, *Br Med J* 2:838-846, 1949.
25. O'Connor PJ: Acephalgic migraine, *Ophthalmology* 88:999-1003, 1981.
26. Fisher CM: Late-life migraine accompaniments as a cause of unexplained transient ischemic attacks, *Can J Neurol Sci* 7:9-17, 1980.
27. Whitty CWM: Migraine without headache, *Lancet* 2:283-285, 1967.
28. Johnson ES, Ratcliffe DM, Wilkinson M: Naproxen sodium in the treatment of migraine, *Cephalalgia* 5:5-10, 1985.
29. Karachalios GN, Fotiadou A, Chrisikos N, Karabetsos A et al: Treatment of acute migraine attack with diclofenac sodium: a double-blind study, *Headache* 32:98-100, 1992.
30. Kloster R, Nestvold K, Vilming ST: A double-blind study of ibuprofen versus placebo in the treatment of acute migraine attacks, *Cephalalgia* 12:169-171, 1992.
31. Subcutaneous Sumatriptan International Study Group: Treatment of migraine attacks with sumatriptan, *N Engl J Med* 325:316-321, 1991.

32. Catarci T, Flacco F, Argentino C, Sette G et al: Ergotomine-induced headache can be sustained by sumatriptan daily uptake, *Cephalalgia* 14(5):374-375, 1994.
33. Thomas SH, Stone CK: Emergency department treatment of migraine, tension, and mixed-type headache, *J Emerg Med* 12(5):657-664, 1994.
34. Lipton SA: Prevention of classic migraine headache by digital massage of the superficial temporal arteries during visual aura, *Ann Neurol* 19:515, 1986.
35. Ziegler DK, Hurwitz A, Hassanein RS: Migraine prophylaxis: a comparison of propranolol and amitriptyline, *Arch Neurol* 44:486, 1987.
36. Drummond PD: Effectiveness of methysergide in relation to clinical features of migraine, *Headache* 25:145-146, 1985.
37. Couch JR, Hassanein RS: Amitriptyline in migraine prophylaxis, *Arch Neurol* 36:695-699, 1979.
38. Daroff RB, Whitney CM: Treatment of vascular headaches, *Headache* 26:470, 1986.
39. Solomon GD, Steel JG, Spaccaventul LJ: Verapamil prophylaxis of migraine: a double-blind, placebo-controlled study, *JAMA* 250:2500-2502, 1983.
40. Meyer JS, Hardenburg J: Clinical effectiveness of calcium entry blockers in prophylactic treatment of migraine and cluster headaches, *Headache* 23:266-277, 1983.
41. Greenberg DA: Calcium channel antagonists and the treatment of migraine, *Clin Neuropharmacol* 9:311-328, 1986.
42. Bickerstaff EB: Cluster headaches. In Vinken PJ, Bruyn GW, eds: *Handbook of clinical neurology*, vol 5, New York, 1968, American Elsevier, 111.
43. Kudrow L: *Cluster headache mechanisms and management*, New York, 1980, Oxford Press.
44. Diamond S, Medina JL: Cluster headaches variant: the spectrum of a new syndrome and its response to indomethacin, *Arch Neuro* 38:705-709, 1981.
45. Watson CP, Evans RS: Chronic cluster headache: a review of 60 patients, *Headache* 27:158-165, 1987.
46. Graham JR: Cluster headache, *Headache* 11:175-180, 1972.
47. Horton BT: Histamine cephalalgia, *Mayo Clin Proc* 31:325, 1965.
48. Diamond S, Frietag FG: The treatment of intractable chronic cluster headache, *Headache* 25:166-167, 1985.
49. Diamond S, Dalessio D: Cluster headache. In Diamond S, Dalessio D, eds: *The practicing physician's approach to headache*, ed 4, Baltimore, 1986, Williams & Wilkins 66-75.
50. The Sumatriptan Cluster Headache Study Group: Treatment of acute cluster headache with sumatriptan, *N Engl J Med* 325(5):322-6, 1991.
51. Kudrow L: Response of cluster headache to episodes of oxygen inhalation, *Headache* 21:1-4, 1981.
52. Kitrelle JP, Grouse DS, Seybold ME: Cluster headache local anesthetic abortive agents, *Arch Neurol* 42:496-498, 1985.
53. Goldor H: Headache and eye pain. In Gay AJ, Burde RM, eds: Clinical concepts in neuro-ophthalmology, *Int Ophthalmol Clin* 7(4)697, 1967.
54. Silberstein S: Tension-type headaches, *Headache* 34(8):2-7, 1994.
55. Diamond S: Depression and headache, *Headache* 23:122-126, 1983.
56. Martin MJ, Rome HP, Swenson WM: Muscle contraction headache: a psychiatric review, *Res Clini Stud Headache* 1:184, 1967.
57. Diamond S, Dalessio D: Muscle contraction headache. In Diamond S, Dalessio D, eds: *The practicing physician's approach to headache*, ed 4, Baltimore, 1986, Williams & Wilkins, 108-111.
58. Ray BS, Parsons H: Subdural abscess complicating frontal sinusitis, *Arch Otolaryngol* 37:536, 1943.
59. Birt D: Headaches and head pain associated with diseases of the ear, nose, and throat, *Med Clin North Am* 62(3):523-531, 1978.
60. Ryan RE, Kern EB: Rhinologic causes of facial pain and headache, *Headache* 18:44-50, 1978.
61. Cameron CE: Cracked tooth syndrome, *J Am Dent Assoc* 68:405, 1964.

62. Reik L, Hale M: The temporomandibular joint pain-dysfunction syndrome: a frequent cause of headache, *Headache* 21:151-156, 1981.
63. Solomon S, Cappa KG: The headache of temporal arteritis, *J Am Geriatr Soc* 35:163, 1987.
64. Biller J, Asconape J, Wienlatt ME, et al: Temporal arteritis associated with normal sedimentation rate, *JAMA* 247:486, 1982.
65. Miller A, Green M: Simple rule for calculating normal erythrocyte sedimentation rate, *Br Med J* 286:266, 1983.
66. Klein RG, Campbell J, Hunder GG, Carney JA: Skip lesions in temporal arteritis, *Mayo Clin Proc* 51:504, 1976.
67. Fromm GH, Terrance CF, Macon JB: Trigeminal neuralgia. Concepts regarding etiology and pathogenesis, *Arch Neurol* 41:1204-1207, 1984.
68. Dalessio DJ: Medical treatment of trigeminal neuralgia, *Clin Neurosurg* 24:579-583, 1977.
69. Sweet WH, Wespic JG: Controlled thermocoagulation of trigeminal ganglion and rootlets for differential destruction of pain fibers: trigeminal neuralgia, *J Neurosurg* 40:143-156, 1974.
70. Diamond S, Dalessio D: Traction and inflammatory headache and cranial neuralgias. In Diamond S, Dalessio D: *The practicing physician's approach to headache,* ed 4, Baltimore, 1986, Williams & Wilkins, 84-88.
71. Troost BT, Glaser JS: Aneurysms, arteriovenous communications, and related vascular malformations. In Glaser JS, ed: *Neuro-ophthalmology,* Philadelphia, 1990, Lippincott, 520.
72. Leblanc R: The minor leak preceding subarachnoid hemorrhage, *J Neurosurg* 66:35, 1987.
73. Troost BT, Newton TH: Occipital lobe arteriovenous malformations: clinical and radiological features in 26 cases with comments on the differentiation from migraine, *Arch Ophthalmol* 93:250, 1975.
74. Jakobsen J, Baadsgaard SE, Thompsen S, et al: Prediction of postconcussional sequelae by reaction time test, *Acta Neurol Scand* 75:341-345, 1987.
75. Baker RS, Carter D, Hendrich EB, et al: Visual loss in pseudotumor cerebri in children, *Arch Ophthalmol* 103:1681, 1985.
76. Speed WG: Posttraumatic headache. In Diamond S, Dalessio D, eds: *The practicing physician's approach to headache,* ed 4, Baltimore, 1986, Williams & Wilkins, 113.
77. Diamond S: Prolonged benign exertional headache: its clinical characteristics and response to indomethacin, *Headache* 22:96-98, 1982.
78. Johns D: Benign sexual headache within a family, *Arch Neurol* 43:1158-1160, 1986.

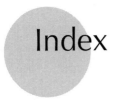

Index

Page numbers in *italic type* refer to figures. Tables are indicated by *t* following the page number.